Skin diseases after organ transplantation

EJD Book Series Editors :
Jean Thivolet
Jean-François Nicolas

ISBN 2-7420-0240-5

Éditions John Libbey Eurotext
127, avenue de la République, 92120 Montrouge, France.
Tél : 01.46.73.06.60

John Libbey and Company Ltd
13, Smiths Yard, Summerley Street, London SW18 4HR, England.
Tel : (1) 947.27.77

John Libbey CIC
Via L. Spallanzani, 11, 00161 Rome, Italy. Tel : (06) 862.289

© John Libbey Eurotext, 1998, Paris.

Il est interdit de reproduire intégralement ou partiellement le présent ouvrage sans autorisation de l'éditeur ou du Centre Français d'Exploitation du Droit de Copie, 20, rue des Grands-Augustins, 75006 Paris.

Skin diseases after organ transplantation

Coordinators

Sylvie EUVRARD
Jean KANITAKIS
Alain CLAUDY

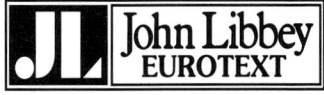

The publication of this book has been made possible through an educational grant from GALDERMA.

Contents

List of contributors VII

Foreword
Jean Thivolet IX

I. General topics

1. Organ transplantation: past, present and putative future
*Jean-Louis Touraine, Anderson Ratsimbazafy, Nicole Lefrançois,
Jeanne-Luce Garnier, Sameh Daoud* 1

2. The skin immune system
Denis Jullien, Robert L. Modlin, Jean-François Nicolas 8

3. Immunosuppressive treatments
Claire Pouteil-Noble 17

4. UV-induced immunosuppression
Iwao Kurimoto, John Wayne Streilein 29

5. Retinoic acid and immune responses: regulation of cutaneous immunomodulation by synthetic retinoid analogs
Michel Démarchez, Xian-Ping Lu 37

6. The skin in chronic renal failure and hemodialysis
Sophie Dalac, Evelyne Collet, Jean-Michel Rebibou, Daniel Lambert .. 43

7. Human papillomavirus and cutaneous carcinogenesis
Slavomir Majewski, Stefania Jablonska 51

8. Hepatitis C virus-related skin disorders
Marie-Sylvie Doutre 62

9. The role of HHV8 in cutaneous tumours
Céleste Lebbé 71

10. Influence of organ transplantation on preexisting dermatoses
Alain Claudy 80

II. Infectious diseases

11. Herpes virus infections and prophylaxis
Gérard Guillet 89

12. Oral hairy leukoplakia in immunocompromised patients
Peter H. Itin 95

13. Cutaneous manifestations of opportunistic infections (excluding viral and parasitic ones)
Jacqueline Chevrant-Breton 102

III. Neoplastic disorders

14. Extracutaneous tumors
Israel Penn 113

15. Cutaneous warts and carcinomas
Jan Nico Bouwes Bavinck, Esther J. Van Zuuren, Jan Ter Schegget 122

16. Kaposi's sarcoma
Camille Francès, Sylvie Lagrange 131

17. Naevi and melanomas
Jane M. McGregor 139

18. Cutaneous lymphomas
Pierre Souteyrand, Lincoln Fabricio, Michel d'Incan 145

19. Anogenital lesions
Michel Faure 150

20. Rare cutaneous tumours
Brigitte Dréno 154

IV. Prevention and treatment of neoplastic disorders

21. Photoprotection
Marie-Thérèse Leccia, Jean-Claude Béani, Pierre Amblard 159

22. Systemic retinoids for the treatment of skin cancer
Christoph C. Geilen, Brigitte Almond-Roesler, Constantin E. Orfanos 167

23. Topical retinoids for the management of dysplastic epithelial lesions
Sylvie Euvrard 175

V. Miscellaneous disorders

24. Porokeratosis
Jean Kanitakis 183

25. Cutaneous complications in bone marrow transplant recipients
Sélim Aractingi 195

26. Graft-*versus*-host disease after solid organ transplantation
Beth A. Drolet, Jennifer S. Peterson, Nancy B. Esterly 204

VI. General guidelines
Sylvie Euvrard 209

Color plates 217

Index 229

List of contributors

Almond-Roesler Brigitte. Department of Dermatology, University Medical Center Benjamin Franklin, The Free University of Berlin, Hindenburgdamm 30, D-12200 Berlin, Germany.

Amblard Pierre. Department of Dermatology, Albert-Michallon Hospital, 38043 Grenoble Cedex, France.

Aractingi Sélim. Department of Dermatology, Tenon Hospital, 4, rue de la Chine, 75020 Paris, France.

Béani Jean-Claude. Department of Dermatology, Albert-Michallon Hospital, 38043 Grenoble Cedex, France.

Bouwes Bavinck Jan Nico. Department of Dermatology, Leiden University Medical Centre, PO Box 9600, 2300 RC Leiden, The Netherlands.

Chevrant-Breton Jacqueline. Deparment of Dermatology, Centre Hospitalier Régional et Universitaire de Rennes-Pontchaillou, 35033 Rennes Cedex, France.

Collet Évelyne. Department of Dermatology, CHU Bocage, 21034 Dijon Cedex, France.

Daoud Sameh. Department of Transplantation and Clinical Immunology, Pavillon P, Hôpital Édouard-Herriot, 69437 Lyon Cedex 03, France.

Dalac Sophie. Department of Dermatology, CHU Bocage, 21034 Dijon Cedex, France.

Démarchez Michel. Galderma R & D, 635, route des Lucioles, BP 87, 06902 Sophia Antipolis Cedex, France.

Doutre Marie-Sylvie. Department of Dermatology, Hôpital Haut-Lévêque, 33604 Pessac, France.

Dréno Brigitte. Department of Dermatology, Nantes, France.

Drolet Beth A. Department of Dermatology, Medical College of Wisconsin, Milwaukee WI, USA.

Esterly Nancy B. Department of Dermatology, Medical College of Wisconsin, Milwaukee WI, USA.

Fabricio Lincoln. Department of Dermatology, FEMPAR, Curitiba, Brazil.

Faure Michel. Department of Dermatology, Hôpital Edouard-Herriot, 69437 Lyon Cedex 3, France.

Francès Camille. Department of Internal Medicine, Pitié-Salpêtrière Hospital, 83, boulevard de l'Hôpital, 75651 Paris Cedex 13, France.

Garnier Jeanne-Luce. Department of Transplantation and Clinical Immunology, Pavillon P, Hôpital Édouard-Herriot, 69437 Lyon Cedex 03, France.

Geilen Christoph C. Department of Dermatology, University Medical Center Benjamin Franklin, The Free University of Berlin, Hindenburgdamm 30, D-12200 Berlin, Germany.

Guillet Gérard. Department of Dermatology, University of Brest, France.

d'Incan Michel. Department of Dermatology, CHU Clermont-Ferrand, France.

Itin Peter H. Department of Dermatology, University of Basel, and Department of Dermatology, Kantonsspital Aarau, Switzerland.

Jablonska Stefania. Department of Dermatology, Warsaw School of Medicine, Koszykowa 82 a, 02-008 Warsaw, Poland.

Jullien Denis. Department of Dermatology, Edouard-Herriot Hospital, 69437 Lyon Cedex 03, France, and INSERM U 999, Laënnec University, 69372 Lyon Cedex 08, France.

Kurimoto Iwao. Department of Dermatology, Osaka University School of Medicine, Osaka, Japan.

Lagrange Sylvie. Department of Internal Medicine, Pitié-Salpêtrière Hospital, 83, boulevard de l'Hôpital, 75651 Paris Cedex 13, France.

Lambert Daniel. Department of Dermatology, CHU Bocage, 21034 Dijon Cedex, France.

Lebbé Céleste. Department of Dermatology, Laboratory of Pharmacology, Hôpital Saint-Louis, Paris, France.

Leccia Marie-Thérèse. Department of Dermatology, Albert-Michallon Hospital, 38043 Grenoble Cedex, France.

Lefrançois Nicole. Department of Transplantation and Clinical Immunology, Pavillon P, Hôpital Édouard-Herriot, 69437 Lyon Cedex 03, France.

Lu Xian-Ping. Galderma Research Inc., 10835 Altman Row, San Diego, CA 92121, USA.

Majewski Slavomir. Department of Dermatology, Warsaw School of Medicine, Koszykowa 82 a, 02-008 Warsaw, Poland.

McGregor Jane M. Department of Photobiology, St Johns Institute of Dermatology, St Thomas' Hospital, London, UK, and Center for Cutaneous Research, Royal London Hospital, London, UK.

Modlin Robert L. Division of Dermatology and Department of Microbiology and Immunology, UCLA School of Medicine, Los Angeles, CA 90095, USA.

Nicolas Jean-François. INSERM U 999, Laënnec University, 69372 Lyon Cedex 08, France, and Clinical Immunology, Centre Hospitalier Lyon-Sud, 69495 Pierre-Bénite, France.

Orfanos Constantin E. Department of Dermatology, University Medical Center Benjamin Franklin, The Free University of Berlin, Hindenburgdamm 30, D-12200 Berlin, Germany.

Penn Israel. Department of Surgery, Transplantation Division, University of Cincinnati Medical Center, and Cincinnati Veterans Affairs Medical Center, Cincinnati, USA.

Peterson Jennifer S. Department of Dermatology, Medical College of Wisconsin, Milwaukee WI, USA.

Pouteil-Noble Claire. Department of Nephrology-Transplantation, Centre Hospitalier Lyon-Sud, 165, chemin du Grand-Revoyet, 69495 Pierre-Bénite Cedex, France.

Ratsimbazafy Anderson. Department of Transplantation and Clinical Immunology, Pavillon P, Hôpital Édouard-Herriot, 69437 Lyon Cedex 03, France.

Rebibou Jean-Michel. Department of Dermatology, CHU Bocage, 21034 Dijon Cedex, France.

Souteyrand Pierre. Department of Dermatology, CHU Clermont-Ferrand, France.

Streilein John Wayne. The Schepens Eye Research Institute and Department of Dermatology, Harvard Medical School, Boston, Massachusetts, USA.

Ter Schegget Jan. Department of Virology, Academic Medical Centre, Amsterdam, The Netherlands.

Touraine Jean-Louis. Department of Transplantation and Clinical Immunology, Pavillon P, Hôpital Édouard-Herriot, 69437 Lyon Cedex 03, France.

Van Zuuren Esther J. Department of Dermatology, Leiden University Medical Centre, PO Box 9600, 2300 RC Leiden, The Netherlands.

Foreword

Renal transplantation has been performed for more than 35 years now. Ever since, transplantation of other organs (heart, bone marrow, lungs, liver, pancreas) has also been successfully carried out, and the number of organ allograft recipients is steadily increasing. A new field in medicine has developed, and organ grafting has allowed numerous patients – that would otherwise be convicted to death or to live under the dependence of artificial organs – to lead a normal life. These techniques (namely haemodialysis) were developed in parallel, since they permit the survival of the patient until a histocompatible graft has been found. However, in several instances (such as for the heart), transplantation is the only possibility to save the life of patients, and in every case it offers them a much higher quality of life.

With the exception of grafts obtained from identical twins, the price to pay for satisfactory graft function is chronic immunosuppression, necessary for organ tolerance. Immunosuppression is achieved through administration of drugs that often bear a non-selective cytotoxic activity, inevitably inducing undesired effects. Most grafted patients develop immunosuppression-induced skin diseases, including infectious (viral, fungal or bacterial) and neoplastic ones. Indeed, immunodeficiency allows for the development of cell lines, mainly epithelial, benign or malignant, that are normally inhibited by the immune system. Remarkably, cutaneous squamous cell carcinomas are the commonest malignancy encountered in organ transplant recipients.

The present textbook reflects the pioneering studies performed since long by Dermatologists and Nephrologists in Lyon, who realized early the benefit of a close collaboration. This work is unique in this field, and has been compiled by internationally-renowned experts. It should be of interest to all physicians who want to keep up-to-date with the advancement of medicine.

Professor Jean THIVOLET

1

Organ transplantation: past, present and putative future

*Jean-Louis TOURAINE, Anderson RATSIMBAZAFY,
Nicole LEFRANÇOIS, Jeanne-Luce GARNIER, Sameh DAOUD
Department of Transplantation and Clinical Immunology, Hôpital Édouard-Herriot, Lyon, France.*

Organ transplantation has gone a long way since the initial successful clinical applications, some four decades ago. It has been a good surprise that, in many cases, a short-term treatment for an acute rejection episode was sufficient not only for the cure of the immunological reaction but also for the acceptance of the transplant without further rejection, despite the fact that the immunosuppressive treatment was back at low dosages.

Major progresses in immunosuppressive therapies have been recorded. However, they have mostly benefited the prevention of early failures and of acute rejection crises, but have proven less remarkable in the suppression of causes for late failures or for complications of immunosuppression itself (especially malignancies and infections).

In spite of considerable experimental research, transplantation tolerance, as initially described by Billingham, Brent, and Medawar [1], has not yet become routinely applicable to the frequent circumstance of clinical organ transplantation.

Past

Basic knowledge

After the discovery that graft failure was a result of an immunological process, several lines of research have led to precious informations on the major histocompatibility complex (MHC). In humans, determinants encoded for by HLA class I and class II genes [2], as well as the expression of ABO molecules are the main targets for the rejection processes. Nevertheless, a full match for all these molecules between donor and recipient is not equivalent to a monozygotic twin situation and does not permit acceptance of the transplant without the help of at least a moderate immunosuppressive therapy. The mechanisms of immunological phenomena leading to rejection have been progressively described; they involve humoral factors including antibodies, and cellular factors including T lymphocytes and macrophages. The recognition of foreign cells can be either direct (MHC molecules expressed by cells of the transplant) or indirect (peptides processed from the donor MHC presented in the groove of MHC molecules of the antigen presenting cells of the host). The latter mechanism is the common mode of recognition of any antigen by the T cell receptor; the former one is specific for recognition in the field of transplantation, *i.e.* in circumstances when the antigen to be recognized by the T cell receptor is a MHC molecule present at the cell surface. That both mechanisms can lead to rejection has been demonstrated by several experimental studies. It can for instance be recalled that transplant rejection does occur in patients with type III of the Bare Lymphocyte Syndrome [3], despite the lack of expression of MHC on host cells, including antigen presenting cells, thus showing that direct recognition of donor MHC can initiate a rejection.

Hyperacute rejection has been shown to occur mostly as a consequence of preformed antibodies [4] but can also result from T cell repeated sensitization to donor antigens [5]. Conversely, acute rejection of a transplanted organ mostly results from T cell sensitization developing after transplantation, but it frequently also involves antibodies, especially anti-HLA ones. Chronic rejection is a complex phenomenon involving several immune injuries on the long-term; it has recently been dissociated from other causes of late failures of organ transplantation, especially the progressive exhaustion of the kidney transplant subjected to hyperfiltration when there is a significantly reduced nephronic mass [6].

It has recently become understood that the initiation of rejection needs two signals to the T lymphocytes, a single signal tending to lead to a form of tolerance. The balance between the various cytokines produced in the recipient following transplantation can also play a major part in the choice between rejection processes or active acceptance of the transplant.

Non-immunological findings have also proven efficient in the improvement of transplantation results. For instance, various measures to prevent ischemic injuries have progressively been applied following basic research along these lines.

Clinical progresses

The first successful organ transplants in humans were kidney transplants between twins. Soon afterwards, transplants of kidneys from related living donors (mostly siblings or parents) were undertaken with various degrees of match and with progressively increasing success rates. Cadaver kidney transplants then developed and were followed by liver, heart, pancreas, lung and other organ transplants.

During all those years, iatrogenic immunosuppression improved: irradiation was rapidly abandoned for azathioprine and steroids, then for cyclosporin and more recently for a large variety of compounds (FK506, mycophenolate mofetil, rapamycin, deoxyspergualin, brequinar, mizoribine, etc.). These new immunosuppressants will be considered in another chapter of this volume; suffice it to say here that the possibility to use several drugs in combination or sequentially permits an improved treatment of the transplant patient. Frequently, at least for an initial period, the patients receive the addition of several drugs, each at a relatively limited dosage so as to avoid individual side-effects of each compound. Careful monitoring usually permits to avoid over-immunosuppression and the many complications associated to it. In any case, when a complication directly related to one drug occurs, it is now possible to readily change it for another immunosuppressant. In addition to these compounds, many transplant patients receive biological treatments for short periods, in the form of anti-lymphocyte globulins or monoclonal antibodies, contributing to a more potent immunosuppression over the induction period or at the time of a severe rejection episode.

All these treatments have been selected in the past by transplant experimentalists, physicians and surgeons, as well as the pharmaceutical industry, based on short-term results (at one or, at the most, three years) and on their capacity to prevent or treat acute rejections. The objective that was looked for has been reached: early failures have nowadays almost disappeared when they were responsible for loss of transplants in approximately one fourth of cases two decades ago. Simultaneously, causes for mortality or severe complications in the early phase after transplantation (such as prevention of *Pneumocystis carinii*, prevention or detection and treatment of CMV infection, prevention and early detection of bacterial infections, prevention of steroid complications, etc.) were eradicated or significanlty reduced.

Improvements in surgical techniques and in post-operative care to the recipient, as well as care to the donor and the transplant itself also contributed to the significant progresses. Even before the use of the new immunosuppressive therapies, the results had been better and better, years after years, based on improved use of the available drugs and the experience in transplantation. Further progresses obviously resulted from introduction of the new and relatively more selective compounds. It was however rapidly felt that great care had to be given to the danger of over-immunosuppression since many treatments are now so effective that given at large doses or in association with other very effective drugs, they can induce a significantly increased risk of EBV-associated lymphoproliferative disorders, of other malignancies, or of other infections.

Present

Organ shortage

Because of increasing successes in organ transplantation, indications for this form of therapy have largely increased. Patients over 60 and even over 70 years are routinely transplanted when necessary. Newborns are also transplanted. Patients with failure of several organs are no longer considered as contra-indication to transplantation. Simultaneous transplantations are also routinely performed (kidney and pancreas, kidney and liver, or kidney and heart, heart and lungs, or heart and liver), as well as the transplantation of three or more organs, up to multivisceral transplants. Sequential transplants are also becoming increasingly frequent since many patients transplanted several decades ago need a second or a third transplant, after long-term failure of their initial transplants. A few patients need a second transplant immediately after the first surgery, due to initial failure. All these reasons and a few others are responsible for a very long waiting list. Few progresses have been very efficient in preventing the development of chronic renal failure. The longer life expectancy has even resulted in more cases. In the face of this increasing need for transplants, the offer does not tend to increase: traffic accidents are fortunately less frequent, intensive cares are able to save more patients, family donors are less often volunteers for organ donations, refusal of organ procurement from a brain-dead cadaver is unfortunately increasing, due to less positive attitudes of some families.

Major efforts have to be made to solve this frustrating organ shortage which results in long waits before transplantation, addition of the complications of dialysis to those of transplantation, death of patients while on the waiting list, ethical, psychological, medical and social difficulties [7]. In some countries, organ traffic has developed as a result of this shortage, and there are patients that travel to other continents to receive a transplant from an unrelated living donor selling one kidney in order to fight poverty. Such attitudes are unacceptable and require an international effort to prevent the traffic of human organs. Education of the population, campaigns of various natures, improved organizations should be helpful and we look forward to seeing the time when possibilities will equal needs and when the main cause of mortality for patients requiring a transplant will no longer be the impossibility of transplantation due to organ shortage.

Long-term results

Most, if not all, of the improvements in transplantation, have led to a dramatic increase in patient and transplant survivals at one and three years. By comparison, very few improvements have been achieved towards long-term results, at ten years or more [8]. Actually, if one plots transplantation results considering only those patients who have a good result at one year, no significant differences are observed in the progressive decline of transplant survival, depending on the fact that the transplant was carried out recently or twenty years ago. If the half-life of the transplant is now longer than in the past, this is due to the fact that early failures were more frequent in the 1960s and 1970s than in the 1980s or 1990s.

Several factors are responsible for this insufficient improvement of long-term results. Research on chronic rejection and its prevention or treatment by drugs have been less intensive than those on early acute rejection; clinical trials with a follow-up of over ten years have been more difficult to develop than shorter term clinical trials; the basic immunological and non-immunological mechanisms responsible for the chronic deterioration of the transplanted organs have proved more difficult to analyze and appear to involve intricated systems; in addition to genuine rejection, recurrence of the initial disease can occur and, in the case of kidney transplantation, progressive exhaustion of the organ develops when the nephronic mass has been reduced as a result of donor age, severe ischemia, initial acute rejection or other factors. The mean age of transplant recipients is higher today than it was some twenty years ago and diseases of the old age can also occur in elderly transplanted patients; some of these complications are favoured by immunosuppressive therapies. Observance of the treatment has also been shown to be deficient on the long-term in some patients and this cause of long-term failure may be more frequent at a time when transplantation is no longer considered as an extraordinary treatment; it should be prevented by more efficient education programs to transplanted patients and their families.

It is well known that the risks of acute rejection and acute failure rapidly decrease with time after transplantation. Several years following surgery and under a chronic immunosuppressive treatment, the transplant patients benefit from organ adaptation (including replacement of donor endothelial cells by recipient ones) and from immunological modifications of the recipient (acceptance of the foreign transplant by the host). If the treatment is discontinued after several years, a good function of the organ is frequently observed for many weeks or months before progressive and slow rejection occurs. In some cases, the transplant can even be definitely accepted, despite discontinuation of treatment on the long-term. It has been postulated that such a phenomenon could result from microchimerism [9]. With sensitive PCR techniques, cells of donor origin are indeed found in various parts of the body of some transplant recipients, especially in lymphoid tissues. It is however uncertain whether such a microchimerism is in any way responsible for the good equilibrium between host and transplant. Alternatively, the microchimerism can be considered as a marker of a good immunological balance, resulting from the long-term immunosuppressive therapy and occasionally continuing many years after discontinuation of the treatment. In this latter hypothesis, when rejection occurs, the first targets of the immunological reaction are these disseminated donor cells which are eliminated before the transplant itself is destroyed; this would then explain the disappearance of microchimerism before the occurrence of the transplant rejection, even without considering that the disappearance of microchimerism is directly responsible for the organ rejection itself. Further research will hopefully answer this question and will unravel whether such phenomena can be used either to monitor or to induce a better acceptance of the transplant organ by the host on the long-term.

Putative future

Transplantation tolerance

The induction of immunological tolerance allowing definite acceptance of a transplant without the chronic use of non-specific immunosuppressive agents has been the goal of all transplantologists for four decades. It will have a number of advantages: avoidance of late immunological failures, lack of need for iterative transplants in a time of organ shortage, and absence of complications associated with chronic immunosuppression (infections of various kinds, malignancies including the most frequent skin cancers and life-threatening lymphomas).

Since 1988, the neonatal type of central tolerance can be induced in humans: it requires injection of stem cells into human fetuses during the first half of pregnancy [10]. Although the analysis of this situation provides interesting and useful information on transplantation tolerance in humans, it does not give the key for tolerance induction in adult organ transplantation. Indeed, replacement of the full lymphoid system of the host, by means of a bone marrow transplant, naturally leads to acceptance of all organs from the same donor. Unfortunately the bone marrow transplant and the large chimerism resulting from it induces mortality and morbidity risks (including GVHD) far superior to those associated with an organ transplant under conventional immunosuppressive therapy. Despite a large number of experiments in the field of tolerance, additional studies are required to define what can be clinically applicable in terms of central or peripheral tolerance, with various degrees of chimerism or other immunological handlings and with a prolonged duration either without chronic treatment after tolerance induction or with a very low maintenance therapy.

Xenotransplantation

Transplantation of animal organs to humans would solve the difficult problem of organ shortage. However, a number of obstacles still remain to be overcome [11]. Natural xenoreactive antibodies result in severe and hyperacute rejection. Such antibodies can be absorbed to decrease the intensity of the immune reaction. In addition, inhibition of the complement activation cascade is possible and interesting results have been obtained using transgenic pigs [12]. Even when these problems are solved, the intensity of rejection of the xenotransplant might be more severe than that of an allotransplant, and xenotransplantation might require more potent immunosuppressive drugs. Complications of immunosuppression could then be more frequent; xenotransplants would be associated with a higher mortality and morbidity rate than allotransplants and it will be ethically difficult to select patients for xeno- rather than allotransplantation. Aside from rare cases when the patient is dying (for instance of fulminating hepatitis) and needs an immediate transplant of the first available organ, allotransplantation will generally be preferred for the next years over xenotransplantation. Finally, the recent medical history has shown us how cautious we should be to protect humans from epidemics due to agents derived from animals. Retroviruses, other viruses, prions, other biological agents have been transmitted from animals to humans and resulted in either small or large epidemics which have proven difficult to control.

Xenotransplants will indeed be the solution for organ procurement to treat human patients. It will however require many years or decades before it is routinely applicable: initially it will be used only in dying recipients unable to wait for human organs. With more experience and more basic knowledge (pending strict avoidance of any transmission of detrimental biological agents, induction of some form of tolerance to the antigens of the xenotransplant, production of appropriate transgenic animals in large numbers, availability of adequately functional organs) xenotransplantation will progressively replace allotransplantation, at least for many of the organ transplants. Not mentioned are the economical aspects of this future field that will require additional resources, difficult to generate in many countries. The years before routine application of clinical xenotransplantation will be sufficiently long to prompt maintenance of efforts to solve current problems of allotransplantation. Organ shortage, immunological aspects of allotransplants, infectious and malignant complications should be faced and prevented at present, in the setting of allotransplantation; it will be helpful to prepare the future use of xenotransplantation, a field in which the additional difficulties will also have to be successfully faced.

Conclusion

Organ transplantation has saved many lives. The quality of life of transplant patients is generally good. It is however frustrating that, at a time when this new therapy is so successful, it cannot benefit all putative patients in any country. To prepare even more satisfactory conditions in the future, efforts should be presently amplified in the following directions: improved immunosuppression for the long-term, reduction of late failures, induction of immunological tolerance, solutions to organ shortage, improvement of xenotransplantation, prevention of malignancies and other complications.

References

1. Billingham RE, Brent L, Medawar PB. Actively acquired tolerance of foreign cells. *Nature* 1953 ; 172 : 603-6.
2. Dausset J, Ivanyi P, Ivanyi D. Tissue alloantigens in humans identification of a complex system (Hu-1). In : *Histocompatibility testing*. Copenhagen : Munksgaard, 1965 : 51-62.
3. Touraine JL. Le syndrome des lymphocytes dénudés. *médecine/sciences* 1987 ; 3 : 270-4.
4. Williams GM, Hume DM, Hudson RP, Morris PJ, Kano K, Milgrom F. Hyperacute renal-homograft rejection in man. *N Engl J Med* 1968 ; 279 : 611-8.
5. Yoshimura R, Touraine JL, Chargui J, Veyron P, Aitouche A. Second-set rejection of skin allografts is mediated by a T cell subset in mice unable to mount a humoral response with cytotoxic antibodies. *Transplant Proc* 1997 ; 29 : 868.
6. Brenner BM, Mackenzie HS. Nephron endowment and the pathogenesis of chronic renal failure. In : Touraine JL, Traeger J, Bétuel H, Dubernard JM, Revillard JP, Dupuy C, eds. *Retransplantation. Transplantation and clinical immunology*, vol. XXVIII. Dordrecht : Kluwer Academic Publishers, 1997 : 93-100.
7. Touraine JL, Traeger J, Bétuel H, Dubernard JM, Revillard JP, Dupuy C. Cancer in transplantation: prevention and treatment. *Transplantation and clinical immunology*, vol. XXVI. Dordrecht : Kluwer Academic Publishers, 1995.
8. Touraine JL, Traeger J, Bétuel H, Dubernard JM, Revillard JP, Dupuy C. *Retransplantation. Transplantation and clinical immunology*, vol. XXVIII. Dordrecht : Kluwer Academic Publishers, 1997.

9. Starzl TE, Demetris AJ, Muarse N, Trucco M, Thomson AW, Rao AS. The lost chord: microchimerism and allograft survival. *Immunol Today* 1996 ; 12 : 577-84.

10. Touraine JL. Treatment of human fetuses and induction of immunological tolerance in humans by *in utero* transplantation of stem cells into fetal recipients. *Acta Haematol* 1996 ; 96 : 115-9.

11. Ferran C, Badrichani AZ, Cooper JT, Stroka DM, Bach FH. Xénotransplantation : en route vers le développement clinique. In : Funck-Brentano JL, Bach JF, Kreis H, Grünfeld JP, eds. *Actualités néphrologiques*. Paris : Flammarion, 1997 : 234-53.

12. Cozzi E, White D. The generation of transgenic pigs as potential organ donors for humans. *Nature Med* 1995 ; 1 : 964-6.

2

The skin immune system

Denis JULLIEN [1,2], Robert L. MODLIN [3], Jean-François NICOLAS [2,4]
1. Department of Dermatology, Edouard-Herriot Hospital, 69437 Lyon Cedex 03, France.
2. INSERM U999, Laënnec University, 69372 Lyon Cedex 08, France.
3. Division of Dermatology and Department of Microbiology and Immunology,
   UCLA School of Medicine, Los Angeles, CA 90095, USA.
4. Clinical Immunology, Centre Hospitalier Lyon-Sud, 69495 Pierre-Bénite, France.

More than being only a mechanical barrier *vis-à-vis* the external environment, the skin functions as an immune organ which allows the body to react to the environment but also to interact with it and to adapt to it. Keratinocytes, fibroblasts, Langerhans cells, dermal dendritic cells, endothelial cells, mast cells, tissue macrophages, skin homing T-cells, vessels, nerves and the humoral system are parts of a network which makes up the skin immune system. In transplantation surgery, immunosuppressive drugs are used to reduce the immune response and prevent graft rejection. Being not tissue-specific, these measures will impair the skin immunological defense system and account for a considerably increased incidence of cutaneous neoplasms and viral infections. The most commonly used regimen to reduce acute and chronic graft rejection is a combination of a very limited number of drugs represented mainly by prednisone, azathioprine, cyclosporin A and mycophenolate mofetil. While all these drugs are aimed to target lymphocyte functions, they do not show a very restricted cellular specificity. For instance, cyclosporin A which is probably the most « T-cell specific » among these drugs affects also keratinocyte and Langerhans cell functions. This chapter will focus on Langerhans cells and T-cells to provide the reader with some clues on how immunosuppressive drug-induced impairment of these cell subsets might affect some essential skin functions.

Langerhans cells

Physiology

Langerhans cells (LC) found in the epidermis are the best characterized dendritic cell population. These powerful antigen-presenting cells form a network able to detect and capture foreign substances such as contact allergens, microbial molecules or tumor-associated protein. They seem to originate from a defined subset of CD34+ circulating precursors cells which express the skin homing receptor cutaneous lymphocyte-associated antigen (CLA) [1]. LC have the ability to process antigen in the periphery and transport it *via* lymphatics to the draining lymph nodes. Migration of the LC is enabled by adhesion molecules which can both maintain LC in the epidermis and allow them to migrate through the basal membrane into the dermis and down to the draining lymph nodes.

Soluble factors, particularly TNFα, could also influence migration of LC to the draining lymph nodes. During migration LC undergo phenotypic and functional changes, including upregulation of costimulatory molecules such as B7.1 and some antigen-presenting molecules. Overall, LC would be particularly efficient for antigen uptake and processing in the epidermis, and when LC have left the epidermis to the draining lymph nodes, antigen processing would be less efficient but on the contrary, antigen presentation capacities would be strongly increased. In the draining lymph nodes, LC are located to the para-cortical area where they are able to cluster with naive antigen-specific T-cells, and activate them to become specific memory T-cells. Specific T-cells emigrate from the lymph nodes and diffuse to the bloodstream through the efferent lymphatic vessels and the thoracic duct on their mission to survey the skin. In the skin, through further antigen presentation, LC will be among the cells able to activate these trafficking specific T-cells.

LC in the skin of graft recipients

Immunosuppressive regimens used in graft recipients are likely to depress both the functions and number of LC. Indeed, *in vitro* data and other results obtained from non-grafted patients support this hypothesis notably for cyclosporin A and steroids [2-6]. However, contradictory data have also been published [7], and the relevance of *in vitro* findings has been questioned [8, 9].

A handful of studies addressed more specifically this question in renal and liver transplant patients. Except for one study [10], they globally demonstrated a marked decrease of dermal and epidermal LC in non sun-exposed skin as compared with controls [11-16]. Results concerning sun-exposed skin were more variable. This reduced number of LC was observed in patients who suffered from skin carcinomas and had been immunosuppressed for over 12 years, but was also present in allograft recipients without skin cancer at 3 to 6 years posttransplant. According to Servitje et al. [12], this change might be more pronounced in patients treated with azathioprine and prednisone than in patients receiving cyclosporin and prednisone. A specific role for azathioprine was similarly pointed out by Bergfelt et al. [15].

In many of these studies, morphological changes of LC were also observed suggesting that LC functions might be impaired too. Indeed, slight differences in the alloantigen-presenting capacity of LC present in epidermal cell suspensions prepared from kidney transplant recipients and controls were reported [11] and a decrease of HLA-DR expression of epidermal LC was demonstrated in a histologic survey spanning pre- and post-transplantation period [17].

Given these data and LC's key functions in cutaneous immunosurveillance, it makes sense that the increase of skin carcinomas and viral infections in graft recipients might be related to the impairment of LC. Therefore, what would happen if we had a way to revert this defect? For

Rook et al. [14], the answer seems to be: good things. Indeed, in a limited, open study these authors observed that the beneficial effect of retinoids on premalignant and malignant skin lesions in renal transplant recipients parallels an increase in the density of LC in the skin, which was proportionate to the duration of therapy. However, increasing LC density may not be enough to restore a fully functional skin immune system. Indeed, in another study, Shuttleworth et al. [18] assessed the delayed-type hypersensitivity response to various antigens in the skin of immunossuppressed renal transplant recipients, and reported that retinoids did not correct the observed anergy.

Lymphocytes

These cells are the other key component of the adaptive immune system in the skin, and are at the same time the main target of immunosuppressive regimens in organ transplantation. Nevertheless, as opposed to LC, almost no study has addressed specifically how these various cell subsets (i.e. $\alpha\beta$ T-cells, $\gamma\delta$ T-cells, B-cells, NK-cells…) are affected in the skin of grafted patients. Actually, it is likely that what these cells undergo in the skin is quite similar to what has been thoroughly described to occur to the same cell subsets *in vitro*, in the bloodstream or in grafted organs. These data will not be reminded here. However, since our understanding of skin-specific T-lymphocyte physiology has increased notably in the last few years, we will present some updated data to allow the reader to envision in which way impairing T-lymphocyte functions may affect the skin immune system.

Trafficking of lymphocytes into the skin

While in normal human skin only a very small number of lymphocytes can be detected around blood vessels, in inflamed skin this number is dramatically increased. Furthermore, there is as much as a 100-fold enrichment of antigen-reactive T-cells at the site of cutaneous inflammation since it has been documented that 1/1,000 to 1/10,000 T-cells in the peripheral blood recognize a given antigen whereas in the skin about 1/50-1/100 T-cells recognize the antigen causing the disease [19]. Except from local proliferation of some resident lymphocytes, the increase in cell numbers is mostly due to the trafficking of circulating lymphocytes to the skin. For some of these T-cells which belong to the memory subset and express CLA, recruitment into the skin is a specific process. CLA is an inducible carbohydrate modification of PSGL-1, a known surface glycoprotein expressed constitutively on all human peripheral-blood T-cells [20]. CLA binds to E-selectin which is induced under inflammation on endothelial cells. This interaction facilitates extravasation of T lymphocytes into the skin by mediating tethering and rolling of T-cells on vascular endothelial cells. Chemokines released by the endothelial cells activate T-cells to express the adhesion molecules LFA-1 and VLA-4. T-cells firmly adhere to the endothelium by the interaction of LFA-1 with ICAM and VLA-4 with VCAM. This strong interaction permits transmigration of T cells into the skin and allows their participation in the inflammatory process. IL8 might play a critical role in this transepithelial migration process [21].

CLA becomes expressed on memory T-cells once antigen-specific naive T-cells have been primed in the draining lymph nodes by activated LC presenting antigens taken up in the skin [22]. Repeated activation in the skin or skin-draining lymph nodes may act to reinforce CLA expression on these T-cells in a TGFβ/IL6 dependent process [23]. Up to 90% of T-cells in various inflammatory skin diseases and primary cutaneous neoplasms are CLA+ [23, 24] and bacterial toxin-induced expansion of skin-homing CLA+ T-cells is thought to contribute to the development of skin rashes in superantigen-mediated diseases [25].

THE SKIN IMMUNE SYSTEM

Studying two well-characterized T-cell-mediated patterns of cutaneous allergic inflammation, atopic and contact dermatitis, it was shown that while blood-derived CLA+ memory T-cells from atopic dermatitis patients preferentially responded to house dust mite or casein and CLA+ memory T-cells from nickel contact dermatitis patients showed an increased response to nickel, CLA− memory T-cells showed very little response in both cases [26, 27].

This CLA-mediated migration allows an efficient distribution of the immune defense to the skin and supports the existence of a regionalization of the SIS. However, recent data suggest that CLA expression may not be an absolute prerequisite for cutaneous T-cell infiltration [28]. It has been proposed that CLA expression may be important for T-cells to extravasate from blood into the skin during immune surveillance or for retention of allergen-specific T-cells in the skin. Besides the CLA, the lymphocyte differentiation antigen CD73 might be involved too in the T-cell specific recruitment in inflamed human skin [29].

It has recently been demonstrated that kidney transplant recipients receiving various combinations of azathioprine, prednisone or cyclosporin A showed dermal depletion for both the CD4+ and the CD8+ T-cell subsets. Impaired proliferation ability or increased cellular death may account for this observation. However, to date there is no available data to show that immunosuppressive regimens do not prevent T-cells from homing into the skin [13].

T-cell populations and antigen presentation in the skin

Based on their expression of cell surface determinants such as the CD4 or CD8 molecules, the kind of T-cell receptor (TCR) heterodimer ($\alpha\beta$ or $\gamma\delta$) they bear or the repertoire of these TCRs in the infiltrate, specific populations of T-cells can be identified that localize to the skin.

In the majority of inflammatory conditions studied, including lichen planus, psoriasis, atopic dermatitis, contact dermatitis and basal cell carcinoma, CD4+ T-cells outnumber CD8+ T-cells, to an extent similar to, or somewhat greater than that present in the peripheral blood. Despite this imbalance, both subsets are sometimes critical in the pathogenesis of the same disease. For instance, a growing body of evidence suggests that both CD4+ and CD8+ hapten-specific T-cells can mediate contact sensitivity. In some instances (such as in leprosy), the specific accumulation of CD4+ T-cells in the skin is associated with one form of the disease (namely tuberculoid leprosy) while CD8+ T-cells are found to be predominant in another form of the same disease (*i.e.* lepromatous leprosy) [30].

T-cells expressing the $\alpha\beta$-TCR are the predominant subset found in skin infiltrates. However, in some conditions, $\gamma\delta$ T-cells can represent as much as 35% of the infiltrating cells [31].

It has been widely accepted that peptide presentation by major histocompatibility complex class I and II molecules respectively to CD8+ and CD4+ T-cells is the basic mechanism by which specific T-cells recognize viruses, bacteria, multicellular parasites and many types of tumors. While most of the peptides presented by class I molecules are derived from the degradation of proteins in the cytoplasm, most of the peptides presented *via* the class II pathway are of extracellular origin.

The most dramatic advance in our understanding of T-cell biology has been the demonstration that T-cells are also able to recognize non-peptide antigens [32]. Indeed, on one hand $\gamma\delta$ T-cells were shown to recognize isopentenyl pyrophosphate and related antigens in a manner independent of antigen presenting molecules [33], while on the other hand CD1 molecules were shown to present lipids and lipoglycans to $\alpha\beta$ T-cells.

While the role of $\gamma\delta$ T-cells present in normal and diseased human skin remains to be clarified [31], the CD1-based system has been demonstrated to contribute to immunologic responses in this organ against mycobacterial infections and is presumably able to play some role in other infectious, tumoral and inflammatory conditions in the skin [34-36].

Since on one hand γδ T-cells and CD1-restricted T-cells do not evade the effects of immunosuppressive drugs [37] and on the other hand LC in the skin are the largest CD1+ cell population, these two antigen presentation systems should be impaired in the same way as the more conventional ones.

The Th1/Th2 paradigm

Cytokine secretion profile is another way to sort various subsets of T-cells in skin infiltrates. Based on murine CD4+ T-cell clone studies, human T-cells producing IL2 and IFNγ are termed « Th1-like cells », and are thought to contribute to cell-mediated immune reactions, whereas T-cells producing IL4, IL5 and IL10 are termed « Th2-like cells » and may promote humoral responses. These cytokine patterns are cross-regulatory. The Th1 cytokine IFNγ downregulates Th2 responses. The Th2 cytokines IL4 and IL10 downregulate both Th1 responses and macrophage function. There is ample evidence that the Th1-Th2 paradigm is not rigid; there are situations in which a mixture of cytokines is found and examples of T-cell clones exist, known as Th0 cells, which secrete a combination of Th1 and Th2 cytokines.

The Th1/Th2 paradigm provides insight into the pathogenesis of many skin diseases in which T-cells have an immunologic role. There are some skin diseases where either a Th1 or Th2 cytokine pattern predominates. For instance, in leprosy and leishmaniasis the Th1 cytokine pattern is characteristic of lesions in which cell-mediated immunity to the pathogen is strong and the lesions involute spontaneously. The Th2 pattern is typical of lesions where immunity to the pathogen is weak and the cutaneous lesions are progressive [30, 38, 39]. Similarly, Th1 responses are involved in immunologic resistance to *Borrellia burgdorferi* [40]. Pathogenic concepts of atopic dermatitis include a central role for allergen-specific T-cells which produce Th2 cytokines including IL4 and IL5. Allergen-specific T-cells which produce this cytokine profile have been demonstrated in the peripheral blood and skin lesions of subjects with active disease [41-43]. In addition, in the lesions of atopic dermatitis abundant expression of IL10 is found, although the source of this cytokine is likely to be tissue macrophages and keratinocytes [44]. The Th2 pattern of cytokines is thought to induce increased immunoglobulin production, particularly IgE, mast cell growth and the infiltration with eosinophils. These cytokines may also downregulate Th1 responses, accounting for the increased susceptibly to cutaneous bacterial infections. In allergic contact dermatitis, sensitization involves the development of a Th1 response. In patients with contact dermatitis, nickel-specific T-cells produce a Th1 cytokine pattern [45]. However, during the elicitation phase of allergic contact dermatitis, IL4 and IL10 are present in the lesions, both in animal models and in human reactions [44, 46]. This Th2 response may act to downregulate and shut off the allergic response [46-48]. Th1/Th2 responses may also be involved in anti-tumor immunity. For example, IL4 and IL10 predominate in basal and squamous cell carcinomas, as compared to the Th1 response present in benign neoplasms [49, 50]. The source of IL10 in these cases is the tumor itself, a mechanism by which the carcinoma can downregulate anti-tumor T-cell responses. Similarly, cutaneous T-cell lymphomas represent a Th1 cytokine response, whereas patients with the more progressive Sézary's syndrome exhibit a Th2 cytokine response [51]. Finally, Th1 cytokine responses predominate in psoriasis skin lesions, including uninvolved skin from psoriatic patients [52, 53].

Of particular interest to immunologists is the delineation of factors which influence the T-cell cytokine pattern. In the skin, cells of the innate immune system which include macrophages, NK cells and mast cells release cytokines which in turn bias the cytokine profile of the acquired T-cell response. For example, in response to an intracellular pathogen, macrophages release

IL12, which acts on NK cells to release IFNγ. The presence of IL12, IL2 and IFNγ, with the relative lack of IL4 facilitates Th1 responses. By contrast, in response to allergens or extracellular pathogens, mast cells or basophils release IL4, which in the absence of IFNγ, leads to differentiation of T-cells along the Th2 pathway. Keratinocytes may also influence the nature of the T-cell cytokine response since they can produce IL10 namely after exposure to UVB [54]. The released IL10 can specifically downregulate Th1 responses thus facilitating the development of Th2 responses.

In organ transplant recipients, the various drugs which compose the immunosuppressive regimen dramatically interfere with the Th1/Th2 secretion ability of T-cells in ways which may vary according to the drug considered.

Other cells

Performing a Medline search provides evidence that the physiology of almost every other cellular components of the skin immune system, from keratinocytes to mast cells and macrophages is impaired by cyclosporin A, steroids, azathioprine and the most recent immunosuppressive drugs. Alterations may concern the cell secretion ability (*i.e.* cytokines, chemokines, enzymes...) the panel of molecules displayed at the cell surface (*i.e.* adhesion molecules, membrane receptors...) or even the cell cycle and cell death.

Conclusion

Immunosuppressive regimens have allowed the development of organ transplantation programs to a large scale. However, since none of the available drugs is able to specifically target the grafted organ, this enormous progress has a payback, *i.e.* the global immune disruption. This side effect is best exemplified in the skin where impairment to the skin immune system results in an increased incidence of viral infections and skin carcinomas. Although their consequences are obvious, many of the mechanisms which account for the skin immune suppression have so far not been clearly assessed. Their better knowledge will hopefully help to design suppressive regimens with fewer cutaneous side effects.

References

1. Strunk D, Egger C, Leitner G, Hanau D, Stingl G. A skin homing molecule defines the Langerhans cell progenitor in human peripheral blood. *J Exp Med* 1997 ; 185 : 1131-6.

2. Braathen LR, Hirschberg H. The effect of short-term corticosteroid incubation on the alloactivating and antigen-presenting capacity of human epidermal Langerhans cells. *Br J Dermatol* 1984 ; 111 : 295-302.

3. Dupuy P, Bagot M, Michel L, Descourt B, Dubertret L. Cyclosporin A inhibits the antigen-presenting functions of freshly isolated human Langerhans cells *in vitro*. *J Invest Dermatol* 1991 ; 96 : 408-13.

4. Haftek M, Urabe A, Kanitakis J, Dusserre N, Thivolet J. Cyclosporin A inhibits DNA synthesis by epidermal Langerhans cells. *Reg Immunol* 1990 ; 3 : 236-41.

5. Teunissen MB, De Jager MH, Kapsenberg ML, Bos JD. Inhibitory effect of cyclosporin A on antigen and alloantigen presenting capacity of human epidermal Langerhans cells. *Br J Dermatol* 1991 ; 125 : 309-16.

6. Petzelbauer P, Wolff K. Effects of cyclosporin A on resident and passenger immune cells of normal human skin and UV-induced erythema reactions. *Br J Dermatol* 1992 ; 127 : 560-5.

7. Urabe A, Haftek M, Kanitakis J, Schmitt D, Thivolet J. Cyclosporin A does not modify Langerhans' cell number and distribution in normal human skin. *Acta Derm Venereol Stockh* 1989 ; 69 : 249-52.

8. Cooper KD, Baadsgaard O, Duell E, Fisher G, Ellis CN, Voorhees JJ. Langerhans cell sensitivity to *in vitro versus in vivo* loading with cyclosporin A. *J Invest Dermatol* 1992 ; 98 : 259-61.

9. Peguet-Navarro J, Slaats M, Thivolet J. Lack of demonstrable effect of cyclosporin A on human epidermal Langerhans cell function. *Arch Dermatol Res* 1991 ; 283 : 198-202.

10. Kelly G, Scheibner A, Murray E, Sheil R, Tiller D, Horvath J. T6+ and HLA-DR+ cell numbers in epidermis of immunosuppressed renal transplant recipients. *J Cutan Pathol* 1987 ; 14 : 202-6.

11. Sontheimer RD, Bergstresser PR, Gailiunas P Jr, Helderman JH, Gilliam JN. Perturbation of epidermal Langerhans cells in immunosuppressed human renal allograft recipients. *Transplantation* 1984 ; 37 : 168-74.

12. Servitje O, Seron D, Ferrer I, Carrera M, Pagerols X, Peyri J. Quantitative and morphometric analysis of Langerhans cells in non-exposed skin in renal transplant patients. *J Cutan Pathol* 1991 ; 18 : 106-11.

13. Galvao MM, Sotto MN, Kihara SM, Rivitti EA, Sabbaga E. Lymphocyte subsets and Langerhans cells in sun-protected and sun-exposed skin of immunosuppressed renal allograft recipients. *J Am Acad Dermatol* 1998 ; 38 : 38-44.

14. Rook AH, Jaworsky C, Nguyen T, Grossman RA, Wolfe JT, Witmer WK, Kligman AM. Beneficial effect of low-dose systemic retinoid in combination with topical tretinoin for the treatment and prophylaxis of premalignant and malignant skin lesions in renal transplant recipients. *Transplantation* 1995 ; 59 : 714-9.

15. Bergfelt L, Larko O, Blohme I. Skin disease in immunosuppressed patients in relation to epidermal Langerhans' cells. *Acta Derm Venereol Stockh* 1993 ; 73 : 330-4.

16. Gilhar A, Enat R, Baruch Y. HLA-DR positive epidermal Langerhans' cells in liver cirrhosis and immunosuppressed liver transplanted patients. *Acta Derm Venereol Stockh* 1994 ; 74 : 93-4.

17. Jontell M, Gabel H, Ohman SC, Brynger H. Class II antigen expression of epidermal Langerhans cells in renal allograft recipients. *Transpl Int* 1988 ; 1 : 186-9.

18. Shuttleworth D, Marks R, Griffin PJ, Salaman JR. Treatment of cutaneous neoplasia with etretinate in renal transplant recipients. *Q J Med* 1988 ; 68 : 717-25.

19. Modlin RL, Melancon-Kaplan J, Young SM, Pirmez C, Kino H, Convit J, Rea TH, Bloom BR. Learning from lesions: patterns of tissue inflammation in leprosy. *Proc Natl Acad Sci USA* 1988 ; 85 : 1213-7.

20. Fuhlbrigge RC, Kieffer JD, Armerding D, Kupper TS. Cutaneous lymphocyte antigen is a specialized form of PSGL-1 expressed on skin-homing T cells. *Nature* 1997 ; 389 : 978-81.

21. Santamaria Babi LF, Moser B, Perez Soler MT, Moser R, Loetscher P, Villiger B, Blaser K, Hauser C. The interleukin 8 receptor B and CXC chemokines can mediate transendothelial migration of human skin homing T cells. *Eur J Immunol* 1996 ; 26 : 2056-61.

22. Butcher EC, Picker LJ. Lymphocyte homing and homeostasis. *Science* 1996 ; 272 : 60-6.

23. Picker LJ, Treer JR, Ferguson-Darnell B, Collins PA, Bergstresser PR, Terstappen LW. Control of lymphocyte recirculation in man. II. Differential regulation of the cutaneous lymphocyte-associated antigen, a tissue-selective homing receptor for skin-homing T cells. *J Immunol* 1993 ; 150 : 1122-36.

24. Gelb AB, Smoller BR, Warnke RA, Picker LJ. Lymphocytes infiltrating primary cutaneous neoplasms selectively express the cutaneous lymphocyte-associated antigen (CLA). *Am J Pathol* 1993 ; 142 : 1556-64.

25. Leung DY, Gately M, Trumble A, Ferguson-Darnell B, Schlievert PM, Picker LJ. Bacterial superantigens induce T cell expression of the skin-selective homing receptor, the cutaneous lymphocyte-associated antigen, *via* stimulation of interleukin 12 production. *J Exp Med* 1995 ; 181 : 747-53.

26. Santamaria Babi LF, Picker LJ, Perez Soler MT, Drzimalla K, Flohr P, Blaser K, Hauser C. Circulating allergen-reactive T-cells from patients with atopic dermatitis and allergic contact dermatitis express the skin-selective homing receptor, the cutaneous lymphocyte-associated antigen. *J Exp Med* 1995 ; 181 : 1935-40.

27. Abernathy-Carver KJ, Sampson HA, Picker LJ, Leung DY. Milk-induced eczema is associated with the expansion of T-cells expressing cutaneous lymphocyte antigen. *J Clin Invest* 1995 ; 95 : 913-8.

28. de Vries IJ, Langeveld-Wildschut EG, van Reijsen FC, Bihari IC, Bruijnzeel-Koomen CA, Thepen T. Nonspecific T-cell homing during inflammation in atopic dermatitis: expression of cutaneous lymphocyte-associated antigen and integrin alphaE beta7 on skin-infiltrating T-cells. *J Allergy Clin Immunol* 1997 ; 100 : 694-701.

29. Arvilommi AM, Salmi M, Airas L, Kalimo K, Jalkanen S. CD73 mediates lymphocyte binding to vascular endothelium in inflamed human skin. *Eur J Immunol* 1997 ; 27 : 248-54.

30. Modlin RL, Hofman FM, Taylor CR, Rea TH. T lymphocyte subsets in the skin lesions of patients with leprosy. *J Am Acad Dermatol* 1983 ; 8 : 182-9.

31. Alaibac M, Morris J, Chu AC. Gamma delta T-cells in human cutaneous immunology. *Int J Clin Lab Res* 1997 ; 27 : 158-64.

32. Porcelli SA, Morita CT, Modlin RL. T-cell recognition of non-peptide antigens. *Curr Opin Immunol* 1996 ; 8 : 510-6.

33. Morita CT, Beckman EM, Bukowski JF, Tanaka Y, Band H, Bloom BR, Golan DE, Brenner MB. Direct presentation of nonpeptide prenyl pyrophosphate antigens to human gamma delta T-cells. *Immunity* 1995 ; 3 : 495-507.

34. Kawano T, Cui J, Koezuka Y, Toura I, Kaneko Y, Motoki K, Ueno H, Nakagawa R, Sato H, Kondo E, Koseki H, Taniguchi M. CD1d-restricted and TCR-mediated activation of valpha14 NKT cells by glycosylceramides. *Science* 1997 ; 278 : 1626-9.

35. Cui J, Shin T, Kawano T, Sato H, Kondo E, Toura I, Kaneko Y, Koseki H, Kanno M, Taniguchi M. Requirement for Valpha14 NKT cells in IL12-mediated rejection of tumors. *Science* 1997 ; 278 : 1623-6.

36. Jullien D, Stenger S, Ernst WA, Modlin RL. CD1 presentation of microbial nonpeptide antigens to T-cells. *J Clin Invest* 1997 ; 99 : 2071-4.

37. Lin T, Matsuzaki G, Umesue M, Omoto K, Yoshida H, Harada M, Singaram C, Hiromatsu K, Nomoto K. Development of TCR-gamma delta CD4−CD8+ alpha alpha but not TCR-alpha beta CD4-CD8+ alpha alpha i-IEL is resistant to cyclosporin A. *J Immunol* 1995 ; 155 : 4224-30.

38. Pirmez C, Yamamura M, Uyemura K, Paes-Oliveira M, Conceicao-Silva F, Modlin RL. Cytokine patterns in the pathogenesis of human leishmaniasis. *J Clin Invest* 1993 ; 91 : 1390-5.

39. Caceres-Dittmar G, Tapia FJ, Sanchez MA, Yamamura M, Uyemura K, Modlin RL, Bloom BR, Convit J. Determination of the cytokine profile in American cutaneous leishmaniasis using the polymerase chain reaction. *Clin Exp Immunol* 1993 ; 91 : 500-5.

40. Yssel H, Shanafelt MC, Soderberg C, Schneider PV, Anzola J, Peltz G. *Borrelia burgdorferi* activates a T-helper type 1-like T-cell subset in Lyme arthritis. *J Exp Med* 1991 ; 174 : 593-601.

41. van Reijsen FC, Bruijnzeel-Koomen CA, Kalthoff FS, Maggi E, Romagnani S, Westland JK, Mudde GC. Skin-derived aeroallergen-specific T-cell clones of Th2 phenotype in patients with atopic dermatitis. *J Allergy Clin Immunol* 1992 ; 90 : 184-93.

42. van der Heijden FL, Wierenga EA, Bos JD, Kapsenberg ML. High frequency of IL4-producing CD4+ allergen-specific T lymphocytes in atopic dermatitis lesional skin. *J Invest Dermatol* 1991 ; 97 : 389-94.

43. Hamid Q, Boguniewicz M, Leung DY. Differential *in situ* cytokine gene expression in acute *versus* chronic atopic dermatitis. *J Clin Invest* 1994 ; 94 : 870-6.

44. Ohmen JD, Hanifin JM, Nickoloff BJ, Rea TH, Wyzykowski R, Kim J, Jullien D, McHugh T, Nassif AS, Chan SC. Overexpression of IL10 in atopic dermatitis. Contrasting cytokine patterns with delayed-type hypersensitivity reactions. *J Immunol* 1995 ; 154 : 1956-63.

45. Kapsenberg ML, Wierenga EA, Stiekema FE, Tiggelman AM, Bos JD. Th1 lymphokine production profiles of nickel-specific CD4+T-lymphocyte clones from nickel contact allergic and non-allergic individuals. *J Invest Dermatol* 1992 ; 98 : 59-63.

46. Gautam SC, Chikkala NF, Hamilton TA. Anti-inflammatory action of IL4. Negative regulation of contact sensitivity to trinitrochlorobenzene. *J Immunol* 1992 ; 148 : 1411-5.

47. Ferguson TA, Dube P, Griffith TS. Regulation of contact hypersensitivity by interleukin 10. *J Exp Med* 1994 ; 179 : 1597-604.

48. Schwarz A, Grabbe S, Riemann H, Aragane Y, Simon M, Manon S, Andrade S, Luger TA, Zlotnik A, Schwarz T. In vivo effects of interleukin 10 on contact hypersensitivity and delayed-type hypersensitivity reactions. *J Invest Dermatol* 1994 ; 103 : 211-6.

49. Yamamura M, Modlin RL, Ohmen JD, Moy RL. Local expression of antiinflammatory cytokines in cancer. *J Clin Invest* 1993 ; 91 : 1005-10.

50. Kim J, Modlin RL, Moy RL, Dubinett SM, McHugh T, Nickoloff BJ, Uyemura K. IL10 production in cutaneous basal and squamous cell carcinomas. A mechanism for evading the local T cell immune response. *J Immunol* 1995 ; 155 : 2240-7.

51. Saed G, Fivenson DP, Naidu Y, Nickoloff BJ. Mycosis fungoides exhibits a Th1-type cell-mediated cytokine profile whereas Sezary syndrome expresses a Th2-type profile. *J Invest Dermatol* 1994 ; 103 : 29-33.

52. Uyemura K, Yamamura M, Fivenson DF, Modlin RL, Nickoloff BJ. The cytokine network in lesional and lesion-free psoriatic skin is characterized by a T-helper type 1 cell-mediated response. *J Invest Dermatol* 1993 ; 101 : 701-5.

53. Schlaak JF, Buslau M, Jochum W, Hermann E, Girndt M, Gallati H, Meyer zum Buschenfelde KH, Fleischer B. T-cells involved in psoriasis vulgaris belong to the Th1 subset. *J Invest Dermatol* 1994 ; 102 : 145-9.

54. Enk AH, Katz SI. Identification and induction of keratinocyte-derived IL10. *J Immunol* 1992 ; 149 : 92-5.

3

Immunosuppressive treatments

Claire POUTEIL-NOBLE
Department of Nephrology-Transplantation, Centre Hospitalier Lyon-Sud, Pierre-Bénite, France.

From the early 1960's, azathioprine and steroids, referred to as « conventional immunosuppression » provided the basis of immunosuppressive therapy in clinical renal transplantation. Since the 1980's, cyclosporine has become the most effective and widely used immunosuppressive agent. Polyclonal antibodies (anti-lymphocyte and anti-thymocyte globulins) have been used since 1965 and monoclonal antibodies, namely OKT3, since 1985. They were both used for rejection prophylaxis and treatment of steroid-resistant rejection.

New immunosuppressive drugs are now available in clinical transplantation, such as mycophenolate mofetil, tacrolimus and sirolimus, while others (deoxyspergualine, brequinar sodium, leflunomide) are still only used in experimental transplantation. Several immunosuppressive protocols now exist; their efficacy, side effects and costs should be evaluated in the trial design, not only in the short term but also at 5-10 years.

Immunosuppressive drugs

Azathioprine

Mode of action
Azathioprine is a purine analogue, a nitro-imidazole derivative of 6-mercaptopurine (6-MP). It is incorporated into cellular DNA and inhibits purine synthesis and metabolism. It does not prevent gene activation, but inhibits gene replication and consequent T cell activation. It inhibits the primary immune response and is effective in preventing the onset of acute rejection but not for the treatment of overt rejection episodes.

Azathioprine is metabolized in the liver before it becomes active; it is rapidly converted *in vivo* into 6-MP that may then be metabolized by S-methylation, catalyzed by thiopurine methyl-transferase (TPMT), oxidized by xanthine oxidase to thiouric acid, or catabolized to 6-thioguanine nucleotides by hypoxanthine-guanine phosphoribosyl-transferase.

6-thioguanine nucleotides are responsible for the cytotoxicity of azathioprine. TPMT activity is either high or low, as determined by an allelic polymorphism. Homozygotes for the low activity allele are at risk for profound bone-marrow suppression with azathioprine while homozygotes for the high allele activity may be insufficiently immunosuppressed [1, 2]. Azathioprine is converted to 6-MP and further to 6-thio-inosine monophosphate. Azathioprine derivatives act by alkylating DNA precursors and by inhibiting various enzyme systems, including the conversion of the central inosine-monophosphate to adenosine monophosphate and guanosine monophosphate. In lymphocytes, 6-MP inhibits lymphocyte proliferation primarily by depletion of adenosine rather than guanosine.

Side effects

The most important side effects of azathioprine are hematologic since the drug is a broad myelocyte suppressant. Delayed hematologic suppression may occur. Blood counts must be performed daily in the first 3 weeks and regularly thereafter. If thrombopenia (< 100,000) or leukopenia (< 2,000) occur, azathioprine must be discontinued; however acute rejection is exceptional when the patient is also on cyclosporine A. Macrocytic anemia is frequent in patients receiving azathioprine for a long time.

Susceptibility to infection and neoplasia are not specific of azathioprine but the drug is potentially mutagenic and may induce chromosome breaks. Hepatotoxicity is frequent in patients with HBV and/or HCV infection and azathioprine should be reduced or avoided in patients with hepatic dysfunction. Pancreatitis is a rare complication. Alopecia may occur.

Allopurinol that inhibits xanthine-oxidase is contraindicated, due to the high risk of aplasia since xanthine-oxidase converts azathioprine to inactive 6-thiouric acid.

Dose and administration

The daily oral dose is 2-3 mg/kg; however, when used as adjunctive therapy with cyclosporine, it should be used at a lower dose (1-2 mg/kg). Following oral intake, the absorption is of 50% and the immunosuppressive activity peaks at 1-2 hours and declines after 12-24 hours. The final inactive metabolites are excreted in the urine and immunosuppressive activity and toxicity are probably unaltered in renal failure.

Steroids

Steroids have widely been used since 1962 as prophylactic and curative treatments for rejection. New immunosuppressive agents should allow their decrease or their discontinuation, to avoid their various side effects.

Mechanism of action

The most important immunosuppressive effect is mediated through blockade of IL1, IL2, IL3, IL6, TNFα and IFNγ expression. The blockade of IL1 and IL6 gene expression by antigen-presenting cells is critical since these cytokines provide costimuli for IL2 expression by activated T cells [3].

Inhibition of IL1 expression is responsible for the fever decrease when high dose steroids are given for acute rejection. They inhibit the antigen-presenting cell function of macrophages and dendritic cells. The inhibition of cytokine gene transcription is mediated by the binding of the steroid-receptor complex to the glucocorticoid response element located in the promoter regions of several cytokine genes, NF-κB a transcription factor. Steroids induce IκBα protein synthesis, which inhibits the nuclear translocation of NF-κB, one of the main transcription factors.

Steroids have also anti-inflammatory effects, by inhibiting phospholipase A2 and thereby the arachidonic acid cascade, including cyclo-oxygenase and 5-lipooxygenase pathways. The migration of monocytes to sites of inflammation is also inhibited. Steroids block the synthesis, release and action of a series of chemotactive factors, permeability-increasing agents and vasodilators.

Glucocorticoids cause lymphopenia through redistribution of lymphocytes to lymphoid tissues, but the total white cell count may increase during high-dose steroid pulse.

Side effects

Their intensity depends on the dose and on the varied concentration of tissue steroid receptors and steroid metabolism. The most common side effects are cushingoid facies, susceptibility to infection, impaired wound healing, osteoporosis, avascular necrosis, growth retardation in children, cataracts, diabetes or glucose intolerance, fluid retention and hypertension, gastritis and peptic ulcer disease, hyperlipidemia, obesity, acne, emotional lability and insomnia. Thus, any steroid sparing immunosuppressive regimen is welcome [4].

Administration and dose

Methylprednisolone is usually given at high dose, in i.v. pulse, at the time of transplantation; thereafter prednisolone is administered at decreasing doses down to 10 mg at the end of the first month. The half-life is in hours but the effect of steroids on lymphokine blockade persists for 24 hours and once daily administration is sufficient. Since steroids are metabolized by hepatic microsomal enzymes, barbiturates, rifampin and phenytoin can lower their plasma levels.

Cyclosporine

Cyclosporine (CSA) is a cyclic undecapeptide isolated from the fungus *Trichoderma polysporum*. Aminoacids at positions 11, 1, 2 and 3 are responsible for the active immunosuppressive site, and the cyclic structure is required for the immunosuppressive effect. The use of CSA has allowed excellent results of kidney and other organ transplants and the development of organ transplantation.

Mechanism of action

The immunosuppressive effect of CSA depends on the formation of a complex with cyclophilin which is an immunophilin, a cytoplasmic receptor, or a cis-transpeptidyl-propyl isomerase « rotamase » [5]. The complex CSA-cyclophilin binds with a very high affinity to the calcineurin-calmodulin complex, inhibits the phosphatase activity of calcineurin, and inhibits the phosphorylation of the cytoplasmic subunit of the transcription factor NF-AT (nuclear factor of activated T cells), which is required for transcription of the IL2 gene and other T cell activation genes, including c-myc, IL3, IL4, GM-CSF, TNFα and IFNγ. The drug is lymphocyte- and T cell-specific. At therapeutic levels, calcineurin activity is reduced by only approximately 50%, thus allowing the maintenance of a certain degree of immune responsiveness in case of a strong signal. Cyclosporine enhances the expression of TGFβ [6] which also inhibits IL2 and the generation of cytotoxic T lymphocytes (CTL) but may be implicated in the development of interstitial fibrosis.

Pharmacokinetics, metabolism and monitoring

CSA is available in two forms, Sandimmune® and the new microemulsion Neoral®. The absorption of CSA from the gastrointestinal tract is variable but incomplete. The time to peak concentration averages 4 hours and the bioavailability is of 30-45%. The steady level of CSA blood level is reached within 4-6 weeks. Bioavailability is better with Neoral® than with Sandimmune® and a better correlation between trough concentration and area under the curve (AUC) exists. The incidence of acute rejection and the dose required to achieve adequate trough levels are reduced by 15% and 10%, respectively.

The parent drug has a half-life of 8 hours and is metabolized by the cytochrome P450 III-A found in the gastrointestinal tract and liver microsomal enzyme system. CSA is excreted in the bile; dosage does not need to be modified in the case of renal failure or dialysis but liver impairement requires a dose reduction. CSA trough levels are measured by high pressure liquid chromatography or radioimmunoassay, and target CSA levels should be around 200 µg/L in the first month and then between 150 and 200 µg/L if associated with steroids and azathioprine. More sophisticated techniques of monitoring are currently evaluated (AUC, T2h...) [7].

Drug interactions

The interactions of CSA with many drugs require that new drugs be introduced with care; a list of drugs likely to interact with CSA metabolism should be handed to patients and their physicians (Table I), and CSA monitoring should be reinforced in the case of new pharmacologic therapy.

Table I. Pharmacological interactions of cyclosporine A (CSA)

1. Drugs decreasing CSA concentration by induction of P450 activity
   – rifampicin, isoniazide
   – barbiturates, phenytoin, carbamazepin
   – IV trimethoprim
2. Drugs increasing CSA levels by inhibition of P450 activity
   – verapamil, diltiazem, nicardipine (drugs of the dihydropyrimine group: nifedipine, isradipine, amlodipine, felodipine have no interaction)
   – ketoconazole, fluconazole, itraconazole
   – macrolide antibiotics
   – corticosteroids in high dose, during pulse steroid therapy
   – oral contraceptives, anabolic steroids, testosterone
3. Drugs enhancing CSA nephrotoxicity
   – amphotericin B
   – aminoglycosides
   – non-steroidal anti-inflammatory drugs
   – angiotensin-converting enzyme inhibitors

Side effects

Nephrotoxicity is the most important side effect of CSA and may be responsible for prolonged delayed graft function and long term chronic renal failure [8]. CSA induces a dose-dependant reversible renal vasoconstriction of the afferent arteriole and induces chronic interstitial fibrosis which may be « striped » and associated with arteriolar lesions. The mechanism involves TGFβ increase, which enhances extracellular matrix accumulation and endothelin production. Acute microvascular disease or thrombotic microangiopathy is rare but raises difficult diagnostic and therapeutic problems. Impaired sodium excretion, hyperkaliema, hyperchloremic acidosis, hypomagnesiemia and hyperuricemia can be seen.

Other side effects include hepatotoxicity, hypertrichosis, gingival hyperplasia, hyperlipidemia, glucose intolerance, neurologic complications (tremor, headache, bone pain), immunologic, infectious and neoplastic complications, mainly skin cancers and EBV lymphoproliferative disorders. The skin is one of the main sites of CSA accumulation; skin thickening, epidermal cysts, pilar keratosis, acne, sebaceous hyperplasia and folliculitis are frequent.

Tacrolimus (Prograf®)

Tacrolimus (or FK 506) is a macrolide lactone synthesized by *Streptomyces tsukubaensis* and is more immunosuppressive than CSA [9].

Mechanism of action

It is similar to that of CSA [10, 11]. Tacrolimus binds intracellularly to an immunophilin, FK-binding protein (BP) 12 (also a rotamase). The FK506-FK-BP12 complex inhibits the calcineurin-calmodulin-induced phosphorylation of the cytoplasmic component of NF-AT transcription factor for IL2 and for other cytokines. FK506 should not be administered simultaneously with CSA because of the synergistic toxicities.

Pharmacokinetics

The bioavailability of FK506 is of 22% and the absorption is rapid (mean T max: 1.5 hour, range: 0.6-7 hours) and not modified by bile salts; it occurs along the gastrointestinal tract, mainly in the duodenum and the jejunum. Absorption is influenced by the food. Half-life is 17 hours and there is a good correlation between AUC and trough levels. The drug accumulates in red blood cells (ratio red blood cells/plasma: 20/1) and binds to $\alpha 1$ glycoprotein and albumin (98.8%). Trough levels correspond to the free and the bound form of tacrolimus; plasma proteins and hematocrit influence the ratio free/bound form. The recommended starting dose is 0.1-0.3 mg/kg/d in 2 daily doses. Target trough blood levels are 10-20 ng/ml during the first 3 months and 5-10 ng/ml after 3 months of transplantation. The drug is metabolized by the liver cytochrome P450 III A and excreted through the biliary system. Renal excretion is negligible and is not dialysable. Drug interactions are similar to those described for CSA.

Side effects

They are similar to those of CSA, *i.e.* nephrotoxicity, hemolytic-uremic syndrome, infections and neoplasia. Neurotoxicity and diabetes are more frequent but hypertension and sodium retention are less frequent; hypertrichosis and gingival hypertrophia have not been described.

Tacrolimus is used as a prophylactic treatment in liver and renal transplantation. In renal transplantation, the American and European multicenter studies showed a significant lower incidence and severity of acute rejection and of corticoresistant rejection under tacrolimus *versus* cyclosporine A, without significant difference in the one year graft survival [12, 13]. Tacrolimus is also used as a rescue therapy for corticoresistant rejection with 74 % of success and with sustained efficacy [14].

Mycophenolate mofetil - MMF (Cellcept®)

The immunosuppressive properties of mycophenolate acid (MPA) were first described by Allison in 1970 and its potential use in transplantation was proposed by Allison, Morris and Engui in 1989 [15]. The active compound is MPA, a fermentation product of *Penicillium species*.

Mechanism of action

MPA is a reversible inhibitor of inosine-monophosphate dehydrogenase (IMPD), a critical rate-limiting enzyme in *de novo* synthesis of purines. As lymphocytes are highly dependent on *de novo* pathway (and cannot use the salvage pathway *via* hypoxanthine-guanine-phosphoribosyl-transferase), the anti-proliferative action is directed mostly to lymphocytes. MPA suppresses mainly IMPD isoform 2 which is expressed in lymphocytes and monocytes, and less isoform 1, the main isoform expressed in neutrophils.

In vitro, MMF inhibits T and B cell proliferation, antibody formation and the generation of cytotoxic T cells, down regulates adhesion molecule expression on lymphocytes (thereby impairing their binding to vascular endothelial cells) and inhibits the proliferation of vascular smooth muscle cells.

Side effects

They are minor, and mainly digestive (diarrhea) and hematologic (anemia). There is no nephrotoxicity.

Administration and dose

The recommended dose is 2 g/day and no blood level monitoring is required [16].

The efficacy on acute rejection incidence and severity has been shown in 3 multicenter randomized, double blind studies in the prevention of renal graft rejection [17]: 16.5% of acute rejection in MMF 3 g, 19.8% in MMF 2 g and 40.8% in the group placebo/azathioprine. However, graft survival at 1 and 3 years is not statistically improved and the beneficial effect of MMF on the prevention of chronic rejection is not proven yet.

Sirolimus

Sirolimus or rapamycine (RPM) is a macrolide antibiotic structurally related to tacrolimus and derived from the actinomycetes *Streptomyces hygroscopicus*. Its immunosuppressive property was discovered in 1977 by Sehgal and its use for controlling rejection in transplantation was described in dogs by Calne in 1989 [18].

Mechanism of action

RPM, like FK 506, binds to FK-BP immunophilin, but has no effect on the calcineurin-calmodulin complex and on the early activation genes of T cells [19, 20]. It inhibits the cytokine-mediated signal transduction pathways in late G1 phase and the progression from the G1-S phase in T cells and in smooth muscle cells. The target molecule of the complex RPM-FK-BP 25 complex is RAFT-1, downstream in the IL2/IL2 receptor pathway. It is antagonist of FK506, but has a synergistic effect with CSA.

In vitro, it inhibits the IL2-IL4 induced proliferation of T cells, but has no action on the synthesis of IL2, IL3, GM-CSF and IFNγ. RPM can differentially modulate distinct intracellular responses to cytokines. It inhibits B cell proliferation and antibody production and the growth factor-induced proliferation of smooth muscle cells. It is active on ongoing rejection.

Pharmacokinetics

The absorption of RPM is rapid (T max: 1 hour) but the bioavailability is weak (15%). It binds strongly to red blood cells (ratio red blood cells/plasma: 36/1); it is metabolized by cytochrome P450 3A4 and has the same drug interactions as CSA and FK 506. Its half-life is long (60 hours) and therefore one daily dose is sufficient. An initial high dose is required to reach rapidly the adequate concentration. There is significant intra-and inter-individual variability. Both RPM and its analog SDZ RAD, a new RPM derivative, are synergistic with CSA [21].

Side effects

RPM is not nephrotoxic but severe hypokaliemia due to tubular dysfunction can be observed. Hypertriglyceridemia (20 g/l), hypercholesterolemia, thrombopenia and cytolysis are dose dependent. Leukopenia is rare; headaches and epistaxis can be seen but no hypertension.

Clinical trials

When administered with CSA (at full or reduced doses), RPM can markedly reduce the incidence of rejection episodes (4% *versus* 32% in the control group). Prophylaxis against *Pneumocystis carinii* is required.

Other experimental immunosuppressive drugs

Leflunomide

This is a promising drug, synergistic with CSA. It blocks T and B cell responsiveness to IL2 and other cytokines; it is able to reverse acute rejection and is efficient in experimental xenotransplantation [22].

Deoxyspergualin (DSG)

DSG is an anti-tumor antibiotic with immunosuppressive activity discovered in 1985. It inhibits the maturation of T and B cells, macrophage activation, the generation of antigen-specific cytotoxic T cells and antigen processing and presentation by antigen presenting cells. It is given IV for 7-10 days (3-5 mg/kg/d). Clinically, DSG reverses steroid-resistant rejection. Its use has been approved in Japan [23].

Brequinar sodium

This is a synthetic antimetabolite, a non competitive inhibitor of dihydro-orotate-dehydrogenase, key enzyme of *de novo* pyrimidine synthesis. Phase I and II clinical trials in organ transplantation are under way. Side effects include thrombocytopenia and mucositis [23].

Polyclonal antibodies

Polyclonal antibodies are produced by immunizing horses or rabbits with human lymphoid tissue. The sera are then collected, heat-inactivated, absorbed on human red blood cells and the IgG fraction is isolated by ultracentrifugation. Anti-lymphocyte (ALG) or anti-thymocyte globulins (ATG) were introduced in the late 1960's. Polyclonal antibodies are effective for rejection prophylaxis in induction regimens and for the treatment of steroid-resistant rejection [24].

Mode of action

After ALG administration, lymphocytes, especially T cells are lysed or cleared into the reticuloendothelial system; their surface antigens (especially the CD3-T cell receptor complex, CD2, CD4, CD8 and LFA1) may be masked by the antibody. Anti-lymphocyte preparations contain different antibodies to HLA-DR, CD 25 as well as to CD4, CD8, CD45, CD18, CD11a and CD5. The amount of antibody activity varies considerably in the different preparations [25].

The rabbit ATG antibodies that persist for the longest time in monkeys include antibodies to CD3, CD4, CD8, CD11a, CD40, CD45, CD54, and to class-I MHC antigens.

Suppressor cells may be involved in the prolonged immunosuppressive effect, without lymphocyte depletion. Following ALG administration, the total lymphocyte count decreases, especially that of T cells.

Dose and administration

ATG are given at 1-10 mg/kg for rabbit preparations and at 10-20 mg/kg for horse preparations, for 10-14 days. The use of peripheral veins is proscribed; the products should be infused in a central vein over 6 hours at least. Methylprednisolone is used before injection to avoid allergic reactions and replaces oral prednisone. Monitoring of T cell numbers, or CD2 and CD3 lymphocytes is useful to adapt the dose and to avoid overimmunosuppression and excessive cost.

Side effects

Large quantities of foreign proteins are administered. Chills, fever and arthralgias are common. Serum sickness may occur and is favoured by a prolonged treatment and the absence of concomitant CSA administration. Occasional cases of anaphylaxis have been described and there is no first dose effect as with OKT3. Thrombopenia and leukopenia may occur because of undesired anti-platelet or anti-leukocyte antibodies. Infectious complications (especially with CMV) and lymphoproliferative disorders are more frequent in patients receiving ALG as an induction treatment, but they are not significantly more frequent as compared with OKT3 prophylactic treatment [26].

Results

The clinical efficacy is difficult to establish because of the variability in the potency of preparations and of dosing regimens, the lack of appropriate controls, the lack of stratification for factors associated with graft survival, and the weak power of some trials [27].

Anti-lymphocyte preparations may be useful to decrease the incidence of delayed graft function and to delay CSA use. Their use leads to a delayed occurrence of the first acute rejection episode and to a slight increase (2%) in the 5 year graft survival [24, 28]. If ALG was in the sixties the most important factor (besides HLA matching) in obtaining long-term graft survival, the cost-effectiveness of ALG as a prophylactic treatment must be reconsidered in the era of new immunosuppressive drugs, in designed clinical studies.

Monoclonal antibodies

OKT3

OKT3 was the first monoclonal antibody introduced into clinical practice in the early 1980's. It is directed against the CD3 antigen complex found on all mature T cells and is highly effective to control steroid-resistant rejection.

Mode of action

OKT3 is an IgG that binds to ε chain of the CD3 complex and induces endocytosis and disappearance from the cell surface of the T-cell receptor. After the first OKT3 injection, T cells completely disappear from the peripheral blood within 30-60 minutes, partially because of cell lysis. Depletion is not complement-dependent but is partially due to phagocytosis secondary to opsonisation. Cell marginalisation occurs through increased adhesiveness on the activated vascular endothelium and opsonisation by the reticuloendothelial system. Remnant cells undergo antigenic modulation of the T-cell receptor/CD3 complex [29]. The absence of CD3+ cells from the circulation is the best parameter for monitoring the efficacy of OKT3. CD3+ functional cells may reappear later, due to the presence of neutralizing anti-CD3 antibodies [30].

Dosage and administration

The standard dose is 5 mg/day, given as an i.v. bolus, for 10 days. The first doses of OKT3 must be administered in the hospital and a high dose of steroids (8 mg/kg i.v.) is given 1/2 hour before the first two administrations, along with paracetamol and diphenhydramine hydrochloride. The patient should be oedema-free and within 3% of dry weight and have a chest-X ray before the treatment. CSA is continued at half dose and is returned to full dose 2 days before completion of the course to reach therapeutic levels at the end of the OKT3 treatment. After 2 doses, prednisone is continued according to the protocol [3]. The presence of OKT3 antibodies must be determined 2 to 3 weeks after the end of the first course and before the second one. During retreatment, CD3 monitoring must be performed every other day and the dose of OKT3 must be doubled if CD3 levels are elevated.

Side effects

During the first days of OKT3 treatment, the release of T cell-derived cytokines (TNFα, IL2 and IFNγ) may induce life-threatening adverse reactions, such as fever and chills, pulmonary oedema, diarrhea, neurologic complications (aseptic meningitis, encephalopathy) and nephrotoxicity [30]. Infections (CMV, EBV) and lympho-proliferative diseases are more frequent in OKT3-treated patients, and antiviral prophylaxis (ganciclovir or acyclovir) or pre-emptive treatment might be recommended during OKT3 treatment for rejection.

Antibodies to the T-cell receptor (TCR)

BMA-031 (a mouse IgG2b) and T10B9-1A-31 (a mouse IgM) have been used for rescue treatments; they are less efficient than OKT3.

Anti-CD4 monoclonal antibodies

These prevent the interaction between TCR and the polymorphic determinants of class-II MHC antigens. In experimental transplantation, tolerance has been induced by anti-CD4 antibodies in combination with blood transfusions [31]. A clinical trial using OKT4A antibody in renal transplantation is ongoing [32].

Anti-CD25 antibodies (anti-IL2R)

In clinical trials, the use of 33B3-1 antibody showed a similar incidence of acute rejection but less bacterial infections than ATG [33]. Anti-CD25 antibodies induced a lower incidence of acute rejection as compared with triple therapy [34].

Antibodies to adhesion molecules

Anti-LFA1 might be useful to decrease the incidence of delayed graft function with the same anti-rejection effect as ATG [35]. The combination of anti-LFA1 and anti-ICAM1 can induce tolerance in fully-mismatched mice heart allografts [36].

Humanized and chimeric monoclonal antibodies

Chimeric monoclonal antibodies are made of rodent variable domains that are linked to the constant domains of human antibodies; they therefore combine a rodent-derived antibody binding site with a human antibody framework. In complementary determining regions (CDR) grafted antibodies, antigen binding loops of rodent monoclonal antibodies are built into human antibodies. The potential advantages are a longer half-life and no development of human anti-mouse antibodies. Humanized anti-CD25 (Zenapax®) binds to the 55p subunit of the IL2R and prevents the formation of the high affinity receptor and its activation by IL2. This product is safe and effective in preventing rejection, in association with standard immunosuppressive agents [37]. A similar study has been performed with a chimeric humanized monoclonal antibody (Simulect®) against IL2R [38].

CTL A4 Ig is an immunoglobulin fusion protein consisting of the CTL A4 receptor and the hinge, CH2 and CH3 regions of Cγ1. It competitively inhibits the CD28 signal by saturating the CD80 and CD86 antigens of antigen-presenting cells. CTL A4 Ig is promising in clinical transplantation since it is able to induce tolerance in rodents [39] and primates.

Immunosuppressive protocols

The conventional immunosuppressive treatment (steroids, azathioprine, CSA) has been used for more than 15 years with good results either in double or triple therapy [40]. With new emerging immunosuppressive drugs, protocols combining different drugs and different sequences of treatment need to be evaluated not only on the incidence of acute rejection during the first 6 months, but also in the long-term, on the incidence of metabolic, infectious and neoplastic complications [41], on the quality of life and on cost-effectiveness. Questions that remain to be answered include the benefits of steroid withdrawal, the regular substitution of azathioprine by MMF, the use of FK506 instead of CSA, the use of RPM or its analogue (RAD) in combination with CSA, the necessity and the type of induction therapy (anti-LFA, anti-IL2R, ATG...) in combination with new immunosuppressive drugs, the treatment of steroid-resistant rejection and the treatment of refractory rejection by FK 506 or MFF. The surrogate markers need to be better determined in clinical trials, since despite a decreased incidence of acute rejection graft survival at 1 or 3 years is not significantly improved in the different protocols.

References

1. Chocair PR, Duley JA, Simmonds HA, Cameron JS. The importance of thiopurine methyltransferase activity for the use of azathioprine in transplant recipients. *Transplantation* 1992 ; 53 : 1051-6.

2. Snow JL, Gibson LE. The role of genetic variation in thiopurine methyltransferase activity and the efficacy and/or side effects of azathioprine therapy in dermatologic patients. *Arch Dermatol* 1995 ; 131 : 193-7.

3. Danovitch G. Immunosuppressive medications and protocols for kidney transplantation. In : Danovitch G, ed. *Handbook of kidney transplantation*, 2nd ed. Little, Brown and Co : 55-94.

4. Grinyo JM, Gil-Vernet S, Seron D, Cruzado JM, Moreso F, Fulladosa X, Castelao AM, Torras J, Hooftman L, Alsina J. Steroid withdrawal in mycophenolate mofetil-treated renal allograft recipients. *Transplantation* 1997 ; 63 : 1688-90.

5. Cardenas ME, Zhu D, Heitman J. Molecular mechanisms of immunosuppression by cyclosporine, FK 506, and rapamycin. *Curr Opin Nephrol Hypertens* 1995 ; 4 : 472-7.

6. Khanna A, Li B, Sehajpal PK, Sharma VK, Suthanthiran M. Mechanism of action of cyclosporine: a new hypothesis implicating transforming growth factor-β. *Transplant Rev* 1995 ; 9 : 41-8.

7. Keown P, Landsberg D, Halloran P, Shoker A, Rush D, Jeffery J, Russell D, Stiller C, Muirehead N, Cole E, Paul L, Zaltman J, Loertscher R, Daloze P, Dandavino R, Boucher A, Handa P, Lawen J, Belitsky P, Parfrey P. A randomized, prospective multicenter pharmacoepidemiologic study of cyclosporine micro emulsion in stable renal graft recipients. *Transplantation* 1996 ; 62 : 1744-52.

8. De Mattos AM, Andoh TF, Bennett WM. Cyclosporine nephropathy: clinical, histological, and functional aspects. *Transplant Rev* 1996 ; 10 : 225-35.

9. Manez R, Jain A, Marino IR, Thomson AW. Comparative evaluation of tacrolimus (FK 506) and cyclosporine A as immunosuppressive agents. *Transplant Rev* 1995 ; 9 : 63-76.

10. Morris RE. Mechanisms of action of new immunosuppressive drugs. *Kidney Int* 1996 ; 53 : S26-38.

11. Halloran P, Miller LW. *In vivo* immunosuppressive mechanisms. *J Heart Lung Transplant* 1996 ; 15 : 959-71.

12. Pirsch JD, Miller J, Deierhoi MH, Vincenti F, Filo RS, for the FK 506 kidney transplant study group. A comparison of tacrolimus (FK 506) and cyclosporine for immunosuppression after cadaveric renal transplantation. *Transplantation* 1997 ; 63 : 977-83.

13. Mayer AD, Dmitrewski J, Squifflet JP, Besse T, Grabensee B, Klein B, Eigler FW, Heemann U, Pichlmayr R, Behrend M, Vanrenterghem Y, Donck J, van Hooff J, Christiaans M, Morales JM, Andres A, Johnson RW, Short C, Buchholz B, Rehmert N, Land W, Schleibner S, Forsythe JL, Talbot D, Pohanka E, *et al*. Multicenter randomized trial comparing tacrolimus (FK 506) and cyclosporine in the prevention of renal allograft rejection. A report of the European tacrolimus multicenter renal study group. *Transplantation* 1997 ; 64 : 436-43.

14. Jordan ML, Naraghi R, Shapiro R, Smith D, Vivas CA, Scantlebury VP, Gritsch HA, McCauley J, Randhawa P, Demetris AJ, McMichael J, Fung JJ, Starzl TE. Tacrolimus rescue therapy for renal allograft rejection; five year experience. *Transplantation* 1997 ; 63 : 223-8.

15. Morris RE, Hoyt EG, Engui EM, Allison AC. Prolongation of rat heart allograft survival by RS 61443. *Surg Forum* 1989 ; 40 : 337-8.

16. Sollinger HN. Mycophenolate mofetil for the prevention of acute rejection in primary cadaveric renal allograft recipients. *Transplantation* 1995 ; 60 : 225-32.

17. Halloran P, Mathew T, Tomlanovich S, Groth C, Hooftman L, Barker C, for the international mycophenolate mofetil renal transplant study group. Mycophenolate mofetil in allograft recipients. *Transplantation* 1997, 63 : 39-47.

18. Calne RY, Collier DS, Lim S, Pollard SG, Samaan A, White DJ, Thines. Rapamycin for immunosuppression in organ allografts. *Lancet* 1989 ; 2 : 227.

19. Sehgal SN, Camardo JS, Scarola JA, Maida BT. Rapamycin (sirolimus, rapamune). *Curr Opin Nephrol Hypert* 1995 ; 4 : 482-7.

20. Morris RE. Rapamycins: antifungal, antitumor, antiproliferative and immunosuppressive macrolides. *Transplant Rev* 1992 ; 6 : 39-87.

21. Schuurman HJ, Cottens S, Fuchs S, Joergenson J, Meerloo T, Sedrani R, Tanner M, Zenke G, Schuler W. SDZ RAD, a new rapamycin derivative. Synergism with cyclosporine. *Transplantation* 1997 ; 64 : 32-5.

22. Waer M. The use of leflunomide in transplantation immunology. *Transplant Immunol* 1996 ; 4 : 181-5.

23. Hayry P. Immunosuppressive drugs. In : Wood K, ed. *The handbook of transplant immunology*. Oxford : Med Sci Publications, 1995 : 135-76.

24. Shield CF, Edwards EB, Davies DB, Daily OP. Antilymphocyte induction therapy in cadaver renal transplantation. *Transplantation* 1997 ; 63 : 1257-63.

25. Bonnefoy-Bérard N, Vincent C, Revillard J. Antibodies against functional leukocyte surface molecules in polyclonal antilymphocyte and antithymocyte globulins. *Transplantation* 1991 ; 51 : 669-73.

26. Raffaele P, Pouteil-Noble C, Lefrançois N, Bosshard S, Betuel H, Aymard M, Dubernard JM, Touraine JL. Influence of a randomized monoclonal or polyclonal therapy on cytomegalovirus infection in kidney transplantation. *Transplant Proc* 1991 ; XXIII : 1361-2.

27. Paul LC, Zaltman JS, Cardella CJ. Prophylactic antilymphocyte antibody therapy in kidney transplantation: *quo vadis? Transplant Rev* 1995 ; 9 : 200-6.

28. Cecka JM, Gjerston D, Terasaki PI. Do prophylactic antilymphocyte globulins (ALG and OKT3) improve renal transplant survival in recipient and donor high risk groups? *Transplant Proc* 1993 ; 25 : 548-9.

29. Chatenoud L. Immunosuppressive biological agents. In : Wood K, ed. *The handbook of transplant immunology*. Oxford : Med Sci Publications, 1995 : 177-222.

30. Chatenoud L, Ferran C, Legendre C, Thourad I, Merite S, Reuter A, Gervaert Y, Kreis H, Franchimont P, Bach JF. *In vivo* cell activation following OKT3 administration. Systemic cytokine release and modulation by corticosteroids. *Transplantation* 1990 ; 49 : 697-702.

31. Pearson TC, Madsen JC, Larsen CP, Morris PJ, Wood KJ. Induction of transplantation tolerance in adults using donor antigen and anti-CD4 monoclonal antibody. *Transplantation* 1992 ; 54 : 475-83.

32. Cooperative clinical trials in transplantation research group. Murine OKT4A immunosuppression in cadaver donor renal allograft recipients. *Transplantation* 1997 ; 63 : 1087-95.

33. Soulillou JP, Cantarovitch D, Le Mauff B, Giral M, Robillard N, Hourmant M, Hirn M, Jacques Y. Randomized controlled trial of a monoclonal antibody against the interleukin-2 receptor (33B3.1) as compared with rabbit antithymocyte globulin for prophylaxis against rejection of renal allografts. *N Engl J Med* 1990 ; 322 : 1175-82.

34. Kirkman RL, Shapiro ME, Carpenter CB, MacKay DB, Milford EL, Ramos EL, Tilney NL, Waldmann TA, Zimmerman CE, Strom TB. A randomized prospective trial of anti-Tac monoclonal antibody in human renal transplantation. *Transplantation* 1991 ; 91 : 107-13.

35. Hourmant M, Bedrossian J, Durand D, Lebranchu Y, Renoult E, Caudrelier P, Buffet R, Soulillou JP. A randomized multicenter trial comparing leukocyte function-associated antigen-1 monoclonal antibody with rabbit antithymocyte globulin as induction treatment in first kidney transplantations.*Transplantation* 1996 ; 62 : 1565-70.

36. Isobe M, Yagita H, Oteumura K, Ihara A. Specific acceptance of cardiac allograft after treatment with antibodies to ILAM 1 and LFA 1. *Science* 1992 ; 255 : 1125-7.

37. Vincenti F, Kirkman R, Light S, Bumgardner G, Pescovitz M, Halloran P, Neylan J, Wilkinson A, Ekberg H, Gaston R, Backman L, Burdick J, for the daclizumab triple therapy study group. Interleukin-2-receptor blockade with daclizumab to prevent acute rejection in renal transplantation. *N Engl J Med* 1998 ; 338 : 161-5.

38. Nashan B, Moore R, Amiot P, Schmidt AG, Abeywickrama K, Soulillou JP, for the CHIB 201 International study group. Randomised trial of basiliximab *versus* placebo for control of acute cellular rejection in renal allograft recipients. *Lancet* 1997 ; 350 : 1193-8.

39. Pearson TC, Alexander DZ, Winn KJ, Linsley PS, Honery RP, Larsen CP. Transplantation tolerance induced by CTLA 4-Ig. *Transplantation* 1994 ; 57 : 1701-6.

40. Kunz R, Neumayer HH. Maintenance therapy with triple *versus* double immunosuppressive regimen in renal transplantation. *Transplantation* 1997 ; 63 : 386-92.

41. Aroldi A, Tarantino A, Montagnino G, Cesana B, Cocucci C, Ponticelli C. Effects of three immunosuppressive regimens on vertebral bone density in renal transplant recipients. *Transplantation* 1997 ; 63 : 380-6.

4

UV-induced immunosuppression

Iwao KURIMOTO [1], John Wayne STREILEIN [2]
1. Osaka University School of Medicine, Department of Dermatology, Osaka, Japan.
2. The Schepens Eye Research Institute and Department of Dermatology,
Harvard Medical School, Boston, Massachusetts, USA.

There is general agreement that excessive exposure to sunlight is the most important environmental cause of skin cancer in man, and that the ultraviolet-B (UVB) region of the solar spectrum is the relevant oncogenic agent [1-4]. The immune system is regionally adapted to create a specialized immunity for pathogens that attack, or arise within, the skin. This specialized cutaneous immune system has been termed skin associated lymphoid tissue (SALT) [5]. Studies of the immunological effects of UVB radiation (UVR) on cutaneous immunity have focused on the deleterious effects of UVR that permit cutaneous tumors to emerge [6-8]. UVR promotes skin cancer by altering DNA within epidermal cells, leading to the loss of the cells' capacity to respond normally to growth-regulating factors [4, 9]. However, UVR also promotes skin cancer because the energy of UVR depresses immune responses within skin and renders the individual unable to mount an immune effector response against neoantigenic malignant cells [5, 10]. The concept of immunologic surveillance has long been accepted, and this concept explains why immune systems damaged by immunosuppressive drugs have been implicated in cancer pathogenesis [11-15]. The interaction in cancer pathogenesis of immunity and UVR is highlighted by reports that the incidence of skin cancer, such as squamous and basal cell carcinomas, is greatly increased in patients placed on continuous immunosuppressive therapy for the maintenance of organ allografts. The first report by Kinlen *et al.* [11] was based on observations in Australia and Southeast Asia, where sunlight is of high intensity and long duration. Thereafter, although the exposure to sunlight is lower than that of subtropical areas, groups in the Netherlands and Sweden also documented that the occurrence of skin cancer in long-term graft survivors is increased [12, 16]. Studies of patients without transplants, who were treated chronically with immunosuppressive drugs, also found that skin cancer is excessive, suggesting that the development of cancer is not due solely to the foreign antigens of the grafts [11, 17]. Recent reports have shown positive and negative associations between certain HLA antigens and skin cancer in renal transplant recipients [18, 19].

Experimental model systems in mice, developed decades ago by Kripke and Daynes [1, 20], revealed that chronic, high dose UVR produced skin cancer. Tumors induced by UVR grew progressively in their hosts but proved to be highly immunogenic when transplanted to syngeneic, non-UVR-exposed recipients. These investigators then demonstrated that even before the appearance of clinically-detectable skin cancer, mice exposed to chronic, high-doses of UVR acquired defect in their immune systems. Their spleens lacked effective professional antigen presenting cells (APC), and application of haptens to their skin failed to induce contact hypersensitivity (CH) [21, 22]. In addition, the spleens of these animals contained suppressor T cells which induced tolerance of tumor-associated antigens and haptens when injected into naive, syngeneic recipients [23, 24]. Curiously, the systemic immune defect was not global. Mice chronically exposed to UVR displayed no increased tendency to autoimmune diseases, their humoral immune response to antigens was intact, and they retained their ability to reject solid organ transplants [1]. Thus, chronic exposure of laboratory mice to high doses of UVR radiation produces cutaneous malignancies in which defects within the cutaneous immune system contribute to the pathogenesis of tumor development. However, the doses of UVR used in these early studies were well beyond doses commonly experienced by human beings. Whether the immune consequences of high-dose chronic UVR are relevant to human skin cancer was unclear, but the principle was established by these studies that UVR is deleterious to the systemic immune system, even though the energy of UVR is largely absorbed within the upper layers of the skin.

Local immunosuppressive effects of UVR

A different model of UVR exposure was developed by Bergstresser and Streilein in the late 1970s, a model that used much lower doses of UVR. In this model, shaved abdominal skin of mice was exposed to UVR ($400J/m^2$) for four consecutive days [25]. This regimen was originally developed to eliminate Langerhans cells from the epidermis, rather than to study the oncogenic properties of UVR. Nonetheless, the findings are relevant to sunlight-induced skin cancer.

When highly reactive haptens, such as dinitrofluorobenzene (DNFB), are applied epicutaneously to a UVR-exposed site immediately after the last exposure, CH fails to develop [26]. By contrast, if the same dose of hapten is applied to unirradiated skin at a site distant to the UVR, intense CH develops. These findings indicated that this acute low-dose UVB regimen achieved its effects on the induction of cutaneous immunity by a strictly local action. This ability of UVR to impair CH induction is genetically determined. Some inbred strains of mice, termed UVB-resistant (UVB-R), are resistant to this effect of UVR. These mice develop CH of comparable intensity whether DNFB is painted on UVB-exposed or unexposed skin. By contrast, other strains of mice, termed UVB-susceptible (UVB-S), are susceptible to the deleterious effects of UVR on CH induction and fail to develop CH when hapten is painted on UVR-exposed skin [27]. It has been shown that intradermally injected tumor necrosis factor α (TNFα) mimics the effects of UVR on CH induction, and that systemically administered neutralizing anti-TNFα antibodies restore CH induction in UVB-S mice following UVR exposure, suggesting that TNFα is the critical mediator of this effect of UVR [28]. In support of this proposal are the findings that alleles at the *Tnfα* and *Lps* (bacterial lipopolysaccharide) loci dictate the UVB-dependent phenotypes. Mice that are homozygous for the LPS-resistant allele (Lps^d) and the $Tnf\alpha^d$ alleles, are UVB-R, whereas mice homozygous for the LPS-susceptible allele (Lps^n) and expressing at least one different $TNF\alpha$ allele are UVB-S [29]. UVB-S and UVB-R mice display a polymorphism within the 5'-untranslated region of the $Tnf\alpha$ gene [30]. Thus, considerable effort has been directed at understanding the relationship between local UVR exposure, TNFα, and failed CH induction in UVB-S mice.

It is reasonable to search for the relevant photoreceptor for UVR within the epidermis since this absorbs more than 95% of the UVB energy. One candidate for the photoreceptor is nucleic acid of epidermal cells. Cyclobutane pyrimidine dimers are one form of DNA damage induced by UVB, and these dimers have the capacity to interfere with cutaneous immunity [31]. Another candidate is urocanic acid (UCA). UCA is present in the *trans* isoform in the upper layer of the epidermis and is naturally converted to the *cis* isoform by UVR [32]. De Fabo and Noonan have shown that *cis*-UCA has systemic immunosuppressive effects [33]. Ross *et al.* [34] have demonstrated that intracutaneous administration of *cis*-UCA induces suppression of delayed hypersensitivity to *Herpes simplex* virus. More to the point, our laboratory has demonstrated that hapten painted on murine skin into which *cis*-UCA had been injected failed to induce CH. In addition, the failed CH observed after intracutaneous injection of *cis*-UCA was abrogated by anti-TNFα antibodies [35]. These findings have led us to propose that UCA is the photoreceptor which plays the key role in the process by which acute, low dose UVR prevents CH induction, and that the mediator of this outcome is locally produced TNFα. However, *cis*-UCA has other effects. Moodycliffe *et al.* [36] proposed that *cis*-UCA also acts as a mediator for some, but not all, of the systemic immunosuppressive effects of UVR. These investigators found that anti-*cis*-UCA monoclonal antibodies injected into mice several hours before exposure to UVR had no effect on UV-induced systemic suppression of CH induction, but restored the ability of these mice to develop delayed hypersensitivity responses.

It has been very recently reported that a third photoreceptor exists in the skin, *i.e.* nerve endings of cutaneous sensory C fibers [37]. Calcitonin gene-related peptide (CGRP), a neuropeptide stored in these nerve termini, is released after UVR radiation [38,39] and plays a central role in the failure of UVR-exposed skin to support CH induction [39]. Moreover, anti-TNFα antibodies injected before CGRP injection into skin surfaces subsequently painted with hapten, restored CH induction. A key finding of these studies was the observation that CGRP induced dermal mast cells to release TNFα, thereby identifying the cellular source of this cytokine after UVR. Remarkably, UVR radiation failed to impair CH induction in mast cell-deficient mice [37]. These findings indicate that mast cells are the important source of TNFα after UVR, and that CGRP from epidermal nerve termini plays an essential role in the multi-step process by which UVB impairs CH induction through local release of TNFα.

Systemic immunosuppressive effects of UVB

Delayed systemic effects of UVB on CH induction

As discussed above, UVR impairs CH induction by a strictly local mechanism. However, even though the acute, low dose UVR regimen used in these studies has a local effect, it also alters the immune system systemically. This becomes apparent when time elapses following the fourth UVR exposure and application of hapten to an unirradiated site. As mentioned above, hapten applied to a cutaneous site distant from the UVR-exposed site immediately after the last dose of UVR readily sensitizes mice. However, if hapten application to a non-UVR-exposed site is delayed for 24 hours or more, CH fails to develop [40, 41]. We refer to this consequence of UVR exposure as « delayed systemic effect ». Unlike the immediate local effect of UVR exposure, the delayed systemic effect occurs in all strains of mice (both UVB-R and UVB-S) and is not reversed by treatment of the mice with anti-TNFα antibodies [41]. These observations indicate not only that the pathway to the delayed systemic effect of UVR is independent of TNFα, but that other mediators must be involved.

To that end, UVR exposure of skin induces the production and release of a wide variety of cytokines and other factors. Some of these factors are known to be immunosuppressive, such as α-melanocyte stimulating hormone (α-MSH) [42, 43], reactive oxygen intermediates [44] and IL10 [45]. Recently, attention has been focused on IL10, since local and systemic administration of IL10 induces immunosuppression, and since transcripts for IL10 mRNA are detected in keratinocytes after UVR. It has been demonstrated that IL10 (2μg) injected intradermally 8 hours before hapten application impairs CH induction [45]. By contrast, Niizeki et al. [46] have demonstrated that intradermal injection of IL10 (200ng) within 30 min of hapten application had the ability to induce tolerance but did not impair CH induction. We suspect that IL10 may be an important mediator of the delayed systemic effects of acute, low dose UVR, but direct experimental verification has yet to be obtained.

Tolerance induced by UVB radiation of skin

The acute low dose regimen of UVR not only impairs CH induction locally, but mice that receive hapten applied to the irradiated site develop specific, long-lasting hapten-specific tolerance. It is relevant that the hapten-specific tolerance induced in this fashion develops in all strains of mice, irrespective of whether they are UVB-S or UVB-R. Intracutaneous injections of cis-UCA also induce a similar form of tolerance, and tolerance evoked by UVB and cis-UCA cannot be reversed by administration of neutralizing anti-TNFα antibodies [47]. These findings indicate that the cellular and molecular bases of UVR-induced tolerance are very likely to be different from the mechanisms responsible for UVR-impaired CH induction. Although locally injected TNFα can induce hapten-specific tolerance, several investigators have reported that IL10 is responsible for the tolerance that follows UVR [46, 48]. In addition, the tolerance induced in mice that received injections of α-MSH is mediated by IL10 [42]. Recent reports reveal that IL10 may promote systemic immunosuppression and tolerance by down-regulating the expression of class II MHC molecules [49], B7-1/2 molecules, and ICAM-1 [50] on the APC responsible for CH induction.

Having implicated professional APC in CH induction, identification of the APC that acquire tolerogenic signals after UVR exposure has been an experimental goal for many laboratories during the past decade. Sullivan et al. [51] demonstrated that dendritic epidermal T cells prepared from normal mouse skin are tolerogenic when hapten-derivatized and injected intravenously into naive mice. Simon et al. [52] reported that epidermal Langerhans cells irradiated in vitro with UVR have the capacity to induce hapten-specific tolerance. The groups of Cooper and Hammerberg [53, 54] have demonstrated that blood-borne monocytic/macrophage cells that enter the dermis and epidermis after UVR exposure have the potential to induce tolerance. We have observed that cells prepared from the dermis of skin exposed to acute, low dose UVR display tolerance-inducing properties [55]; in addition, injection into UVR-exposed skin of macrophage-depleting dichloromethylene diphosphonate (Cl_2MDP) containing liposomes did not abolish the ability of dermal cells to induce tolerance, suggesting that non-phagocytic cells (perhaps dermal dendritic cells) acquire tolerance-inducing activities [56]. It has been very recently reported that dendritic cells generated from human blood progenitor cells induce tolerance after treatment with IL10 [57].

If anything, there are too many candidates for the role of « tolerance-conferring APC » after UVR exposure of the skin. What we have recently learned in our laboratory is that the aberrant APC that are responsible for the delayed systemic effects of UVR are located in lymph nodes and spleen. More importantly, cutaneous APC, especially Langerhans cells, display normal APC function if the cells are harvested from non-UVR-exposed skin.

How systemic tolerance emerges after UVR exposure is thus unknown. Our recent studies suggest that UVR exposure fails to promote tolerance in mice from which the spleen was removed prior to irradiation. Moreover, CD8+ T cells are essential for the expression of UVR-induced tolerance. Understanding these immunoregulatory forces is a formidable challenge to immunodermatologists interested in this problem.

Effects of UVR on cutaneous immunity in humans

Since sunlight induces skin cancer in humans, but not in mice, it is important to know the relevance to humans of the experimental findings in mice. To that end, Yoshikawa et al. [58] demonstrated that, similarly to mice, human beings also display the UVB-S and UVB-R phenotypes when hapten is applied to skin exposed to acute low dose UVB radiation protocol. When 2mg of dinitrochlorobenzene (DNCB) is applied to UVR-exposed skin within an hour after completion of UVR, 40% of normal adult volunteers fail to develop CH (UVB-S) when challenged with diluted hapten 30 days later. The remaining 60% develop vigorous CH. More importantly, almost all patients with biopsy-proven skin cancer, basal/squamous cell cancers and malignant melanoma, turned out to be UVB-S. Moreover, when UVB-S human subjects were re-exposed to sensitizing doses of DNCB, 50% displayed unresponsiveness. Thus, both local and systemic abnormalities of the cutaneous immune system, originally described in mice, also develop in humans exposed to doses of UVR that resemble what human beings typically experience in their daily lives. The hope is that insights into the pathogenesis of UVR-impaired cutaneous immunity will help to prevent and treat the patients suffering from the oncogenic effects of sunlight exposure.

References

1. Kripke ML. Immunobiology of photocarcinogenesis. In : Parish JA, ed. *The effect of ultraviolet radiation on immune system*. New Brunswick : Johnson and Johnson Products, 1983 : 87-106.
2. Green AES, Findley GB, Klenk W, Wilson W, Mo T. The ultraviolet dose dependence of non-melanoma skin cancer incidence. *Photochem Photobiol* 1976 ; 24 : 353-62.
3. Vitasa BC, Taylor HY, Sticklands PT, Rosenthal FS, West S, Abbey H, Ng SK, Bunoz B, Emmett EA. Association of non-melanoma skin cancer and actinic keratosis with cumulative solar ultraviolet exposure in Maryland watermen. *Cancer* 1990 ; 65 : 2811-7.
4. Harver JC, Bickers DR. Ultraviolet carcinogenesis In : *Photosensitivity diseases*. Philadelphia : WB Saunders, 1981 : 246-57.
5. Streilein JW. Skin associated lymphoid tissues (SALT). *J Invest Dermatol* 1983 ; 80 : 12S-6S.
6. Kripke ML, Fisher MS. Systemic alteration induced in mice by ultraviolet light irradiation and its relationship to ultraviolet carcinogenesis. *Proc Natl Acad Sci USA* 1977 ; 74 : 1688-92.
7. Fisher MS, Kripke ML. Suppressor T lymphocytes control the development of primary skin cancers in ultraviolet-irradiated mice. *Science* 1982 ; 216 : 1133-4.
8. Spellman CW, Daynes RA. Properties of ultraviolet light-induced suppressor lymphocytes within a syngeneic tumor system. *Cell Immunol* 1978 ; 36 : 383-7.
9. Nomura T, Nakajima H, Hongyo T, Taniguchi E, Fukuda K, Li LY, Kurooka M, Sutoh K, Hande PM, Kawaguchi T, Ueda M, Takatera H. Induction of cancer, actinic keratosis, and specific p53 mutations by UVB light in human skin maintained in severe combined immunodeficient mice. *Cancer Res* 1997 ; 57 : 2081-4.

10. Kripke ML, Lofgreen JS, Beard J, Jessup J.M, Fisher MS. *In vivo* immune responses of mice during carcinogenesis by ultraviolet irradiation. *J Natl Cancer Inst* 1977 ; 59 : 1227-41.

11. Kinlen LJ, Sheli AG, Peto J, Doll R. Collaborative United Kingdom-Australasian study of cancer in patients treated with immunosuppressive drugs. *Br Med J* 1979 ; 2 : 1461-6.

12. Hartevelt MM, Bouwes Bavinck JN, Kootte AMM, Vermeer BJ, Vandenbroucke JP. Incidence of skin cancer after renal transplantation in the Netherlands. *Transplantation* 1990 ; 49 : 506-9.

13. Ferrandiz C, Fuente MJ, Ribera M, Bielsa I, Fernandez MT, Lauzurica R, Roca J. Epidermal dysplasia and neoplasia in kidney transplant recipients. *J Am Acad Dermatol* 1995 ; 33 : 590-6.

14. King GN, Healy CM, Glover MT, Kwan JT, Williams DM, Leigh IM, Worthington HV, Thornhill MH. Increased prevalence of dysplastic and malignant lip lesions in renal-transplant recipients. *N Engl J Med* 1995 ; 332 : 1052-7.

15. Espana A, Redondo P, Fernandez AL, Zabala M, Herreros J, Llorens R, Quintanilla E. Skin cancer in heart transplant recipients. *J Am Acad Dermatol* 1995 ; 32 : 458-65.

16. Blöhme I, Larko O. Premalignant and malignant skin lesions in renal transplant patients. *Transplantation* 1984 ; 37 : 165-7.

17. Kinlen LJ. Incidence of cancer in rheumatoid arthritis and other disorders after immunosuppressive treatment. *Am J Med* 1985 ; 78 : 44-9.

18. Bouwes Bavinck JN, Vermeer BJ, van der Woude FJ, Vandenbroucke JP, Schreuder GM, Thorogood J, Persijn GG, Class FH. Relation between skin cancer and HLA antigens in renal-transplant recipients. *N Engl J Med* 1991 ; 325 : 843-8.

19. Bouwes Bavinck JN, Class FH, Hardie DR, Green A, Vermeer BJ, Hardie IR. Relation between HLA antigens and skin cancer in renal recipients in Queensland, Australia. *J Invest Dermatol* 1997 ; 108 : 708-11.

20. Daynes RA, Bernhard EJ, Gurish MF, Lynch DH. Experimental photoimmunology: immunologic ramifications UV-induced carcinogenesis. *J Invest Dermatol* 1981 ; 77 : 77-85.

21. Schwartz RP. Role of UVB-induced serum factors in suppression of contact hypersensitivity in mice. *J Invest Dermatol* 1984 ; 83 : 305-7.

22. Noonan FP, Kripke ML, Pedersen GM, Greene MI. Suppression of contact hypersensitivity in mice by ultraviolet irradiation is associated with defective antigen presentation. *Immunology* 1981 ; 43 : 527-33.

23. Grabbe S, Bruvers S, Gallo RL, Knisely TL, Nazareno R, Granstein RD. Tumor antigen presentation by murine epidermal cells. *J Immunol* 1991 ; 146 : 3656-61.

24. Elemet CA, Bergstresser PR, Tigelaar RE, Wood PJ, Streilein JW. Analysis of the mechanism of unresponsiveness produced by haptens painted on skin exposed to low dose ultraviolet radiation. *J Exp Med* 1983 ; 158 : 781-94.

25. Bergstresser PR, Towes GB, Streilein JW. Natural and perturbed distributions of Langerhans cells: responses to ultraviolet light, heterotopic skin grafting, and dinitrofluorobenzene sensitization. *J Invest Dermatol* 1980 ; 75 : 73-7.

26. Toews GB, Bergstresser PR, Streilein JW. Epidermal Langerhans cell density determines whether contact hypersensitivity or unresponsiveness follows skin painting with DNFB. *J Immunol* 1980 ; 124 : 445-53.

27. Streilein JW, Bergstresser PR. Genetic basis of ultraviolet-B effects on contact hypersensitivity. *Immunogenetics* 1988 ; 27 : 252-8.

28. Yoshikawa T, Streilein JW. Genetic basis of the effects of ultraviolet light B on cutaneous immunity. Evidence that polymorphisms at the Tnfα and Lps loci governs susceptibility. *Immunogenetics* 1990 ; 32 : 398-405.

29. Kurimoto I, Streilein JW. Characterization of the immunogenetic basis of ultraviolet-B light effects on contact hypersensitivity induction. *Immunology* 1994 ; 81 : 352-8.

30. Vincek V, Kurimoto I, Medema JP, Prieto E, Streilein JW. Tumor necrosis factor-α polymorphism correlates with deleterious effects of ultraviolet B light on cutaneous immunity. *Cancer Res* 1993 ; 53 : 728-32.

31. Kripke ML, Cox PA, Alas G, Yarosh DB. Pyrimidine dimers in DNA initiate systemic immunosuppression in UV-irradiated mice. *Proc Natl Acad Sci USA* 1992 ; 89 : 7516-20.
32. Noonan FP, De Fabo EC. Immunosuppression by ultraviolet B radiation: initiation by urocanic acid. *Immunol Today* 1992 ; 13 : 250-4.
33. De Fabo EC, Noonan FP. Mechanism of immune suppression by ultraviolet irradiation *in vivo*. I. Evidence for the existence of a unique photoreceptor in skin and its role in photoimmunology. *J Exp Med* 1983 ; 157 : 84-98.
34. Ross JA, Howie SEM, Norval M, Maingay J, Simpson TJ. Ultraviolet-irradiated urocanic acid suppresses delayed-type hypersensitivity to *Herpes simplex* virus. *J Invest Dermatol* 1986 ; 87 : 630-3.
35. Kurimoto I, Streilein JW. Cis-urocanic acid suppression of contact hypersensitivity induction is mediated *via* tumor necrosis factor-α. *J Immunol* 1992 ; 148 : 3072-8 .
36. Moodycliffe AM, Bucana CD, Kripke ML, Norval M, Ullrich SE. Differential effects of a monoclonal antibody to cis-urocanic acid on the suppression of delayed and contact hypersensitivity following ultraviolet irradiation. *J Immunol* 1996 ; 157 : 2891-9.
37. Niizeki H, Alard P, Streilein JW. Calcitonin gene-related peptide is necessary for ultraviolet B-impaired induction of contact hypersensitivity. *J Immunol* 1997 ; 159 : 5183-6.
38. Hosoi J, Murphy GF, Egan CL, Lerner EA, Grabbe S, Asahina R, Granstein RD. Regulation of Langerhans cell function by nerves containing calcitonin gene-related peptide. *Nature* 1993 ; 363 : 159-63.
39. Benrath J, Eschenfelder C, Zimmermann M, Gillardon F. Calcitonin gene-related peptide, substance P and nitric oxide are involved in cutaneous inflammation following ultraviolet irradiation. *Eur J Pharmacol* 1995 ; 293 : 87-96.
40. Noonan FP, De Fabo EC. Ultraviolet-B dose-response curves for local and systemic immunosuppression are identical. *Photochem Photobiol* 1990 ; 52 : 801-10 .
41. Shimizu T, Streilein JW. Local and systemic consequences of acute, low-dose ultraviolet B radiation are mediated by different immune regulatory mechanisms. *Eur J Immunol* 1994 ; 24 : 1765-70.
42. Grabbe S, Bhardwaj RS, Mahnke K, Simon MM, Schwarz T, Luger TA. α-melanocyte-stimulating hormone induces hapten-specific tolerance in mice. *J Immunol* 1996 ; 156 : 473-8.
43. Shimizu T, Streilein JW. Influence of alpha-melanocyte stimulating on induction of contact hypersensitivity and tolerance. *J Dermatol Sci* 1994 ; 8 : 187-93.
44. Nakamura T, Pinnell SR, Darr D, Kurimoto I, Itami S, Yoshikawa K, Streilein JW. Vitamine C abrogates the deleterious effects of UVB radiation on cutaneous immunity by a mechanism that does not depend on TNFα. *J Invest Dermatol* 1997 ; 109 : 20-4.
45. Enk AH, Saloga J, Becker D, Mohamadzadeh M, Knop J. Induction of hapten-specific tolerance by interleukin-10 *in vivo*. *J Exp Med* 1994 ; 179 : 1397-402.
46. Niizeki H, Streilein JW. Hapten-specific tolerance induced by acute, low-dose ultraviolet B radiation of skin is mediated *via* interleukin-10. *J Invest Dermatol* 1997 ; 109 : 25-30.
47. Shimizu T, Streilein JW. Evidence that ultraviolet B radiation induces tolerance and impairs induction of contact hypersensitivity and tolerance. *Immunology* 1994 ; 82 : 140-8.
48. Ullrich SE. Mechanism involved in the systemic suppression of antigen-presenting cell function by UV irradiation: keratinocyte-derived IL10 modulates antigen-presenting cell function of splenic adherent cells. *J Immunol* 1994 ; 152 : 3410-6.
49. de Waal Malefyt RW, Haanen J, Spits H, Roncarolo MG, te Velde A, Figdor C, Johnson K, Kastelein R, Yssel H, de Vries JE. Interleukin-10 (IL10) and viral IL10 strongly reduce antigen-specific human T cell proliferation by diminishing the antigen-capacity of monocytes via downregulation of class II major histocompatibility complex expression. *J Exp Med* 1991 ; 174 : 915-24.
50. Willems F, Marchant A, Delville JP, Gerard C, Delvaux A, Velu T, de Boer M, Goldman M. Interleukin-10 inhibits B7 and intercellular adhesion molecule-1 expression on human monocytes. *Eur J Immunol* 1994 ; 24 : 1007-9 .
51. Sullivan S, Bergstresser PR, Tigelaar RE, Streilein JW. Induction and regulation of contact hypersensitivity by resident bone marrow derived, dendritic epidermal cells: Langerhans cells and Thy-1+ epidermal cells. *J Immunol* 1986 ; 137 : 2460-7.

52. Simon JC, Tigelaar RE, Bergstresser PR, Edelbaum D, Cruz PDJ. Ultraviolet B radiation converts Langerhans cells from immunogenic to tolerogenic antigen-presenting cells. Induction of specific clonal anergy in CD4+ T helper 1 cells. *J Immunol* 1991 ; 146 : 485-91.

53. Cooper KD, Duraiswarmy N, Hammerberg C, Allen E, Kimbrough-Green C, Dillon W, Thomas D. Neutrophils, differentiated macrophages, and monocyte/macrophage antigen presenting cells infiltrate murine epidermis after UV injury. *J Invest Dermatol* 1993 ; 101 : 155-63.

54. Hammerberg C, Duraiswarmy N, Cooper KD. Active induction of unresponsiveness (tolerance) to DNFB by *in vivo* ultraviolet-exposed epidermal cells is dependent upon infiltrating class II MHC+ CD11b (bright) monocytic/macrophagic cells. *J Immunol* 1994 ; 153 : 4915-24.

55. Kurimoto I, Arana M, Streilein JW. Role of dermal cells from normal and ultraviolet B-damaged skin in induction of contact hypersensitivity and tolerance. *J Immunol* 1994 ; 152 : 3317-24.

56. Kurimoto I, van Rooijen N, Dijkstra CD, Streilein JW. Role of phagocytic macrophages in induction of contact hypersensitivity and tolerance by hapten applied to normal and ultraviolet B irradiated skin. *Immunology* 1994 ; 82 : 281-7 .

57. Steinbrink K, Wolfl M, Jonuleit H, Knop J, Enk AH. Induction of tolerance by IL10 treated dendritic cells. *J Immunol* 1997 ; 159 : 4772-80.

58. Yoshikawa T, Rae V, Bruins-Slot W, Van Den Berg JW, Taylor JR, Streilein JW. Analysis of effects of UVB radiation on induction of contact hypersensitivity as a risk factor for skin cancer in humans. *J Invest Dermatol* 1990 ; 95 : 530-6.

5

Retinoic acid and immune responses: regulation of cutaneous immunomodulation by synthetic retinoid analogs

Michel DÉMARCHEZ [1], Xian-Ping LU [2]
1. Galderma R & D, Sophia Antipolis, France.
2. Galderma Research Inc., Princeton, USA.

It is now established and well documented that retinol (vitamin A) and its natural metabolites have an important role in the development, growth and differentiation of various tissues and in maintaining reproduction and visual function in vertebrates [1-3]. On the other hand, while epidemiological and experimental studies have clearly shown that vitamin A deficiency appears to be associated with impaired immunity and that vitamin A supplementation affects immune responses, the underlying mechanisms involved in these responses are still poorly understood. Recent studies have shown that the major biologically active forms of vitamin A are retinoic acid isoforms (*e.g.*, all-*trans*-retinoic acid, 13-*cis*-retinoic acid, and 9-*cis*-retinoic acid). The molecular basis of vitamin A action was well established with the discovery of two classes of retinoid nuclear receptors, retinoic acid receptors (RAR) and retinoid X receptors (RXR), belonging to the steroid/thyroid hormone receptor superfamily of ligand-activated transcription factors [4].

During the past fifteen years, our laboratory and several others around the world have developed research programs to generate new analogs of retinoic acid with better therapeutic indices and novel pharmacological profiles. From these studies, novel compounds with agonist or antagonist activity selective for a given RAR or RXR subtype, and with new biological profiles, have been identified. In the first instance, they are useful experimental tools for the investigation of the mechanism of action of retinoids. Moreover, several of them are promising candidates for treating immune diseases.

In this review, starting with recent findings that have provided new insights in the signaling transduction of nuclear hormone receptors and then presenting data generated on the role of vitamin A and its metabolites in immune responses (for review see [5, 6]), we discuss the potential of new synthetic analogs to treat immune diseases in the skin.

Molecular basis for retinoid activity in immune response

Two classes of nuclear retinoid receptors, retinoic acid receptors (RAR) and retinoid X receptors (RXR), have been identified and are each composed of α, β, and γ subtypes. RAR and RXR bind as heterodimers to specific DNA sequences (retinoic acid response elements, RARE) in regulatory regions of target genes. The RARs are activated by all-*trans* retinoic acid and by 9-*cis* retinoic acid whereas the RXRs, which can also form homodimers between themselves, are exclusively activated by 9-*cis* retinoic acid. In addition to forming heterodimers with RAR, RXR can also heterodimerize with many other nuclear receptors, including the vitamin D3 receptor (VDR), the thyroid hormone receptor (TR), the liver X receptor (LXR), the farnesoid X-activated receptor (FXR), the nerve growth factor induced B (NGFI-B) (Nur77), and the peroxisome proliferator activated receptor (PPAR) [4].

While gene activation appears to be the major mode of action of retinoids, RARs or RXR may also interact in a ligand-dependent manner with other transactivation factors, such as AP1 (activator protein 1), NFAT (nuclear factor of activated T cells), or NF-IL6 (nuclear factor-interleukin 6), this interaction leading to repression of gene expression mediated by those factors [7-13]. The AP-1 transcription complex plays an important role in inflammation and immune responses by controlling the expression of a subset of genes which are immediately and early expressed in response to extracellular mitogenic stimuli or to stress. RAR and RXR were also shown to downregulate the transforming growth factor-beta 1 promoter by antagonizing AP1 activity [7]. Retinoids with selective anti-AP1 activity have been identified [8]. Recently, it was demonstrated that CD 2409, an anti-AP1-selective retinoid with no RARE transcriptional activity, inhibited TPA-induced vascular endothelial growth factor (VEGF) mRNA expression [9]. VEGF is the major angiogenesis factor and its expression is upregulated in certain skin diseases such as psoriasis, delayed-type hypersensitivity reactions, bullous diseases and Kaposi's sarcoma.

Recently, it was proposed that the immunosuppressive activity of $1\alpha,25$-dihydroxyvitamin D3 could be partly due to diminished activity of the transcription factor NFAT [10, 11]. NFAT belongs to a family of transcription factors which cooperatively bind to Fos and Jun family members. The immunosuppressive activity of cyclosporin A and FK 506 is due to the inhibition of calcineurin, a Ca^+-activated serine/threonine phosphatase necessary for nuclear translocation of cytoplasmic NFAT proteins. Recent data suggest that the VDR-RXR heterodimer blocks NFAT/AP1 complex formation, then links with an important positive regulatory element, NFAT-1 and eventually inhibits transcriptional activation of genes such as IL2. In addition, IL3, IL4, TNFα, and GM-CSF are other cytokine genes that have NFAT responsive elements in their promoters [12].

Nuclear factor-interleukin 6 is another transcription factor, in addition to AP1, whose activity is inhibited by RAR in a ligand-dependent manner. NF-IL6 regulates the expression of interleukin 6 and of migration inhibitory factor protein 8 (MRP8) which are involved in the pathophysiology of several cutaneous diseases including psoriasis in which they are highly expressed [13].

Apoptosis, which plays a major role in shaping the T cell repertoire, is another mechanism through which retinoids may affect immune functions. It has been shown that retinoic acid can induce apoptosis, increase the rate of dexamethasone-induced death and inhibit activation-induced death of thymocytes and T lymphocytes. T lymphocyte apoptosis could be regulated through an interplay between RAR and RXR receptors [14]. However, the biological relevance of these results is debatable since retinoic acid at physiological concentrations is not able to induce thymocyte apoptosis [15].

All these studies clearly illustrate the complexity of the interactive network between transcription factors through which retinoids might interfere with the immune system. Therefore, synthetic retinoids that are able to interact with other transcription factors through RARs or RXRs represent novel effectors on the immune system.

Vitamin A deficiency and supplementation

Epidemiological studies have linked vitamin A status to increased childhood mortality in developing countries where children with vitamin A deficiency are more susceptible to infectious diseases. Supplementation with vitamin A reduces mortality by 30-50%, and more in preschool children [6, 16, 17]. In animal models, it appears that vitamin A deficiency is associated with loss of lymphoid tissue and reduced immune responses and that these abnormalities are improved by vitamin A supplementation. More recently, it has been observed that repeated oral administrations of RAR antagonists could also induce tissue involution in lymphoid organs, such as spleen, thymus, and lymph nodes (our unpublished data). However, excessively high doses of vitamin A appear to have similar effects with a decrease of lymphoid tissue and immune deficiency [18]. In vitamin A-deficient animals, the production of antigen-specific antibody was severely decreased both in mice and rats, and such decreases were reversed by dietary supplementation of retinol and its derivatives [19]. It was further shown that vitamin A is a key regulator for cell growth, cytokine production and differentiation in normal and activated B cells [20, 21]. All-*trans* RA as well as several other RAR agonists inhibit polyclonal expansion initiated by LPS *in vitro*, and the inhibitory effect on B cell proliferation induced by a mitogen is reversed by an RAR antagonist [22]. Retinoids can also inhibit natural killer cell activity, reduce interferon production and reverse some of the effects of interferon [23]. On the other hand, administration of pharmacological doses of vitamin A increases resistance to infections in animals as well as in humans. Retinol and retinoic acid can act as adjuvants for the development of both humoral immunity and antigen specific, T lymphocyte-mediated cytotoxicity. However, the level of retinol inside the animal body does not always correlate with humoral immune response. For example, antibody production is not decreased in vitamin A-deficient rodents in the presence of LPS antigen [19].

From the above observations, it appears that an optimal level of vitamin A is essential for optimal immune responses. Such a conclusion is in line with the notion that a critical level of retinoic acid is required for optimal epidermal differentiation [24]. It further suggests that application of an RAR agonist or an RAR antagonist could be an effective way to shift the balance of the physiological retinoid level *in vivo*, thus, generating a pharmacological response for therapeutical applications.

Functionally, T cells can be defined by their capacity to modulate immune responses by helper or suppressor functions or by exerting cytotoxic immune responses. T cells can also be classified by the profile of cytokines they produce. T cells that produce predominantly IL2, IFNγ, and tumor necrosis factor α (TNFα) are referred to as Th1 cells, and T cells that produce predominantly IL4, IL5, IL9, IL10, and IL13 are referred to as Th2 cells [25]. Interestingly, it was reported that vitamin A deficiency induced a state of imbalance between Th1 and Th2 cells. Specifically, the overproduction of IFNγ by Th1 cells and the small number of Th2 cells as well as low production of IL4, IL5, and IL10 are prominent features in vitamin A-deficient animals, resulting in an impairment of Th2-dependent humoral immunity in response to antigen challenge [23]. These disturbed patterns were normalized by the application of retinoids *in vivo* or *in vitro* [23]. It appears that transcriptional regulation by all-*trans* RA is involved in IFNγ and IL12 production in Th1 cell development [26]. These *in vivo* and *in vitro* findings, *i.e.* that retinol as well as retinoic acid modulate the balance in the development and function of both Th1 and Th2 cells, are further upheld by the observation that, in an experimental allergic encephalomyelitis model, retinoid-induced improvement of clinical symptoms are correlated with IL4 production [27]. Altogether, these data strongly suggest that retinoids might regulate the balance of Th1 and Th2 function in favor of a development of Th2-dominant response *in vivo*, probably mediated through transcriptional modulation by nuclear retinoid receptors.

Future implication of retinoids in the management of cutaneous immune diseases

Skin is an unique and distinct immunologic organ providing both specific and non specific protective immunity against invasion by pathogenic microorganisms and other environmental antigens. The skin is also an important target for a variety of allergic and autoimmune skin responses such as atopic dermatitis, allergic contact dermatitis and psoriasis [28-31].

Although glucocorticoids and immunomodulators such as cyclosporin A and FK 506 are proposed for the treatment of contact allergy or atopic dermatitis, no retinoids or retinoid-like compounds have yet been developed in this domain. The above data demonstrate a crucial role of vitamin A or its metabolite, retinoic acid, in the development of immune responses, by modulating the balance between the regulatory T cell subsets and directing the immune system to cell-mediated or antibody-mediated response pathways. It was therefore tempting to hypothesize that compounds that would modulate the activity of endogenous retinoic acid could have immunomodulatory activity. In line with this thinking, two RAR antagonists, CD 2665 and CD2848, have been tested in a model of chronic eczema induced in mice [32]. In this model, topical applications of 0.2% oxazolone, once a day, for eleven days onto the back of hairless mice lead to the development of an inflammatory response characterized by a dramatic enhancement of transepidermal water loss (TEWL), extensive desquamation, erythema, epidermal hyperplasia and dermal infiltrates. The test compounds were administered either orally or topically and their activity was determined by clinical score, TEWL measurement, and by histological score. Topically applied, CD 2665 and CD 2848 (0.1%) were slightly less active than Dermoval® (0.05% clobetasol), Diprosone® (0.05% betamethasone), and FK 506 (0.1%) but more active than Locapred® (0.1% desonide) and Parfenac® (5% bufexamac). Orally, CD 2665 and CD 2848 were also active in a dose-dependent manner. At a dose of 30 mg/kg, their activity was superior to that of Dermoval® or Diprosone® and equivalent to that of FK 506. These results confirm that endogenous retinoic acid is probably involved in the development of the inflammatory response in chronic eczema and suggest that an RAR antagonist could represent an alternative to the use of glucocorticoids or immunosuppressive drugs for the treatment of chronic eczema, but possibly also atopic dermatitis or other cutaneous immune diseases. In psoriasis, oral treatments with the retinoid etretinate or its active metabolite acitretin have been shown to be effective, not only because of their activity on epidermal cell proliferation and differentiation, but probably also because of their anti-inflammatory and immunomodulatory activities. However, acitretin and etretinate have demonstrated both immunosuppressive and immunostimulating activities [33]. Immunosuppression induced by these molecules was demonstrated in the delayed murine hypersensitivity inhibitory test and in the model of arthritic rats, by the modulation of the reaction of peripheral blood lymphocytes to different stimuli and by inhibition of PMN migration. Immunostimulating activities were revealed by the increased number of Langerhans cells in normal and psoriatic skin after acitretin treatment, by the immunostimulation of natural killer cells and by tumor growth inhibition in an animal model of neoplasia. Once more, these results suggest that the retinoid level is crucial to determine the immune response type. Recently, a new retinoid, AGN 190168 or tazarotene, an RARβ/RARγ selective agonist, was developed for the topical treatment of psoriasis and showed therapeutic activity [34]. Liarozole, an inhibitor of cytochrome P-450, able to induce an increase of retinoic acid by the inhibition of retinoic acid 4-hydroxylation, was also shown to be active in patients with chronic plaque-like type psoriasis [35].

In conclusion, retinoids have clearly demonstrated their usefulness in dermatology for orally or topically treating acne and psoriasis. The research for new synthetic retinoids presenting less side effects has lead to the discovery of molecules such as adapalene for acne. New retinoids such as tazarotene have been proposed recently for the topical treatment of psoriasis. A new era could be opened with molecules such as RAR antagonists, RXR agonists, or inhibitors of retinoic acid metabolism that would interact locally or systemically with the activity of endogenous retinoic acid. The data presented above clearly favor a potential for the use of such compounds in the treatment of cutaneous immune diseases. Future clinical studies will address this question.

References

1. Morriss-Kay GM, Sokolova N. Embryonic development and pattern formation. *FASEB J* 1996 ; 10 : 961-8.
2. Marshall H, Morrison A, Studer M, Popperl H, Krumlauf R. Retinoids and hox genes. *FASEB J* 1996 ; 10 : 969-78.
3. Chambon P. A decade of molecular biology of retinoic acid receptors. *FASEB J* 1996 ; 10 : 940-54.
4. Mangelsdorf DJ, Thummel C, Beato M, Herrlich P, Schutz G, Umesono K, Blumberg B, Kastner P, Mark M, Chambon P, Evans RM. The nuclear receptor superfamily, the second decade. *Cell* 1995 ; 83 : 835-9.
5. Ross AC, Hammerling UG. Retinoids and the immune system. In : Sporn, MB, Roberts AB, Goodman DS, eds. *Retinoids: biology, chemistry, and medicine*. New York : Raven Press, 1994 : 521-43.
6. Blomhoff HK, Smeland EB. Role of retinoids in normal hematopoiesis and the immune system. In : Blomhoff R, ed. *Vitamin A in health and disease*. New York, Basel, Hong Kong : Marcel Dekker, 1994 : 451-84.
7. Salbert G, Fanjul A, Piedrafita FJ, Lu XP, Kim SJ, Tran P, Pfahl M. Retinoic acid receptors and retinoic X receptor-alpha down-regulate the transforming growth factor-beta 1 promoter by antagonizing AP-1 activity. *Mol Endocrinol* 1993 ; 7 : 1347-56.
8. Fanjul A, Dawson MI, Hobbs PD, Jong L, Cameron JF, Harlev E, Graupner G, Lu XP, Pfahl M. A new class of retinoids with selective inhibition of AP-1 inhibits proliferation. *Nature* 1994 ; 372 : 107-11.
9. Vega-Diaz B, Ladoux A, Frelin C, Démarchez M, Michel S. Regulation of vascular endothelial growth factor mRNA expression in human keratinocytes by retinoids. *J Invest Dermatol* (accepted).
10. Alroy I, Towers TL, Freedman LP. Transcriptional repression of the interleukin-2 gene by vitamin D3: direct inhibition of NFATp/AP-1 complex formation by a nuclear hormone receptor. *MCB* 1995 ; 15 : 5789-99.
11. Takeuchi A, Reddy GS, Kobayashi T, Okano T, Park J, Sharma S. Nuclear factor of activated T cells (NFAT) as a molecular target for 1a,25-dihydroxyvitamin D3-mediated effects. *J Immunol* 1998 ; 160 : 209-18.
12. Rao A. NF-Atp: a transcription factor required for the co-ordinate induction of several cytokine genes. *Immunol Today* 1994 ; 15 : 274-81.

13. DiSepio D, Malhotra M, Chandraratna RAS, Nagpal S. Retinoic acid receptor-nuclear factor-interleukin 6 antagonist. A novel mechanism of retinoid-dependent inhibition of a keratinocyte hyperproliferative differentiation marker. *J Biol Chem* 1997 ; 272 : 25555-9.

14. Szondy Z, Reichert U, Fésüs L. Retinoic acid regulate apoptosis of T lymphocytes through an interplay between RAR and RXR receptors. *Cell Death Diff* 1998 ; 5 : 4-10.

15. Ashwell JD. When complex worlds collide: retinoic acid and apoptosis. *Cell Death Diff* 1998 ; 5 : 1-3.

16. Scrimshaw NW, Taylor CE, Gordon JE. *Interactions of nutrition and infection*. Monogr. Ser n° 57. Geneva : WHO, 1968.

17. Bellagio report. *Bellagio meeting on vitamin A deficiency and children mortality*. New York : Helen Keller Internationals Inc, 1993.

18. Dennert G, Lotan R. Effects of RA on the immune system: stimulation of T killer cell induction. *Eur J Immunol* 1978 ; 8 : 23-9.

19. Pasatiempo AMG, Kinoshita M, Taylor CE, Ross AC. Antibody production in vitamin A-depleted rats is impaired after immunization with bacterial polysaccharide or protein antigens. *FASEB J* 1990 ; 4 : 2518-27.

20. Blomhoff HK, Smeland EB, Erikstein B, Rasmussen AM, Strede B, Skjonsberg C, Blomhoff R. Vitamin A is a key regulator for cell growth, cytokine production and differentiation in normal B cells. *J Biol Chem* 1992 ; 267 : 23988-92.

21. Buck J, Ritter, G, Dannecker L, Katta V, Cohen SL, Chait BT, Hammerling U. Retinol is essential for growth of activated human B cells. *J Exp Med* 1990 ; 171 : 1613-24.

22. Apfel C, Bauer F, Crettaz M, Forni L, Kamber M, Kaufmann F, Lemotte P, Pirson W, Klaus M. A retinoic acid receptor alpha antagonist selectively counteracts retinoic acid effects. *Proc Natl Acad Sci USA* 1992 ; 89 : 7129-33.

23. Hayes CE, Nashold F, Chun TY, Cantorna M. Vitamin A: a regulator of immune function. In : Livrea MA, Vidali G, eds. *Retinoids: from basic science to clinic applications*. Basel : Birkhauser Verlag, 1994 : 215-31.

24. Asselineau D, Bernard B, Bailly C, Darmon M. Retinoic acid improves epidermal morphogenesis. *Dev Biol* 1989 ; 133 : 322-35.

25. Huston DP. The biology of the immune system. *JAMA* 1997 ; 278 : 1804-14.

26. Cantorna MT, Nashold FE, Hayes CE, Vitamin A deficiency results in a priming environment conducive for Th1 cell development. *Eur J Immunol* 1995, 25 : 1673-9.

27. Racke MK, Burnett D, Pak SH, Albert PS, Cannella B, Raine CS, McFarlin DE, Scott DE. Retinoid treatment of experimental allergic encephalomyelitis. IL4 production correlates with improved disease course. *J Immunol* 1995 ; 154 : 450-8.

28. Leung DYM, Diaz LA, DeLeo V, Soter NA. Allergic and immunologic skin disorders. *JAMA* 1997 ; 278 : 1914-23.

29. Cooper KD. Atopic dermatitis: recent trends in pathogenesis and therapy. *J Invest Dermatol* 1994 ; 102 : 128-37.

30. Baker SB, Fry L. The immunology of psoriasis. *Br J Dermatol* 1992 ; 126 : 1-9.

31. Strange P, Cooper KD, Hansen ER, Fisher G, Larsen JK, Fox D, Krag C, Voorhees JJ, Baadsgaard O. T-lymphocytes clones initiated from lesional psoriatic skin release growth factors that induce keratinocyte proliferation. *J Invest Dermatol* 1993 ; 101 : 695-700.

32. Jomard A, Feraille G, Dessauvages H, Démarchez M. RAR antagonists inhibit the inflammatory response in a model of chronic eczema in the mouse (in preparation).

33. Gollnick HPM, Dümmler U. Retinoids. *Clin Dermatol* 1997 ; 15 : 799-810.

34. Weinstein GD. Safety, efficacy and duration of therapeutic effect of tazarotene used in the treatment of plaque psoriasis. *Br J Dermatol* 1996 ; 135 (Suppl. 49) : 32-6.

35. Dockx P, Decree J, Degreef H. Inhibition of the metabolism of endogenous retinoic acid as treatment for severe psoriasis: an open study with oral liarozole. *Br J Dermatol* 1995 ; 133 : 426-32.

6

The skin in chronic renal failure and hemodialysis

Sophie DALAC, Évelyne COLLET, Jean-Michel REBIBOU, Daniel LAMBERT
Department of Dermatology, CHU Bocage, Dijon, France.

Chronic renal failure (CRF), hemodialysis and peritoneal dialysis are associated with several dermatologic manifestations that are, however, of relatively weak specificity.

Skin lesions in chronic renal failure and hemodialysis (excluding allergic manifestations)

Xerosis

Xerosis is frequently severe; cutaneous biopsies show atrophic eccrine sweat glands and a poor vascularization. Decreased sweating and thermal disorders are observed [1, 2]. Local emollient therapy is often necessary for patients on hemodialysis.

Pruritus

Pruritus is the most common cutaneous symptom in CRF (10% to 30% of patients) and hemodialysis (20% to 90%). The prevalence is the same in hemodialysis and continuous ambulatory peritoneal dialysis. Pruritus may be the first sign of renal disease [3, 4] but appears usually 6 months after starting hemodialysis. Pruritus manifests with non specific lesions; it is usually generalized, variable in intensity and often paroxysmal during hemodialysis (2/3). The etiology remains unclear, but multiple factors have been incriminated, including:
– *xerosis of the skin*;
– *metabolic disorders*: in uremic patients, there is a decrease of 25 (OH) D3 synthesis with hyperphosphoremia, hypocalcemia and metabolic acidosis. Complications comprise

hyperparathyroïdism, renal osteodystrophy with increased calcium x phosphate product and subclinical skin deposits of calcium. In some cases, parathyroïdectomy induces remission of pruritus. Hyposideremia, hypermagnesemia, hyperalbuminemia are other factors of pruritus [5];
– *mast cells and histamine*: parathormone provokes mast cell proliferation with increased release of histamine [6-10]. Plasma histamine is increased during and after the hemodialysis session;
– *vitamin A*: serum levels of vitamin A and retinol-binding protein are increased in patients with CRF and the renal clearance of the latter is decreased. There is also a decrease in the conversion of retinol to retinoic acid. The clinical manifestations of hypervitaminosis A are similar, *i.e.* xerosis, pruritus, and osteodystrophy; however in one study no difference between serum vitamin A levels in patients on hemodialysis with or without pruritus was found [11, 12]. Epidermal retinol is also increased in the epidermis of patients on hemodialysis. UVA and B therapy reduces epidermal retinol (retinol absorption: 280-380 nm);
– *neuropathy*: Stahle-Backdall suggests that hemodialysis patients can develop abnormal cutaneous innervation [13, 14].

Since the origin of pruritus is multifactorial different therapeutic approaches exist [15, 16]. The best treatment is kidney transplantation. It is necessary to comfort patients with emollients. Sedatives, H1 and H2 anti-histamines, cholestyramine, heparin, topical capsaicin, nicergoline, lidocaine, erythropoietin and calcium carbonate are used with moderate efficiency. Subtotal parathyroidectomy may relieve pruritus [17-20]. UVB therapy is successfully used, but in patients waiting for transplantation, the total dose of UVB must be limited to prevent the development of carcinomas in sun-exposed areas [21-23]. Modifications of hemodialysis can be necessary to treat the itchy patient. However, the results of treatment are disappointing in many cases [24, 25].

Cutaneous calcifications and necrosis

Calcium deposits occur in various tissues, in the following order of decreasing frequency: blood vessels, eyes (cornea, conjunctiva), periarticular tissue, skin and subcutaneous tissue, viscera [26] (*Figure 1, page 217*). Deposits of hydroxy-apatite crystals are found in the dermis or hypodermis of patients with CRF, with or without clinical manifestations.

Metastatic calcifications and calciphylaxis can be individualized. The lesions include papules, nodules, ulcerations, livedo reticularis or cutaneous necrosis and are often associated with severe pruritus. There are two clinical forms depending on whether necrosis occurs (diffuse panarteritis, acral calcifications or panniculitis) or not.

In calcifying panniculitis, sensitization results from high levels of parathormone and the challenger is a minor injury or drug injection [27]. The patient's condition deteriorates rapidly with extensive and painful cutaneous necrosis over the trunk or proximal extremities and the prognosis is ominous [28, 29]. Calciphylaxis is a rare and life-threatening complication estimated to occur in 1% of patients on hemodialysis. Typically, extensive microvascular calcifications and occlusions/thromboses lead to violaceous skin lesions, which progress to ulcers and sepsis; secondary infection is frequent. Most calciphylaxis patients have abnormalities of calcium, *i.e.* hypercalcemia, hyperphosphoremia and elevated levels of parathyroid hormone; however, these abnormalities do not appear to be fundamental to the physiopathology of the disorder and the etiology still remains unclear. There are similarities between calciphylaxis and warfarin-induced skin necrosis. Reduced functional protein C levels may be involved in the pathogenesis [30, 31] (*Figure 2, page 217*).

Calciphylaxis patients have a tendency to improve after parathyroidectomy. In metastatic calcifications without necrosis, where hyperphosphatemia appears to play a major pathogenic role, parathyroidectomy is also often successful.

In secondary cutaneous oxalosis due to long-term hemodialysis, cutaneous deposits of calcium oxalate dihydrate are observed and miliary deposits occur frequently on the fingers [32].

Perforating disorders

Kyrle's disease, perforating folliculitis, reactive perforating collagenosis and elastosis perforans serpiginosa share a common pathogenic mecanism, *i.e.* transepithelial elimination [33, 34]. These conditions, collectively referred to as « acquired perforating disease », are observed in 5% to 10% of uremic patients. Clinically, the disease manifests with hyperkeratotic, umbilicated and pruriginous papules on the trunk and the extremities (*Figure 3, page 217*) that occur singly or as linear plaques. Pruritus is present and is often severe. Histologically, early lesions show a concave depression of the epidermal surface. Traversing the acanthotic epidermis, transepidermal channels are seen, filled with keratin, pyknotic nuclear debris, inflammatory cells, elastin and collagen. As the lesions mature, the transepidermal channels widen, forming large cup-shaped plugs within the epidermis, that are eliminated through the surface. As the plugs mature, elastin disappears and collagen acquires a more basophilic staining. Koebner's phenomenon is often described [35-38]. Diabetes mellitus and chronic renal disease are frequently associated with acquired perforating dermatoses. The pathogenesis of these disorders is unknown. Acquired perforating dermatoses may improve spontaneously, with topical retinoids or topical/intradermal steroids, or after renal transplantation.

Bullous dermatoses

Bullous dermatoses include mainly pseudo-porphyria cutanea tarda (PPCT), and phototoxic drug reactions due to certain drugs such as furosemide, nalidixic acid and tetracyclins. True PCT is rare and may be associated with hepatitis C virus infection.

PPCT is observed in 4% to 18% patients on hemodialysis or peritoneal dialysis. PPCT is clinically and histologically indistinguishable from PCT. It manifests clinically with bullous lesions on the back of the hands (*Figure 4, page 217*), but also on the face and neck (sun-exposed areas), skin fragility with erosions, photosensitivity, atrophic scars and milia, pigmentation, rarely malar hypertrichosis. Histologically, a subepidermal cleavage is found; by direct immunofluorescence hyaline deposits of IgG and/or IgM, IgA and C3 around blood vessels and at the dermal-epidermal junction are seen [39-41]. The majority of patients on hemodialysis have plasma porphyrin levels higher than those of normal persons due to inadequate clearance of porphyrins, but the titres are independent from the presence of clinically overt blistering disease. Conventional hemodialysis whith lower blood flow rates (less than 250 ml/mn) and cuprophan or cellulose acetate membranes is ineffective in removing significant amounts of porphyrins. In high-flux hemodialysis with a polysulfone dialyser, predialysis plasma porphyrins fell by 37%. High-flux hemodialysis with more permeable membranes may be a useful adjunct in treating dialysis patients with PPCT [42-44].

The treatment of PCT and PPCT is very difficult: chloroquine is ineffective and venesection, the conventional treatment, is not always a satisfactory option because of anemia of end-stage renal disease. Erythropoietin treatment may be used with success. Only kidney transplantation can lead to complete resolution [45-47].

Amyloidosis

Long-term hemodialysis may result in systemic β2-microglobulin-induced amyloidosis. The amyloid-producing potential of β2-microglobulin has been well documented.

The most common manifestations include carpal tunnel syndrome, bone cysts, destructive spondylarthropathy, arthropathy and fractures. Fifty percent of patients who have been on hemodialysis for more than 12 years develop carpal tunnel syndrome. Skin lesions are rare and include lichenoid eruptions, pigmentation and subcutaneous nodules or tumors. Histology shows amyloid deposition within dermal papillae and in the reticular dermis around sweat ducts, hair follicles and blood vessels [48, 49].

Pigmentary disorders

Melanoderma (of Bright) develops slowly, after several months on sun-exposed regions, sparing mucosal surfaces. Skin color changes from yellowish to light brown. The factors responsible are mainly anemia, accumulation of pigments (carotenoids, lipochromes) and βMSH increase (which is poorly dialyzable), inducing an increase of melanogenesis [50].

Nail and hair changes

Nail changes are very frequent in uremic patients and include leuconychia, half-and-half nails (35%), striped nails, Beau's lines, splinter hemorrhages and photoonycholysis (*Figures 5 and 6, page 217*). Alopecia, hair discoloration, fine, dry and brittle hair have been reported [51-54].

Allergic cutaneous manifestations

Thirty percent of patients on hemodialysis or peritoneal dialysis present allergic manifestations, such as immediate hypersensitivity reactions or contact dermatitis. When dermatitis is present, tests for delayed hypersensitivity should be carried out for the numerous substances that come into contact with patient's blood or skin during dialysis sessions [55, 56].

Immediate hypersensitivity reactions

Pruritus, urticaria and angioneurotic edema can be severe, associated with bronchospasm or anaphylactic shock in 5% to 15 % of patients on hemodialysis. They usually occur at the beginning of each session. Specific IgE and anaphylactic mecanisms (histamine, anaphylatoxins C3a and C5a, kinins...) are implicated [57].

Ethylene oxide is used during sterilization. There is no correlation between the presence of IgE antibodies against ethylen-oxide and clinical manifestations.

Formaldehyde, phtalates and *isocyanates* are other allergens in IgE-mediated reactions.

Membranes of dialysis: pruritus is sometimes less when high permeability membranes are used instead of cuprophane membranes [58].

Contact dermatitis

Dermatitis is observed in 30% of hemodialysis patients, on the arterio-venous shunt and may secondarily become generalized [59]. The responsible agents include mainly:
– *formaldehyde* (used for sterilization),
– *thiuram* (two possible ways of contact with rubber chemicals exist during dialysis, *i.e.* contact with the small rubber parts of the dialysis equipment and with rubber gloves [60-62],
– *nickel* of the needles [63],
– *epoxy* of the glue at the tube-needle joint [64],
– *collophane* of glues,
– *local antiseptics* (*e.g.* iodine solution) used to clean the skin.

Local complications in dialysis

Complications of the arterio-venous shunt include extravasation with hematoma, phlebitis, aneurysms, sepsis and contact dermatitis (*Figures 7 and 8, page 218*).

Arterio-venous shunt dermatitis is described without positive patch-tests (standard ICDRG battery and a « dialysis » battery). The mean duration on hemodialysis is longer in patients with irritant contact dermatitis than in those without dermatitis. Patients with atopy are more susceptible to have an irritant contact dermatitis than non-atopics [65].

Pseudo-Kaposi's sarcoma has been described in the vicinity of arterio-venous fistula. Venous pressure and skin surface temperature are increased around the lesions and may play an important role in the development of lesions. Patients present with erythematous patches or plaques on the hands. Histologic findings include a proliferation of small vessels with narrow lumina lined by spindle cells, extravasated erythrocytes and hemosiderin deposits [66].

Conclusion

Among the various dermatologic troubles that are associated with advanced chronic renal failure or hemodialysis, pruritus is the most disturbing one. Treatment is difficult as reflected by the variety of treatments that have been tried. UVB therapy is efficient but must be limited in anticipation of a future transplantation. Renal transplantation is the best treatment for these various cutaneous manifestations.

References

1. Yosipovitch G, Reis J, Tur E, Sprecher E, Yarn T. Sweat secretion, stratum corneum hydratation, small nerve function and pruritus in patients with advanced chronic renal failure. *Br J Dermatol* 1995 ; 133 : 561-4.

2. Bencini PL, Montagnino G, Citterio A, Graziani G, Crosti C, Caputo R, Ponticelli C. Cutaneous abnormalities in uremic patients. *Nephron* 1985 ; 40 : 316-21.

3. Gilchrest BA, Stren RS, Steimann TI, Brown RS, Arndt KR, Anderson WW. Clinical features of pruritus among patients undergoing maintenance hemodialysis. *Arch Dermatol* 1982 ; 118 : 154-6.

4. Gupta AK, Gupta MA, Cardella CJ, Haberman HF. Cutaneous associations of chronic renal failure and dialysis. *Int J Dermatol* 1986 ; 25 : 498-504.

5. Ponticelli C, Bencini PL. Uremic pruritus: a review. *Nephron* 1992 ; 6 : 1-5.

6. Matsumoto M, Ichimaru K, Horie A. Pruritus and mast cell proliferation of the skin in end stage renal failure. *Clin Nephrol* 1985 ; 23 : 285-8.

7. Cohen EP, Russel TJ, Garancis JC. Mast cells and calcium in severe uremic itching. *Am J Med Sci* 1992 ; 303 : 360-5.

8. Dimkovic N, Djukanovic L, Radmilovic A, Bojic P, Juloski T. Uremic pruritus and skin mast cells. *Nephron* 1992 ; 61 : 5-9.

9. Gill DS, Fonseca VA, Barradas MA, Balliod R, Moorhead JF, Dandona P. Plasma histamin in patients with chronic renal failure and nephrotic syndrome. *J Clin Pathol* 1991 ; 44 : 243-5.

10. De Marchi S, Cecchin E, Villalta D, Sepiacci G, Santini G, Bartoli E. Relief pruritus and decrease in plasma histamine concentrations during erythropoietin therapy in patients with uremia. *N Engl J Med* 1992 ; 326 : 969-74.

11. De Kroes S, Smeek G. Serum vitamin A levels and pruritus in patients on hemodialysis. *Dermatologica* 1983 ; 166 : 199-202.

12. Kelleher J, Humphrey CS, Homer D, Davidson AM, Giles GR, Losowsky MS. Vitamin a and its transport proteins in patients with chronic renal failure receiving maintenance hemodialysis and after renal transplantation. *Clin Sci* 1983 ; 65 : 619-26.

13. Stahle-Backdahl M. Pruritus in hemodialysis patients. *Skin Pharmacol* 1992 ; 5 : 14-20.

14. Fantini F, Baraldi A, Sevignani C, Spattini A, Pincelli C, Giannetti A. Cutaneous innervation in chronic renal failure patients. *Acta Derm Venereol* 1992 ; 72 : 102-5.

15. Tan JK, Haberman HF, Coldman AJ. Identifying effective treatment for uremic pruritus. *J Am Acad Dermatol* 1991 ; 25 : 811-8.

16. Masi CM, Cohen EP. Dialysis efficacy and itching in renal failure. *Nephron* 1992 ; 62 : 257-61.

17. Francos GC, Kauh YC, Gittlen SD, Schulman ES, Besarab A, Goyals, Burke JF. Elevated plasma histamin in chronic uremia. Effects of ketotifene on pruritus. *Int J Dermatol* 1991 ; 30 : 884-9.

18. Breneman DL, Cardone JS, Blumsack RF, Lather RM, Searle EA, Pollack VE. Topical capsaicin for treatment of hemodialysis-related pruritus. *J Am Acad Dermatol* 1992 ; 26 : 91-4.

19. Tercedor J, Lopez-Hernandez B, Rodenas JM, Herranz MT, Serrano-Ortega S. Erythropoietin therapy for uremic pruritus. *N Engl J Med* 1992 ; 327 : 734.

20. Balaska EV, Uldall RP. Erythropoietin treatment does not improve uremic pruritus. *Perit Dial Int* 1992 ; 12 : 330-1.

21. Gilchrest BA, Rowe JW, Brown RS, Steinman TI, Arndt KA. Ultraviolet phototherapy of uremic pruritus. Long-term results and possible mechanism of action. *Ann Intern Med* 1979 ; 91 : 17-21.

22. Taylor R, Taylor AE, Diffey BL, Hindson TC. A placebo controlled trial of UVA phototherapy for the treatment of uraemic pruritus. *Nephron* 1983 ; 33 : 14-6.

23. Berne B, Vahlquist A, Fisher T, Danielson BG, Bern C. UV-treatment of uraemic pruritus reduces the vitamin A content of the skin. *Eur J Clin Invest* 1984 ; 14 : 203-6.

24. Carmichael AJ, Hugh MI, Martin AM. Itch unrelated to adequacy of hemodialysis. *Br J Dermatol* 1992 ; 126 : 95.

25. Robertson KE, Mueller BA. Uremic pruritus. *Am J Health Syst Pharm* 1996 ; 53 : 2159-70.

26. Tada J, Torigoe R, Shimoe K, Ohara S, Arata J, Ashizawa K. Calcium deposition in the skin of a hemodialysis patient with widespread necrosis. *Am J Dermatopathol* 1991 ; 13 : 605-10.

27. Grob JJ, Legre R, Bertocchio P, Payan MJ, Andrac L, Bonerandi JJ. Calcifying panniculitis and kidney failure. Considerations on pathogenesis and treatment of calciphylaxis. *Int J Dermatol* 1989 ; 28 : 129-31.

28. Tork L, Kozepessy L. Uraemic gangrene syndrome. *Acta Derm Venereol* 1991 ; 71 : 455-7.

29. Buchet S, Blanc D, Humbert PH, Derancourt C, Arbey-Gindre F, Atallah L, Agache P. La panniculite calcifiante. *Ann Dermatol Venereol* 1992 ; 119 : 659-66.

30. Mehta RL, Scott G, Sloand J, Francis JW. Skin necrosis associated with acquired protein C deficiency in patients with renal failure and calciphylaxis. *Am J Med* 1990 ; 88 : 252-7.

31. Kant KS, Glueck HI, Coots MC, Tonne VA, Brubaker R, Penn I. Protein S deficiency and skin necrosis associated with cutaneous ambulatory peritoneal dialysis. *Am J Kidney Dis* 1992 ; 19 : 264-71.

32. Ohtake N, Uchiyama H, Furue M, Tamaki K. Secondary cutaneous oxalosis: cutaneous deposition of calcium oxalate dihydrate after long-term hemodialysis. *J Am Acad Dermatol* 1994 ; 31 : 368-72.

33. Randle HW. Keratotic papules of chronic renal failure: the process of transepithelial elimination. *Arch Dermatol* 1983 ; 119 : 874-5.

34. Patterson JW. The perforating disorders. *J Am Acad Dermatol* 1984 ; 10 : 561-81.

35. Bank DE, Cohen PR, Hohn SR. Reactive perforating collagenosis in a setting of double disaster. Acquired immunodeficiency syndrome and end-stage renal disease. *J Am Acad Dermatol* 1989 ; 21 : 371-4.

36. Chang P, Fernandez V. Acquired perforating disease associated with chronic renal failure. *Int J Dermatol* 1992 ; 31 : 117-8.

37. Morton CA, Henderson IS, Jones MC, Lowe JG. Acquired perforating dermatosis in a british dialysis population. *Br J Dermatol* 1996 ; 135 : 671-7.

38. Farrell AM. Acquired perforating dermatosis in renal and diabetic patients. *Lancet* 1997 ; 349 : 895-6.

39. Thivolet J, Euvrard S, Perrot H, Moskovtchenko JF. La pseudo-porphyrie cutanée tardive des hémodialysés. *Ann Dermatol Venereol* 1977 ; 104 ; 12-7.

40. Day RS, Eales L. Porphyrins in chronic renal failure. *Nephron* 1980 ; 26 : 9-5.

41. Amblard P, Cordonnier D, Reymond JL, Beani JC, Elsener M, Cuffon MP. La pseudo-porphyrie cutanée tardive chez l'hémodialysé. *Ann Dermatol Venereol* 1981 ; 108 : 1019-20.

42. Poh-Ftzpatrick MB, Sosin AE, Bemis J. Porphyrins levels in plasma and erythrocytes of chronic hemodialysis patients. *J Am Acad Dermatol* 1982 ; 6 : 100-4.

43. Carson RW, Dunningan EL, Dubose TD, Goeger DE, Anderson KE. Removal of plasma porphyrins with high-flux hemodialysis in porphyria cutanea tarda associated with end-stage renal disease. *J Am Soc Nephrol* 1992 ; 2 : 1445-50.

44. Gibson GE, Mc Ginnity E, Mc Grath P, Carmody M, Wrlshe J, Donohoe J, O'Moore R, Murphy GM. Cutaneous abnormalities and metabolic disturbance of porphyrins in patients on maintenance hemodialysis. *Clin Exp Dermatol* 1997 ; 22 : 124-7.

45. Hebert AA, Farmer KL, Poh-Ftzpatrick MB. Peritoneal dialysis does not reduce serum porphyrin levels in porphyria cutanea tarda. *Nephron* 1992 ; 60 : 240.

46. Piazza V, Villa G, Galli F, Segagni S, Bovio G, Poggio F, Piccardi L, Bianco L, Salvadeo A, Barosi G. Erythropoietin as treatment of hemodialysis-related prophyria cutanea tarda. *Nephrol Dial Transplant* 1992 ; 7 : 438-42.

47. Stevens BR, Fleisher AB, Piering F, Crosby DL. Porphyria cutanea tarda in the setting of renal failure. Response to renal transplantation. *Arch Dermatol* 1993 ; 129 : 337-9.

48. Floege J, Brandis A, Nonnast-Daniel B, Westhoff-Bleck M, Tiedow G, Kinke RP, Hoch KM. Subcutaneous amyloid-tumor of beta-2-microglobulin origin in a long-term hemodialysis patient. *Nephron* 1989 ; 53 : 73-5.

49. Sato KC, Kumakiri M, Koizumi H, Ando M, Ohkawara A, Fujioka Y, Kon T. Lichenoid skin lesions as a sign of B2-microglobulin-induced amyloidisis in a long-term hemodialysis patient. *Br J Dermatol* 1993 ; 128 : 686-9.

50. Comaish JJ, Ashhcroft T, Ken DNS. The pigmentation of the renal failure. *Nephron* 1980 ; 26 : 90-5.

51. Leyden JJ, Wood MG. The half and half nail. A uremic onychopathy. *Arch Dermatol* 1972 ; 105 : 591-2.

52. Kint A, Bussels L, Fernandes M. Skin and nail disorders in relation to chronic renal failure. *Acta Derm Venereol* 1974 ; 54 : 137-40.

53. Bencini PL, Graziani G, Crosti C. Hair shaft abnormalities in uremia, a SEM study. *Eur J Dermatol* 1992 ; 2 : 119-21.

54. Guillaud V, Moulin G, Bonnefoy M, Cognat T, Balme B, Barrut D. Photoonycholyse bulleuse au cours d'une pseudoporphyrie des hémodialysés. *Ann Dermatol Venereol* 1990 ; 117 : 723-5.

55. Kessler M, Moneret Vautrin DA, Cau Huu T, Mariot A, Chanliau J. Dialysis pruritus and sensitivation. *Nephron* 1992 ; 6 : 241.

56. Lemke HD. Hypersensitivity reactions during hemodialysis. *Nephrol Dial Transplant* 1994 ; 9 : 120-5.

57. Nicholls AJ, Platts MM. Anaphylactoid reactions due to hemodialysis, haemofiltration or membrane plasma separation. *Br Med J* 1982 ; 285 : 1607-9.

58. Montagnac R, Schillinger F, Milcent T, Croix JC. Réaction d'hypersensibilité au cours de l'hémodialyse. Rôle de la haute perméabilité, de la rétrofiltration et de la contamination bactérienne du dialysat. *Nephrologie* 1988 ; 9 : 29-32.

59. Mariot A, Moneret Vautrin DA, Kessler M, Chanliau J, Cao Huu T, Mouton C. Les hypersensibilités retardées aux réactogènes chimiques chez les hémodialysés. *Rev Fr Allergol* 1986 ; 26 : 15-8.

60. Penneys NS, Edwards NS, Katsikas JL. Allergic contact sensitivity to thiuram compounds in a hemodialysis unit. *Arch Dermatol* 1976 ; 112 : 811-3.

61. Buxton K, Coing SM, Hunter JAA, Winney RJ. Allergic reaction due to rubber chemicals in hemodialysis equipment. *Br Med J* 1983 ; 287 : 1513-4.

62. Kruis De Vries MH, Coenraads PJ, Nater JP. Allergic contact dermatitis due to rubber chemicals in hemodialysis equipment. *Contact Dermatitis* 1987 ; 17 : 303-5.

63. Olerud JE, Lee M, Uvelli DA, Goble GJ, Babb AL. Presumptive nickel dermatitis from hemodialysis. *Arch Dermatol* 1984 ; 12 : 1066-8.

64. Brandao M, Pinto J. Allergic contact dermatitis to epoxy resin in hemodialysis needles. *Contact Dermatitis* 1980 ; 6 : 218-9.

65. Goh CL, Phay KL. Arterio-venous shunt dermatitis in chronic renal failure patients on maintenance hemodialysis. *Clin Exp Dermatol* 1988 ; 13 : 379-81.

66. Kim TH, Kim KH, Kang JS, Kim JH, Wang IY. Pseudo-Kaposi's sarcoma associated with acquired arterio-venous fistula. *J Dermatol* 1997 ; 24 : 28-33.

7

Human papillomavirus and cutaneous carcinogenesis

Slavomir MAJEWSKI, Stefania JABLONSKA
Department of Dermatology, Warsaw School of Medicine, Warsaw, Poland.

The association of genital tumors with HPV is well documented, and in cervical cancers HPV DNA is found in almost 96% of cases [1]. Precursor lesions also contain HPV DNA in more than 90% of biopsies [2]. This fact provides the most significant epidemiological evidence of the link between HPVs and cancerogenesis. In other genital malignancies HPV DNA is not invariably detected, however, the association is confirmed in up to 70% of cases [1].

Specific HPVs have been found to be a risk factor, persist in tumor cells, become integrated into the host genome, and their transforming proteins E6 and E7 interfere with cellular factors involved in the control of cell proliferation (*Table I*). E6 protein of high risk HPVs interacts with the *p53* antioncogene and leads to its degradation, while E7 oncoprotein binds to cellular

Table I. Role of genital HPV proteins in viral DNA replication and keratinocyte transformation

E1 and E2 proteins:
 – bind a set of cellular transcription factors necessary for HPV DNA replication
 – E2 is a main viral protein in the process of viral integration into the host genome

E6 protein:
 – binds to p53 leading to its degradation
 – main factor in keratinocyte transformation

E7 protein:
 – binds to pRb protein leading to its inactivation
 – releases E2F transcription factor
 – induces proliferation and immortalization of keratinocytes

protein pRb (*Table II*). E6 and E7 proteins are also able to stimulate keratinocyte proliferation upon transfection. Thus the criteria of zur Hausen concerning the etiologic role of specific HPVs in cancerogenesis [3] are fulfilled for cervical cancer, and the role of HPVs in this cancer is widely accepted.

Table II. Role of EV HPV proteins in cutaneous carcinogenesis

E2 protein:
– may stimulate or inhibit (SIL) viral DNA replication
– does not induce viral integration into host genome

E6 protein:
– does not bind to p53 and does not degrade this protein
– does not transform and immortalize keratinocytes
– displays unusual heterogeneity due to numerous transcripts of the E6 gene; E6 variants could serve as a target for immune response

E7 protein:
– stimulates keratinocyte proliferation
– does not induce keratinocyte transformation and immortalization

In the multistep process of carcinogenesis, several genetic alterations affect host cell genes. This process may last several years, up to 20 [3], and the degradation of p53 leads to accumulation of damaged DNA and to tumor formation. However, the intracellular control of viral oncogene expression and host defense mechanisms are responsible for the spontaneous regression of about 70% of benign lesions associated with high-risk HPV16, and/or disappearance of these HPVs in latent infections. The malignant progression of cells infected with high-risk HPVs requires interruption of the signaling pathways regulating the function of viral oncoproteins and genes suppressing viral transcription. The integration of HPV DNA by interruption of intragenomic viral regulation leads to a partial or complete escape from intracellular control mechanisms suppressing HPV E6-E7 transcription [3].

Contrasting with genital malignancies, the relationship of HPVs with cutaneous tumors is not very clear. Strong evidence for the link between HPVs and skin cancers exists only in a rare genetic disorder, epidermodysplasia verruciformis (EV), associated with HPVs specific for this disease (EV-HPVs) [4, 5].

Epidermodysplasia verruciformis

This genodermatosis is a model of cutaneous oncogenesis; it is characterized by life-long persistence of wart-like and macular benign lesions, induced by EV-specific HPVs [6]. About half of the patients develop in fourth-fifth decade skin cancers associated with potentially oncogenic EV-HPVs. Benign EV lesions harbor several EV HPV types (over 20 have been cloned and characterized and new types and variants are regularly detected) [7]. Carcinomas in EV are associated exclusively with specific oncogenic HPVs, predominantly HPV5 and HPV8, and only rarely with HPV types 14, 17, 20 or 47 [5, 8, 9].

The main limitation of studying the role of EV HPVs in cell transformation is the lack of an *in vitro* system for replication of HPVs. Alternative models include xenograft skin transplantation and transgenic animal systems. Using experimental systems *in vivo*, we were able to propagate skin fragments of EV lesions transplanted under the kidney capsule of nude mice for up to 12 months [10]. After several months the grafts contained multiple copies of

HPV5 and HPV8 DNA and EV HPV particles, as detected by specific antibodies. Also transplantation of an EV squamous cell carcinoma tissue into SCID mice allowed the *in vivo* propagation of this tumor for up to 10 generations [11]. In the model of transgenic mice, the E7 oncogene of HPV16 was expressed in the basal layer of the epidermis under the control of human keratin 14 [12] or keratin 1 [13] gene promoters. In this system, HPV16 oncoproteins induced epidermal hyperplasia and development of skin tumors (SCC and sebaceous gland epitheliomas), however, the activity of E6/E7 of EV HPVs was not studied.

Evidence for the role of EV HPVs is provided by the (weak) transforming potential of E6 gene of HPV5 and HPV8 and the detection of E6/E7 transcripts in skin cancers (*Table II*). The cell-transforming potential of E6 of high-risk HPVs reflects the *in vivo* association of these EV HPVs with skin cancers, whereas E7 is able to transform rodent cells exclusively in collaboration with an activated H-*ras* gene [14].

In contrast to genital cancers associated with high-risk HPVs, where viral sequences are integrated into the host genome, the DNA of oncogenic EV HPVs remains extrachromosomal [15]. Unlike anogenital HPVs, E6 and E7 transforming proteins of oncogenic EV HPVs do not bind the p53 or pRb proteins. Positive immunostaining with monoclonal anti-p53 antibody was reported in over 90% of benign lesions of EV, whereas it was negative in all non-EV warts [16]. However, no p53 mutations were detected in exons 5-8 of the *p53* gene in 4 analyzed lesions. The authors concluded that the immunostaining was probably due to accumulation of the wild type p53. Overexpressed p53 protein might not be functional; alternatively, its suppressor function may be overcome by unknown mechanisms in EV leading to malignant transformation. In a recent study (presented by Padlewska *et al.* at the Human Papillomavirus Workshop, Siena 1997) on a large series of EV cases we found mutations of p53 both in sun-exposed and non sun-exposed skin in exons differing from those mutated in skin cancers of the general population, related mainly to sun exposure [17]. Thus, it is conceivable that, in addition to sun-induced mutations, EV HPVs might contribute to degradation of p53.

It has been suggested that EV HPVs interfere with the growth control of human keratinocytes by mechanisms that differ from those of anogenital HPVs [18]. One possibility is a function derangement of E2-coded transactivator of regulatory elements within the LCR (long control region) of HPV8. It has been shown that loss of E2 transactivating function results in the loss of the transforming function of this gene. Recently, a negatively acting oligonucleotide (SIL for silence) was cloned from HPV8 sequences and shown to be a *cis*-acting element down-regulating the transcription [19]. Moreover, it was found that SIL region contains the sequence P1 which binds the viral transactivator protein E2. Therefore it was suggested that the viral factor E2 can relieve repression by SIL leading to an elevated transcription of HPV8 genes in the process of malignant progression [19]. In about half of EV cancers there are deletions in EV HPV DNA [9], including those affecting sequences homologous to the SIL [20]. The sequencing data of the regions flanking the deletions and the E6 genes of HPV5 and HPV8, however, did not support the involvement of point mutations in EV tumor progression [20].

Oncogenic EV HPVs show an unusual genomic heterogeneity, even within isolates from the same skin lesion of a EV patient suggesting that the E6 gene codes for different forms of E6 proteins [20]; these different allelic forms could show different affinities for their target proteins or DNA sequences as well as other biological functions [15]. Some EV HPV oncogene products may not only be involved in cell transformation, but may also serve as a source of specific antigens recognized by host immune mechanisms.

Immunosuppression and malignancy

The role of immunosuppression for HPV infection and HPV-associated cancerogenesis is best evidenced in transplant recipients, requiring chronic immunosuppressive therapy for preservation of graft. The prevalence of cutaneous warts and skin malignancies parallels the duration of immunosuppression, reaching 48-92% after 5 years [21-26]. The persistence of warts increases with the duration of immunosuppression and graft life. Renal transplant recipients are simultaneously at high risk of developing cutaneous malignancies, mainly actinic keratoses (AK) transforming themselves into squamous cells carcinomas (SCC), and more rarely basal cell carcinomas (BCC). The prevalence of malignant cutaneous tumors in immunosuppressed population depends, as for warts, on graft life, and SCC have been linked with warts [25, 27, 28]. After 9 years of transplantation SCC were found in 40% of patients, in whom the prevalence of warts was as high as 89% [29]. Another group reported a cumulative incidence of non-melanoma skin cancer of 23% at 10 years and 40% at 25 years post-transplant [24]. The difference might be due to the age of patients at transplantation, the intensity of immunosuppressive therapy, and to multiple exogenous factors, mainly sun exposure, that appears to be one of the strongest co-carcinogens [25].

Epidemiological data on the prevalence of particular HPVs in cutaneous tumors of immunosuppressed patients must be cautiously evaluated since the employed techniques varied in sensitivity from dot-blot to the extremely sensitive nested PCR [30], as well as in the primers used for detection. Some studies used only genital probes [31], others used only probes for the commonest cutaneous and mucosal HPVs, and only HPV5 as a EV HPV [32]. Thus the techniques might be not sensitive enough to detect a low copy number of HPV DNA in the specimens studied.

The use of nested PCR with degenerate primers designed to detect EV HPVs, and also able to amplify DNA of genital and cutaneous HPVs, with sequencing of the PCR-amplified products revealed a great variety of HPVs in the immunosuppressed population [23, 30, 33, 34]. Multiple HPVs were detected in proportion of the lesions, with high prevalence of EV HPVs and EV-related HPVs, whereas in previous studies only cutaneous and mucosal types had been detected using molecular *in situ* hybridization or PCR [32]. Thus every technique detects a different spectrum of HPVs; this reason, along with the presence of multiple HPV types in the lesions may account for the discrepancy of results obtained by various investigators.

The most sensitive nested PCR technique reveals mainly EV- or EV-related HPVs in immunosuppressed population somewhat more often than in immunocompetent patients with non-melanoma skin cancers, since the amount of HPV DNA is higher in immunosuppressed patients. In contrast to EV cancers, associated with high risk EV-HPVs, mainly HPV5 and HPV8, cancers and precancerous lesions in immunosuppressed population are associated with several EV HPVs and other HPVs, but not with HPV5 and HPV8.

Factors affecting HPV cancerogenesis in immunosuppressed patients

The host immune system

There is growing evidence that the host immune system plays a crucial role in limiting the growth and progression of HPV-associated tumors [35-37] (*Table III*). Immunosurveillance against HPV-infected or HPV-transformed keratinocytes is operative both at the early induction phase and at the effector phase leading to cell death. These mechanisms involve, in general, natural-killer (NK) cell mediated cytotoxicity, generation of specific T cytotoxic lymphocytes as well as production of various humoral responses [reviewed in 36, 37]. Inhibition of these mechanisms results in an increased frequency of HPV infections and HPV-associated

Table III. Factors enhancing or suppressing HPV-associated cutaneous carcinogenesis

Enhancement	Suppression

• EV HPVs
• EV-related HPVs?
• Ultraviolet light (UVB, PUVA)
  – induction of p53 mutations
  – induction of immunosuppression:
    . local
    . systemic
• Stimulation of viral DNA expression by some growth factors (EGF, PDGF and others)
	• Non specific immunity:
	  – NK cell activity
	  – cytokines (e.g. TNFα, IFNs, TGFβ, etc.):
	    . inhibition of E6 and E7 oncoprotein expression
	    . inhibition of keratinocyte proliferation
	    . induction of apoptosis
	    . stimulation of non-specific and specific anti-viral immunity (e.g. ICAM-1, MHC class I and II expression)
	• Specific immunity:
	  – cytotoxic T lymphocytes
	  – neutralizing antibodies

tumors. It is believed that a defect of cell mediated immunity (CMI) is mainly responsible for an increased susceptibility to infection with HPVs, especially with oncogenic types. In EV, NK cell-mediated immunity against EV HPV-harboring keratinocytes (specific target cells) was found to be dramatically decreased, as compared to the NK cell activity against non-specific target cells [38]. Similar findings were reported for patients suffering from HPV16-associated tumors whose NK cells were unable to kill HPV16-harboring keratinocytes, and the degree of this specific immune defect correlated with tumor progression [39].

Immunogenetics in the progression of HPV-associated tumors

The role of immunogenetic factor in controlling HPV infection and HPV-induced tumors is strongly supported by the fact that in rabbit Shope papilloma-carcinoma complex MHC polymorphism is linked to wart regression or progression [40]. Similar negative or positive associations of specific class II MHC haplotypes have been reported in patients with EV [41]. HPV-associated cervical cancer [42] and recurrent respiratory papillomatosis [43] are also associated with MHC alleles. These results suggest that some MHC alleles involved in antigen presentation could be permissive for HPV infection and be associated with specific immunotolerance.

Abnormal cytokine production

Many immunosuppressants inhibit the production of various immunostimulatory cytokines (e.g. IFNγ, IL1, IL2, IL6, leading to downregulation of some adhesion molecules (e.g. ICAM-1, class I MHC) crucial for T cell cytotoxicity and NK cell activity against HPV-harboring cells in both anogenital and cervical cancers [44]. In addition, immunosuppression affects the production of main cytokines characteristic of Th1-dependent immune reactions (e.g. IL2, IFNγ) resulting in decreased T cell proliferation and CD4 counts in peripheral blood. Under these conditions Th2 cells predominate, favoring generation of immunosuppressive cytokines (IL10, IL4, IL13), as shown for non-melanoma skin cancers [45].

A decreased production of some cytokines could result in upregulation of HPV gene expression, since it has been shown that interferons, TNFα and MCP-1 (monocyte chemotactic protein-1) inhibit transcription of E6/E7 genes in HPV-immortalized or HPV-transformed keratinocytes

[46, 47] (*Table III*). Moreover, TNFα, TGFβ and other cytokines are involved in the process of apoptosis. In an experimental system of rabbit uterine cell cultures it was shown that TGFβ1 inhibited cell proliferation with a concomitant induction of apoptosis [48]. In a model of rabbit Shope papillomas Hagari *et al.* [49] found that TNFα stimulated regression of the cutaneous lesions by enhancing apoptosis, probably due to decrease of cell cycle regulatory proteins (cyclins). We have shown that both TGFβ1 and TNFα are overexpressed in the lesional epidermis of patients with EV [50] in which an enhanced apoptosis could be detected (unpublished). Another important mechanism controlling the balance between tumor cell proliferation and apoptosis is related to the Fas-Fas-ligand expression on both tumor cells and infiltrating immunocompetents cells [51], however, this was not studied in HPV-associated malignancy.

It should be remembered that some immunosuppressive factors (such as steroid hormones) transregulate HPV genes and induce growth of oncogenic HPV-harboring keratinocytes [52].

Growth factors

Several immunosuppressive compounds bind a number of cellular receptors thus interfering with a wide range of signal transduction systems, especially those related to calcium and phosphorylation. Therefore it seems probable that immunosuppressive compounds are capable of affecting directly mechanisms of HPV-associated carcinogenesis, especially those related to the activity of various growth factors (*e.g.* EGF, TGFα, TGFβ, etc.). It is tempting to speculate that growth factors are in part responsible for a massive infection with HPVs in immuno-suppressed patients (*Table III*). It has been shown that proliferation of malignant HPV16- or HPV18-harboring cells can be stimulated by IL1α and TNFα in an EGF-dependent pathway [53]. Another important mechanism regulating HPV infection and persistence of HPV-associated lesions seems to be related to the expression of cellular receptors for HPV. Such receptors were recently detected and identified as α6β4 integrin, *i.e.* a cell surface molecule acting as laminin receptor [54]. We have found overexpression of α6β4 in the lesional epidermis of EV patients infected with HPV5 and HPV8 (presented by Majewski *et al.* at the Papillomavirus Workshop, Amsterdam 1994) suggesting that an upregulation of this receptor may, at least in part, facilitate HPV infection and persistence within keratinocytes.

p53 gene mutations

The role of *p53* gene mutations in posttransplant cancers is not clear. immunohistochemical studies with the use of antibodies to the wild and the mutated p53 oncoprotein have given equivocal results. It is doubtful whether they truly represent one or other type of mutations [55]. The detection rate of p53 mutations in cancers from transplant patients appear to be less frequent (42-43%) than in cancers in the general population [56], and might be due to the direct effect of interaction between HPV E6 and p53. Another immunohistochemical study of benign and (pre)malignant skin lesions from grafted persons showed p53 accumulation in 70% of precancerous lesions and malignant tumors, with no clear correlation with the presence of potentially oncogenic or non-oncogenic HPVs [57]. p53 accumulation could result from an interaction of p53 with HPV E6 protein. Since carcinomas develop in sun-exposed areas, it is likely that UV-type mutations could also coexist with mutations due to the viral effect. The role of p53 in tumors of grafted patients must be further studied with the use of molecular techniques based on sequencing of PCR products.

Ultraviolet (UV) radiation

In addition to its mutagenic effect on DNA, UV radiation (especially UVB), is capable of inducing both local and systemic immunosuppression, partially due to induction of TNFα synthesis [58], a cytokine found to be overexpressed in epithelial cells harboring cutaneous [50] and genital [59] HPV types. One of the immunosuppressive mechanisms of action of TNFα in the initiation phase of CMI is its effect on Langerhans cells (LC), despite the fact that these cells in EV did not show significant changes in their number and morphology [60, 61]. The immunosuppressive effect of UVB exposure in EV does not seem to be related to a down-regulatory effect on ICAM-1 expression as reported for normal keratinocytes [62], since this adhesion molecule was found upregulated in lesional skin of the patients (unpublished). In addition to TNFα, cis-urocanic acid generated in the stratum corneum upon UVB exposure, known to exert a strong immunosuppressive activity, was also detected in large amounts in the epidermis of EV patients [63]. The abnormal isomerization of urocanic acid in EV patients seems to have a genetic background since its increased levels were found in uninvolved and sun-protected skin areas of these patients as well as in healthy members of their families.

Several other factors and cytokines released or produced upon UV exposure, mainly TGFβ1, IL1ra (IL1 receptor antagonist), IL10 and αMSH, contributing to immunosuppression, may enhance the progression of HPV-associated tumors. Interestingly, αMSH antagonizes the effects of proinflammatory cytokines such as IL1, IL6, IFNγ, and selectively induces the production of Th2-associated IL10 [64]. Its involvement in HPV infections and cancerogenesis requires further studies.

HPV-associated cancers in the general population

With the same highly sensitive technique of nested PCR used in the immunosuppressed population, a high prevalence of HPVs, especially EV-HPVs, DNA has also been found in NMSC of the general population [30]. As in immunosuppressed persons, there is a great diversity of EV HPVs, but DNA is present in a very small amount (less than one genome per cancer cell). The role of these viruses in cancerogenesis is not documented, since no transcripts were found in cancers, no single predominant type was disclosed, and the prevalence of high risk EV HPVs is extremely rare. Therefore cofactors such as UV, X-rays or immunosuppression are necessary for cancer induction. UVB, inducing p53 mutations, stimulates viral transcription and inactivates cellular genes which downregulate virus expression. It should be remembered that, in addition to UVB, PUVA therapy is a potent mutagenic factor [65] exerting also immunosuppressive effects and enhancing the process of cutaneous carcinogenesis [66]. It seems that both HPVs and PUVA could act as cocarcinogens.

The detection of EV HPVs in various premalignant and malignant lesions in immuno-competent patients [67], and also in a high proportion of hair follicles, both in immunosuppressed and immunocompetent population [68], strongly suggest that EV HPVs are widely distributed. Although their presence in skin cancers is well documented, their role in malignant transformation remains to be established.

References

1. zur Hausen H. Roots and perspectives of contemporary papillomavirus research. *J Cancer Res Clin Oncol* 1996 ; 122 : 3-13.
2. Matsukara T, Sugase M. Identification of genital human papillomaviruses in cervical biopsy specimens: segregation of specific virus types in specific clinicopathological lesions. *Int J Cancer* 1995 ; 61 : 13-22.

3. zur Hausen H. Molecular pathogenesis of cancer of the cervix and its causation by specific human papillomavirus types. *Curr Top Microbiol Immunol* 1994 ; 186 : 131-56.

4. Jablonska S, Dabrowski J, Jakubowicz K. Epidermodysplasia verruciformis as a model in studies on the role of papillomavirus in oncogenesis. *Cancer Res* 1972 ; 32 : 585-9.

5. Orth G. Epidermodysplasia verruciformis: a model for understanding the oncogenicity of human papillomaviruses. In : *Papillomaviruses*. Ciba Foundation Symposium 120. Chichester : Wiley, 1986 : 157-74.

6. Majewski S, Jablonska S. Epidermodysplasia verruciformis as a model of human papillomavirus-induced genetic cancer of the skin. *Arch Dermatol* 1995 ; 131 : 1312-8.

7. Majewski S, Jablonska S, Orth G. Epidermodysplasia verruciformis. Immunological and nonimmunological surveillance mechanisms: role in tumor progression. *Clin Dermatol* 1997 ; 15 : 321-34.

8. Orth G, Jablonska S, Favre M, Croissant O, Jarzabek-Chorzelska M, Rzesa G. Characterization of two types of human papillomaviruses in lesions of epidermodysplasia verruciformis. *Proc Natl Acad Sci USA* 1978 ; 75 : 1537-41.

9. Orth G. Epidermodysplasia verruciformis. In : Salzman HP, Howley PM, eds. *The papillomaviruses*. New York, London : Plenum Press, 1987 : 199-243.

10. Majewski S, Breitburd F, Skopinska M, Croissant O, Jablonska S, Orth G. A mouse model for studying epidermodysplasia verruciformis-associated carcinogenesis. *Int J Cancer* 1994 ; 56 : 7727-30.

11. Adachi A, Kiyono T, Hayashi Y, Ohashi M, Ishibashi M. Detection of human papillomavirus type 47 DNA in malignant lesions from epidermodysplasia verruciformis by protocols for precise typing of related HPV DNAs. *J Clin Microbiol* 1996 ; 34 : 369-75.

12. Herber R, Liem A, Pitot H, Lambert PF. Squamous epithelial hyperplasia and carcinoma in mice transgenic for the human papillomavirus type 16 E7 oncogene. *J Virol* 1996 ; 70 : 1873-81.

13. Greenhalgh DA, Wang XJ, Rothnagel JA, Eckhardt JN, Quintanilla MI, Barber JL, Bundman DS, Longley MA, Schlegel R, Roop DR. Transgenic mice expressing targeted HPV-18 E6 and E7 oncogenes in the epidermis develop verrucous lesions and spontaneous rasH-activated papillomas. *Cell Growth Diff* 1994 ; 5 : 667-75.

14. Yamashita T, Segawa K, Fujinaga Y, Nishikawa T, Fujinaga K. Biological and biochemical activity of E7 genes of the cutaneous human papillomavirus type 5 and 8. *Oncogene* 1993 ; 8 : 2433-41.

15. Favre M, Ramoz N, Orth G. Human papillomaviruses: general features. *Clin Dermatol* 1997 ; 15 : 181-98.

16. Pizarro A, Gamallo C, Castresana JS, Ganez L, Palacios J, Benito N, Espada J, Fanseca E, Contraras F. p53 protein expression in viral warts from patients with epidermodysplasia verruciformis. *Br J Dermatol* 1995 ; 132 : 513-9.

17. Brash DE, Rudolph JA, Simon JA, Lin A, McKenna GJ, Baden HP, Walperin AJ, Ponten J. A role of sunlight in skin cancer: UV-induced p53 mutations in squamous cell carcinoma. *Proc Natl Acad Sci USA* 1991 ; 88 : 10124-8.

18. Fuchs G, Pfister H. Molecular biology of HPV and mechanism of keratinocyte transformation. In : Gross G, von Krogh G, eds. *Human papillomavirus infections in dermatology*. Boca Raton : CRC Press, 1997 : 15-46.

19. May M, Dong XP, Beyer-Finkler E, Stubenrauch F, Fuchs PG, Pfister H. The E6/E7 promoter of extrachromosomal HPV16 DNA in cervical cancers escapes from cellular repression by mutation of target sequences for YY1. *EMBO J* 1994 ; 13 : 1460-6.

20. Deau MC, Favre M, Orth G. Genetic heterogeneity among papillomaviruses (HPV) associated with epidermodysplasia verruciformis: evidence for multiple allelic forms of HPV and HPV 8 E6 genes. *Virology* 1991 ; 184 : 492-503.

21. Barr BBB, Benton EC, Mc Laren K, Bunney MH, Smith IW, Blessing MW, Hunter JAA. Human papilloma virus infection and skin cancer in renal allograft recepients. *Lancet* 1989 ; ii : 124-9.

22. Blohme I, Larko O. Skin lesions in renal transplant patients after 10-23 years of immunosuppressive therapy. *Acta Derm Venerol (Stockh)* 1990 ; 70 : 491-4.

23. De Jong-Tieben LM, Berkhout RJM, Smits HI, Bouwes Bavinck JN, Vermeer BJ, van der Woude FJ, ter Schegget J. High frequency of detection of epidermodysplasia verruciformis-associated human papillomavirus DNA in biopsies from malignant and premalignant skin lesions from renal transplant recipients. *J Invest Dermatol* 1995 ; 105 : 367-71.

24. Bouwes Bavinck JN, Berkout RJM, Tieben LM, Vermeer BJ, Schegget J. DNA of EV-associated human papillomavirus in skin cancers from non-immunosuppressed patients. In : *Abstract book of the international conference of papillomavirus*. Quebec 1995 : 93.

25. Bouwes-Bavinck JN, Berkhout RJM. HPV infections and immunosuppression. *Clin Dermatol* 1997 ; 15 : 427-37.

26. Euvrard S, Kanitakis J, Pouteil-Noble C, Dureau G, Touraine JL, Faure M, Claudy A, Thivolet J. Comparative epidemiologic study of premalignant and malignant epithelial cutaneous lesions developing after kidney and heart transplantation. *J Am Acad Dermatol* 1995 ; 33 : 222-9.

27. Boyle J, MacKie RM, Briggs JD, Junor BJ, Aitchison TC. Cancer, warts and sunshine in renal transplant patients. *Lancet* 1984 ; 1 : 702-5.

28. Noel JC, Detremmerie O, Peny MO, Candaele M, Verhest A, Heenen M, de Dobeleer G. Transformation of common warts into squamous cell carcinoma on sun-exposed areas in an immunosuppressed patient. *Dermatology* 1994 ; 189 : 308-11.

29. Proby CM, Shamanin IV, Rausch C, Glover MT, de Villiers EM, Leigh IM. Novel human papillomaviruses identified in skin cancers and keratinocyte cell lines from renal transplant recipients. *Br J Dermatol* 1995 ; 132 : 644.

30. Berkhout RJ, Tieben LM, Smiths HI, Bouwes Bavinck JN, Vermeer BJ, Schegget J. Nested PCR approach for detection and typing of epidermodysplasia verruciformis-associated human papillomavirus types in cutaneous cancers from renal transplant recipients. *J Clin Microbiol* 1995 ; 33 : 690-5.

31. Weinstock MA, Coulter S, Bates J, Bogaars HA, Larson PL, Bourmer GC. Human papillomavirus and widespread cutaneous carcinoma after PUVA photochemotherapy. *Arch Dermatol* 1995 ; 131 : 701-4.

32. Soler C, Chardonnet Y, Allibert P, Euvrard S, Schmitt D, Mandrand B. Detection of mucosal human papillomavirus types 6/11 in cutaneous lesions from transplant recipients. *J Invest Dermatol* 1993 ; 101 : 286-91.

33. Shamanin V, Glover M, Rausch C, Proby C, Leigh IM, zur Hausen H, de Villiers EM. Specific types of human papillomavirus found in benign proliferations and carcinomas of the skin in immunosuppressed patients. *Cancer Res* 1994 ; 54 : 4610-3.

34. Shamanin V, zur Hausen H, Lavergne D, Proby C, Leigh IM, Neumann C, Hamm H, Goos M, Haustein UF, Jung EG, Plewig G, Wolff H, de Villiers EM. HPV infections in non-melanoma skin cancers from renal transplant recipients and non-immunosuppressed patients. *J Natl Cancer Inst* 1996 ; 88 : 802-11.

35. Tindle RW, Frazer IH. Immune response to human papillomaviruses and the prospects for human papillomavirus-specific immunisation. *Curr Top Microbiol Immunol* 1994 ; 186 : 218-53.

36. Malejczyk J, Majewski S, Jablonska S. Cellular immunity in cutaneous and genital HPV infections. *Clin Dermatol* 1997 ; 15 : 261-74.

37. Malejczyk J, Majewski S, Jablonska S. The regulatory influence of immunological host responses. In : Gorss G, von Krogh G, eds. *Human papillomavirus infections in dermatology*. Boca Raton : CRC Press, 1997 : 203-26.

38. Majewski S, Malejczyk J, Jablonska S, Misiewicz J, Rudnicka L, Obalek S, Orth G. Natural cell-mediated cytotoxicity against various target cells in patients with epidermodysplasia verruciformis. *J Am Acad Dermatol* 1990 ; 22 : 423-7.

39. Malejczyk J, Malejczyk M, Majewski S, Orth G, Jablonska S. NK-cell activity in patients with HPV16-associated anogenital tumors: defective recognition of HPV16-harboring keratinocytes and restricted unresponiveness to immunostimulatory cytokines. *Int J Cancer* 1993 ; 54 : 917-21.

40. Han R, Breiburd F, Marche PN, Orth G. Linkage of regression and malignant conversion of rabbit viral papillomas to MHC class II genes. *Nature* 1992 ; 156 : 66-8.

41. Favre M, Ramoz N, Jablonska S, Majewski S, Rueda LA, Blanchet-Bardon C, Orth G. Search for a gene predisposing to epidermodysplasia verruciformis within the major histocompatibility complex. In : 14th International Papillomavirus Conference. Abstract Book. Quebec 1995 : 198.

42. Apple JR, Erlich HA, Klitz W, Manos MM, Becker TM, Wheeler CM. HLA DR-DQ associations with cervical carcinoma show papillomavirus-type specificity. *Nature Genet* 1994 ; 6 : 157-67.

43. Bonagura VR, O'Reilly ME, Abramson AL, Steinberg BM. Recurrent respiratory papillomatosis (RRP): enriched HLA DQw3 phenotype and decreased class I MHC expression. In : Steinberg BM, ed. *Immunology of papillomaviruses*. London : Plenum Press, 1993.

44. Majewski S, Breitburd F, Orth G, Jablonska S. Regulation of MHC class I, class II and ICAM-1 expression by cytokines and retinoids in HPV-harboring keratinocyte lines. In : Stanley MA, ed. *Immunology of human papillomaviruses*. New York : Plenum Press 1994 : 207-10.

45. Kim J, Modlin RL, Dubinett SM, McHugh T, Nicoloff BJ, Uyemura K. IL10 production in cutaneous basal and squamous cell carcinomas. *J Immunol* 1995 ; 155 : 2240-7.

46. Delvenne P, al-Saleh W, Gilles C, Thiry A, Boniver J. Inhibition of growth of normal and human papillomavirus-transformed keratinocytes in monolayer and organotypic cultures by interferon-gamma and tumor necrosis factor-alpha. *Am J Pathol* 1995 ; 146 : 589-98.

47. Kleine K, Knig G, Kreutzer J, Komitowski D, zur Hausen H, Rsl F. The effect of the JE (MCP-1) gene, which encodes monocyte chemoattractant protein-1 on the growth and derived somatic cell hybrids of HeLa-cells in nude mice. *Mol Carcinogen* 1995 ; 14 : 179-89.

48. Rotello RJ, Lieberman RC, Purchio AF, Gerschenson LE. Coordinated regulation of apoptosis and cell proliferation by transforming growth factor 1 in cultured uterine cells. *Proc Natl Acad Sci USA* 1991 ; 88 : 3412-5.

49. Hagari Y, Budgeon LR, Pickel MD, Kreider JW. Association of tumor necrosis factor-gene expression and apoptotic cell death with regression of Shope papillomas. *J Invest Dermatol* 1995 ; 104 : 526-9.

50. Majewski S, Hunzelmann N, Nischt R, Eckes B, Rudnicka L, Orth G, Krieg T, Jablonska S. TGFβ-1 and TNF expression in the epidermis of patients with epidermodysplasia verruciformis. *J Invest Dermatol* 1991 ; 97 : 862-7.

51. Strand S, Hofmann WJ, Hug H, Moller M, Otto G, Strand D, Mariani SM, Stremmel W, Krammer PH, Galle PR. Lymphocyte apoptosis induced by CD95 (APO-LFas) ligand-expressing tumor cells. A mechanism of immune evasion? *Nature Med* 1996 ; 2 : 1361-6.

52. von-Knebel-Doeberitz M, Bauknecht T, Bartsch D, zur Hausen H. Influence of chromosomal integration on glucocorticoid-regulated transcription of growth stimulating papillomavirus genes E6 and E7 in cervical carcinoma cells. *Proc Natl Acad Sci USA* 1991 ; 88 : 1411-5.

53. Woodworth CD, Lichti U, Simpson S, Evans CH, DiPaolo JA. Leukoregulin and gamma-interferon inhibit human papillomavirus type 16 gene transcription in human papillomavirus-immortalized human cervical cells. *Cancer Res* 1992 ; 52 : 456-61.

54. Evander M, Frazer JH, Payne E, Qi YN, Hengst K, McMillan NA. Identification of the alpha 6 integrin as a candidate receptor for papillomaviruses. *J Virol* 1997 ; 71 : 2429-56.

55. Battifora H. p53 immunohistochemistry: a word of caution. *Human Pathol* 1994 ; 25 : 435-7.

56. McGregor JM, Farthing A, Crook T, Yu CC, Dublin EA, Levison DA, MacDonald DM. Posttransplant skin cancer: a possible role for p53 gene mutation but not for oncogenic human papillomaviruses. *J Am Acad Dermatol* 1994 ; 30 : 701-6.

57. Pelisson I, Chardonnet Y, Euvrard S, Schmitt D. Immunohistochemical detection of p53 protein in cutaneous lesions from transplant recipients harbouring human papillomavirus DNA. *Virchows Arch* 1994 ; 424 : 623-30.

58. Streilein JW. Sunlight and skin-associated lymphoid tissues (SALT): if UVB is the trigger and TNF is its mediator, what is the message? *J Invest Dermatol* 1993 ; 100 : 47S-52S.

59. Malejczyk J, Malejczyk M, Kock A, Urbanski A, Majewski S, Hunzelmann N, Jablonska S, Orth G, Luger TA. Autocrine growth limitation of human papillomavirus type 16-harboring keratinocytes by constitutively released tumor necrosis factor. *J Immunol* 1992 ; 149 : 2702-8.

60. Haftek M, Jablonska S, Szymanczyk J, Jarzabek-Chorzelska M. Langerhans cells in epidermodysplasia verruciformis. *Dermatologica* 1987 ; 174 : 173-9.

61. Cooper KD, Androphy EJ, Lowy DR, Katz SI. Antigen presentation and T cell activation in epidermodysplasia verruciformis. *J Invest Dermatol* 1990 ; 94 : 769-76.

62. Krutmann J, Bohnert E, Jung EG. Evidence that DNA damage is a mediator in ultraviolet B radiation-induced inhibition of human gene expression: ultraviolet B radiation effects on intercellular adhesion molecule-1 expression. *J Invest Dermatol* 1994 ; 102 : 428-32.

63. Jablonska S, Majewski S. Epidermodysplasia verruciformis: immunological and clinical aspects. *Curr Top Microbiol Immunol* 1994 ; 186 : 157-75.

64. Hiltz ME, Catania EA, Lipton JM. α-MSH peptides inhibit acute inflammation induced in mice by rIL1beta, rIL6, rTNFα and endogenous pyrogen but not that caused by LTB4, PAF and rILIa. *Cytokine* 1992 ; 4 : 320-8.

65. Nataraj AJ, Wolf P, Cerroni L, Ananthaswamy HN. p53 mutation in squamous cell carcinomas from psoriasis patients treated with psoralen +UVA (PUVA). *J Invest Dermatol* 1997 ; 109 : 238-43.

66. Stern RS. Risks of cancer association with long-term exposure to PUVA in humans: current status-1991. *Blood Cells* 1991 ; 18 : 91-9.

67. Astori G, Lavergne D, Benton C, Höckmayr B, Egawa K, Garbe C, de Villiers EM. Human papillomaviruses are commonly found in normal skin of immunocomponent hosts. *J Invest Dermatol* 1998 ; 110 : 752-5.

68. Boxman ILA, Berkhout RJM, Mudler LHC, Wolkers MC, Bouwes Bavinck JN, Vermeer BJ, ter Schegget J. Detection of human papillomavirus DNA in plucked hairs from renal transplant recipients and healthy volunteers *J Invest Dermatol* 1997 ; 108 : 712-5.

8

Hepatitis C virus-related skin disorders

Marie-Sylvie DOUTRE
Department of Dermatology, Hôpital Haut-Lévêque, Pessac, France.

Hepatitis C virus (HCV) infection is a major public health problem in numerous countries. In the United-States and Western and Southern Europe, the prevalence of HCV markers varies from 0,5% to 2%. In France, an estimate of 5×10^5-2×10^6 subjects are infected [1].

Infection becomes chronic in 70% to 80% of cases and is complicated by cirrhosis within 20 years of contamination in about 20% of them. Once the cirrhotic process has begun, the incidence of hepatocellular carcinoma ranges from 1% to 4%. Some factors leading to more severe liver injury have been identified such as excessive alcohol comsumption, older age at the time of initial age infection, immunosuppression and specific genotypes [2].

HCV infection is common in immunocompromised patients such as transplant recipients [3]. These patients combine several risk factors such as multiple hospital admissions, nosocomial transmission, multiple transfusions and contamination through the graft (that was possible prior to elimination of positive donors). Several studies have confirmed the high prevalence of HCV in renal transplant recipients both before and after transplantation. The markers of the hepatitis are also frequently found in patients with bone marrow grafts, cardiac transplants and above all liver transplant recipients. When the cause of liver transplantation is an infection due to HCV, reinfection of the graft is particularly frequent [4].

Several extra-hepatic clinical manifestations, in particular cutaneous diseases are associated with HCV infection [5-7]. HCV is clearly involved in patients with mixed cryoglobulinemia and porphyria cutanea tarda [8]. Other cutaneous diseases, such as lichen planus, are possibly or probably associated to HCV infection [9].

Before considering the various studies of the literature, two points should be made clear:
– on the one hand, HCV markers must be detected by comparable techniques such as second and third-generation assays [enzyme linked immunosorbent assay (ELISA) and immunoblot (RIBA)] for detection of anti-HCV antibodies and polymerase chain reaction (PCR) for

detection of HCV RNA. In patients on systemic immunosuppressive therapy, antibody tests underestimate the prevalence of HCV infection and detection of viral RNA is often necessary for establishing the diagnosis;
– on the other hand, the prevalence of HCV infection should always be compared with that in a control population, given the differences observed according to the geographic origin of the patients studied.

Vasculitis

Cryoglobulin-associated vasculitis

The syndrome of mixed cryoglobulinemia (MC) is characterized by palpable purpura, arthralgias and general weakness associated with cryoglobulins composed of different immunoglobulins with a monoclonal component (rheumatoid factor) in type II and polyclonal immunoglobulins in type III. This is observed in the course of infections, auto-immune diseases, lymphoproliferative disorders, etc. In the absence of such disorders, this syndrome has been designated « essential mixed cryoglobulinemia » (EMC).

Recent evidence has incriminated HCV infection as the culprit in many patients who, in the past, would have been consigned to the diagnosis of EMC.

Since the initial observations in 1990 [10], single case reports and subsequently several studies on large populations were reported. However, the initial studies came from countries where HCV prevalence was extremely high and anti-HCV antibodies were often traced by tests of first generation.

Presently, several reports have described MC in about half of all patients with chronic hepatitis [11-15]. Patients with cryoglobulinemia had cirrhosis more frequently and had a longer history of hepatitis [16]. In parallel, about 50% to 90% of patients with MC had anti-HCV antibodies and liver dysfunction.

Affected patients often present with signs and symptoms attributable to vasculitis involving one or more organ systems. An increasing number of recent reports suggests that cutaneous lesions are a major presenting feature in some patients and even lead to the discovery of occult HCV infection [17]. Palpable purpura is the most frequent cutaneous lesion, localized most frequently on the lower limbs (Figure 9, page 218). A correlation was found between the presence of purpuric palpable lesions and cryoglobulin levels. Other cutaneous manifestations include urticaria, Raynaud's phenomenon, livedo reticularis, leg ulcers, nodules and digital necrosis. Skin biopsy specimens reveal leukocytoclastic vasculitis, and occasionally lymphocytic vasculitis. Variable features attributable to MC include arthralgias, peripheral neuropathy and glomerular disease including proteinuria, hematuria and hypertension.

Several findings suggest that HCV is the etiologic agent for the disease and that the virus may be involved in the pathogenesis of the vasculitis:
– HCV RNA sequences and anti-HCV antibodies are found in sera and cryopreci-pitates and are more concentrated in cryoprecipitates than in supernatants [18];
– by immunohistochemical methods or *in situ* hybridization, HCV was found in association with IgM and IgG in the cutaneous vasculitic lesions of some patients [19-21].

One possible mechanism for the development of vasculitis is that immune complexes initiate activation of endothelials cells, leading to altered vascular permeability, neutrophil infiltration and vessel wall damage that allow complex formation *in situ*. An alternative mechanism was suggested by the finding of HCV in vascular endothelial cells. Antibody or sensitized T cells to HCV-containing endothelial cells may initiate the process.

Regarding HCV genotypes, no predominance of a genotype has been noted [22] except in two Italian studies: HCV 1b subtype is the one found more often in the series of Sirico [23] whereas HCV 2a/III had a significantly higher prevalence in the series of Zignego [24].

The efficacy of IFNα in EMC had been reported before knowledge of HCV infection [25]. Recent studies confirm the efficacy of IFNα with improvement in cryoglobuli-nemia occurring in parallel to that of liver function tests [26, 27]. In non-responders serum aminotransferase levels do not decrease and cryoglobulins remain detectable. The parallelism between the course of cryoglobulinemia and the serologic markers of HCV infection under IFNα administration suggests a direct role for HCV in the development of EMC. However, in few cases, the clinical manifestations of MC improve despite unchanged hepatitis or vasculitis worsens despite improvement of hepatitis [28, 29].

Recently cases have been reported where exacerbation or appearance of cryoglobulinemia occurred after orthotopic liver transplantation with cutaneous vasculitis and/or renal manifestations [30, 31]. HCV-associated cryoglobulinemia could become clinically overt only after transplantation, possibly due (at least in part) to the post-transplant increase in viremia as reflected by HCV RNA levels.

Other forms of vasculitis

Some cases of leukocytoclastic vasculitis have been reported with no detectable cryoglobulins [32].

Polyarteritis nodosa (PAN) is a systemic necrotizing vasculitis involving small and medium sized arteries. Ten to fifty percent of patients with PAN are carriers of hepatitis B surface antigen. By contrast, PAN is rarely observed in patients with chronic hepatitis C: in a French study, anti-HCV antibodies were detected in the serum of 2 of 38 patients using first generation tests [33] and 3 of these 38 patients using two second generation tests [34]. In another study, anti-HCV antibodies were found in 7 of 50 patients using ELISA 2, confirmed by RIBA 2 in 6 of 50 patients [35]. In the series of Carson [36], a minority of patients (5%) had HCV specific antibodies.

Theilman et al. [37] tested sera from 21 patients with Wegener's granulomatosis (group I) and 35 patients with microscopic polyarteritis (group II) and found only one patient of each group positive for anti-HCV antibodies.

HCV does not seem to play a significant role in the pathogenesis of systemic necrotizing vasculitis.

Porphyria cutanea tarda

Porphyria cutanea tarda (PCT) is caused by reduced uroporphyrinogen decarboxylase activity; it is either acquired (sporadic form) or inherited as an autosomal dominant trait (familial form). Extrinsic factors such as various drugs or alcohol abuse are required for the disease to become clinically manifest with photosensitivity, cutaneous fragility, blisters (*Figure 10, page 218*), milia, pigmentation and hypertrichosis. Hepatitis B virus (HBV) infection, human immuno-deficiency virus (HIV) infection and HCV infection may also precipitate PCT [38].

A very strong association between sporadic PCT and HCV infection (50-90%) has been demonstrated especially in patients originating from the European Mediterranean basin (Italy, Spain, France) but also in patients from Scotland and Japan. In others countries, Germany, Ireland and New Zealand, the prevalence is low, indicating that there is no significant association between HCV and PCT (*Table 1*). Virologic studies (presence of RNA-VHC in serum) show that in most cases, the viral disease is active.

Table I. Porphyria cutanea tarda and HCV infection

Authors	Country	Patients	Anti HCV antibodies	HCV/RNA
Piperno [39]	Italy	12	7 (58%)	–
Fargion [40]	Italy	74	56 (76%)	47/56
De Castro [41]	Spain	34	24 (71%)	–
Herrero [42]	Spain	(95 sporadic PCT 5 familial PCT)	75 (79%)	18/18 tested
D'Alessandro Gondolfo [43]	Italy	110	58 (50%)	–
Lacour [44]	France	15	10 (66%)	–
Murphy [45]	Ireland	20	2 (10%)	2/2
Ferri [46]	Italy	23	(91%)	17/22
Hussain [47]	Scotland	12	11 (92%)	11/11
Stolzel [48]	Germany	108	8 (8%)	8/8
Navas [49]	Spain	34	31 (91%)	21/31
Lim [50]	USA	4	3 (75%)	–
Cribier [51]	France	13 (12 sporadic PCT 1 familial PCT)	7 (58%)	7/7
Salmon [52]	New-Zealand	25	1 (4%)	0/1
Malina [53]	Czech Republic	92	21 (22,8%)	18/21
Kondo [54]	Japan	26	22 (85%)	7/26

The mean age at the onset of PCT is significantly lower in HCV-infected patients than in non-infected patients; however, the clinical manifestations and the course of PCT were identical in both groups. The prevalence of HCV infection is associated with an increased severity of liver histologic changes, chronic hepatitis and cirrhosis. Some cases of hepatocellular carcinoma complicating PCT may be linked to HCV infection.

Coinfection with both HBV and HCV is frequent in PCT: in one study, HBV DNA and HCV RNA were simultaneously detected in the serum of 10 of 32 (31%) patients [49]. In another study, 30% of 110 patients had anti-HBV and anti HCV antibodies [43]. In HIV-positive patients, both HIV and HCV are etiologic factors for PCT. However, HCV probably plays the major role.

Only few reports on the treatment of patients with chronic hepatitis C and PCT with INFα are available: one study suggested a favorable response on cutaneous manifestations [51] but further studies are necessary to determine the effect of antiviral therapy on PCT.

Porphyrin metabolism, however, appears normal in patients with chronic HCV infection but no PCT.

Lichen planus

Lichen planus (LP) is characterized clinically by pruritic violaceous papules and histologically by hydropic degeneration of basal cell layer keratinocytes and a dense infiltration of lymphocytes in the upper dermis « hugging » the epidermis. Mucosal involvement is frequent.
Since the earliest report en 1978 by Rebora et al. [55], many authors reported on the relationship between LP and hepatic diseases, such as primary biliary cirrhosis, chronic active hepatitis or virus B hepatitis. In 1991, LP was described in a patient with chronic hepatitis and

HCV antibodies [56]. Since then, several cases of LP associated with HCV infection have been published in the literature.

LP manifestations may be cutaneous, mucous membrane or both. However, HCV infection is more frequently in patients with erosive oral LP (*Figure 11, page 218*). The onset of skin and hepatic manifestations is variable, with liver disease as the most frequent revealing pathology.

Several studies have been performed in order to gather information on the prevalence of HCV infection in patients with LP. In most studies, a high prevalence was reported. However, the reported prevalence rates of HCV infection in patients with LP show wide geographical variations (*Table II*). Only two studies reported the genotype distribution of HCV infected patients with LP: this was similar to that of patients with chronic hepatitis C without LP [66, 67].

Table II. Lichen planus and HCV infection

Authors	Country	Patients	Anti HCV antibodies	HCV/RNA	Controls
Divano [57]	Italy	46	–	–	–
Cribier [58]	France	52	2 (3,8%)	–	3/112 (2,6%)
Santander [59]	Spain	50	19 (38%)	15/19	1/27 (3,8%)
Bellman [60]	USA	30	7 (23%)	5/7	2/41 (4,8%)
Nagao [61]	Japan	45	28 (62%)	27/28	20/253 (7,9%)
Sanchez Perez [62]	Spain	78	16 (30%)	13/16	2/82 (2,4%)
Dupin [63]	France	102	5 (4,9%)	–	13/306 (4,5%)
Carrozzo [64]	Italy	70	16 (27,1%)	15/16	2/70 (4,3%)
Dupond [65]	France	29	8 (27,6%)	5/8	–
Imhof [66]	Germany	84	13 (16%)	12/13	1/87 (1,1%)

In most cases, HCV RNA is evidenced by polymerase chain reaction in the serum samples of these patients suggesting that LP could be related to HCV infection. However, the role of HCV remains unclear: alteration of epidermal antigenicity by HCV? replication of virus in skin and mucosal LP lesions?

The effect of INF treatment remains also unclear: in several patients, LP clears with INF therapy but it is aggravated or develops after the introduction of INF in other patients [68].

Chronic lichenoid cutaneous graft-*versus*-host disease (GVHD) is a frequent problem in patients undergoing bone marrow transplantation (BMT). Cutaneous manifestations share numerous clinical, histologic and immunologic characteristics with LP, making possible a relationship between HCV infection and GVHD. In one study a similar incidence of chronic GVHD in HCV positive and HCV negative patients was found; however, patients chronically infected before BMT could be at higher risk for this complication [69].

Other cutaneous manifestations

Sporadic or single case reports of various skin manifestations have been described with acute or chronic HCV.

One case of acute urticaria was associated with seroconversion to HCV after transfusion [70]. Some cases of chronic urticaria were also described with HCV infection [71]. Moreover, Kanazawa *et al.* detected antibodies to HCV in 24% of 79 Japanese patients with urticaria (*versus*

1,1% of 1,692 healthy blood donors) [72]. However, these tests were consistently negative in 50 English patients [73] and one single case was positive among 50 French patients [74].

Pruritus may be the presenting sign of hepatitis C [75]. HCV infection could be also a significant cause of prurigo. In one study, it was found that 11 (39%) in 28 patients with prurigo had evidence of HCV infection [76].

One case of erythema multiforme has been recorded during post-transfusion jaundice due to hepatitis C [77]. Cutaneous lesions disappeared in 3 weeks. A case of persistant erythema multiforme during several months associated with chronic HCV infection has been reported. Two courses of IFNα treatment were rapidly efficient on cutaneous lesions and relapse occurred after discontinuation [78].

One case of erythema nodosum has been reported during the acute course of HCV infection [79]. The association of hepatitis C with chronic panniculitis has been also described [80]. Treatment with IFNα led to remission of cutaneous lesions and normalisation of hepatic function but both reappared upon treatment withdrawal.

In seven patients, a necrolytic acral erythema was observed to occur almost exclusively with hepatitis C. It occurred in the form of well circumscribed dusky erythematous areas that develop flaccid blisters, then a hyperkeratotic surface on the dorsa of the feet. Microscopically, the lesions were similar to those of other necrolytic erythemas [81].

A case of cutaneous malakoplakia has also been described with chronic hepatitis [82].

Some cases of dermatomyositis with positivity for HCV have been reported [83] but these results need to be confirmed. Until now, no study including a systemic search for HCV serological markers has been carried out.

It remains unclear whether these reported associations are clinically important or not.

References

1. Giral P, Serfaty L, Loria A, Poupon R. L'hépatite C. *Rev Med Intern* 1994 ; 15 : 487-93.

2. Martin P. Hepatitis C genotypes: the key to pathogenicity? *Ann Intern Med* 1995 ; 122 : 227-8.

3. Garcia G, Terrault N, Wright L. Hepatitis C virus infection in the immunocompromised patients. *Semin Gastro Enterol Dis* 1995 ; 6 : 35-45.

4. Collier J, Heathcote J. Hepatitis C viral infection in the immunosuppressed patient. *Hepatology* 1998 ; 27 : 2-6.

5. Doutre MS, Beylot C, Beylot-Barry M, Couzigou P, Beylot J. Les manifestations dermatologiques associées au virus de l'hépatite C. *Rev Med Intern* 1995 ; 16 : 666-72.

6. Pawlotsky JM, Dhumeaux D, Bagot M. Hepatitis C virus in dermatology. A review. *Arch Dermatol* 1995 ; 131 : 1185-93.

7. Willson RA. Extra-hepatic manifestations of chronic viral hepatitis. *Am J Gastroenterol* 1997 ; 92 : 4-17.

8. Durand JM. Affections extra-hépatiques certainement liées au virus de l'hépatite C. *Presse Med* 1997 ; 26 : 1014-22.

9. Durand JM. Affection extra-hépatiques chez les malades infectés par le virus de l'hépatite C. Associations probables ou possibles. *Presse Med* 1997 ; 26 : 1023-8.

10. Pascual M, Perrin L, Giostra E, Schifferli JA. HCV in patients with cryoglobulinemia type II. *J Infec Dis* 1990 ; 162 : 569-70.

11. Ferri C, Greco F, Longombardo G, Palla P, Moretti A, Marzo E, Fosella PV, Pasero G, Bombardieri S. Antibodies to hepatitis C virus in patients with mixed cryoglubulinemia. *Arthritis Rheum* 1991 ; 34 : 1606-10.

12. Dammacco F, Sansonno D. Antibodies to hepatitis C virus in essential mixed cryoglobu-linaemia. *Clin Exp Immunol* 1992 ; 87 : 352-6.

13. Pechere-Berthschi A, Perrin L, De Saussure P, Widmann JJ, Giostra E. Hepatitis C: a possible etiology for cryoglobulinaemia type II. *Clin Exp Immunol* 1992 ; 89 : 419-22.

14. Cacoub P, Lunel-Fabiani F, Musset L, Perrin M, Frangeul L, Leger JM, Huraux JM, Piette JC, Godeau P. Mixed cryoglobulinemia and hepatitis C virus. *Am J Med* 1994 ; 96 : 124-32.

15. Levey JM, Bjornsson B, Banner B, Kuhns M, Malhotra R, Lohitman N, Romain PL, Cropley TG, Bonkowsky H. Mixed cryoglobulinemia in chronic hepatitis C infection; a clinicopathologic analysis of 10 cases and review of recent literature. *Medicine* 1994 ; 73 : 53-67.

16. Lunel F, Musset L, Cacoud P, Frangeul L, Cresta P, Perrin M, Grippon P, Hoang C, Piette JC, Huraux JM, Opolon P. Cryoglobulinemia in chronic liver diseases: role of hepatitis C virus and liver damage. *Gastroenterology* 1994 ; 106 : 1291-300.

17. Dupin N, Chosidow O, Lunel F, Cacoub P, Musset L, Cresta P, Frangeul L, Piette JC, Godeau P, Opolon P, Frances C. Essential mixed cryoglobulinemia. A comparative study of dermatologic manifestations in patients infected or non infected with hepatitis C virus. *Arch Dermatol* 1995 ; 131 : 1124-7.

18. Agnello V, Chung RT, Kaplan LM. A role for hepatitis C virus infection in type II cryoglobulinemia. *N Engl J Med* 1992 ; 327 : 1490-5.

19. Agnello V, Abel G. Localization of hepatitis C virus in cutaneous vasculitic lesions in patients with type II cryoglobulinemia. *Arthritis Rheum* 1997 ; 40 : 2007-15.

20. Durand JM, Kaplanski G, Richard MA, Lefevre P, Quiles N, Trepo C, Soubeyrand J. Cutaneous vasculitis in a patient infected with hepatitis C virus. Detection of hepatitis C virus RNA in the skin by polymerase chain reaction. *Br J Dermatol* 1993 ; 128 : 359-60.

21. Sansonno D, Cornacchiulo V, Iacobelli AR, Di Stefano RD, Lospalluti M, Dammacco F. Localization of hepatitis C virus antigens in liver and skin tissues of chronic hepatitis C virus-infected patients with mixed cryoglobulinemia. *Hepatology* 1995 ; 21 : 305-12.

22. Pawlotsky JM, Roudot-Thoraval F, Simmonds P, Mellor J, Ben Yahia M, Andre C, Voisin MC, Intrator L, Zaffranie S, Duval J, Dhumeaux D. Extrahepatic immunologic manifestations in chronic hepatitis C and hepatitis C virus serotypes. *Ann Intern Med* 1995 ; 122 : 169-73.

23. Sirico RA, Ribero ML, Fomasieri A. Hepatitis C viraemia and hepatitis C virus genotypes in patients with essential mixed cryoglobulinemia. *Arthritis Rheum* 1994 ; 37 : S427.

24. Zignego AL, Ferri C, Giannini C, Monti M, La Civita L, Careccia G, Longombardo G, Lombardini F, Bombardieri S, Gentilini P. Hepatitis C virus genotype analysis in patients with type II mixed cryoglobulinemia. *Ann Intern Med* 1996 ; 124 : 31-4.

25. Casato M, Lagana B, Antonelli G, Dianzani F, Bonomo L. Long-term results of therapy with interferon a for type II essential mixed cryoglobulinemia. *Blood* 1991 ; 78 : 3142-7.

26. Misiani R, Bellavita P, Fenili D, Vicari O, Marchesi D, Sironi PL, Zilio P, Vernocchi A, Massazza M, Vendramin G, Tanzi E, Zanetti A. Interferon alfa-2a therapy in cryoglobulinemia associated with hepatitis C virus. *N Engl J Med* 1994 ; 330 : 751-6.

27. Musset L, Lunel F, Cacoub P, Opolon P. Cryoglobulinémies mixtes lors de l'infection par le virus de l'hépatite C. *Presse Med* 1996 ; 25 : 598-8.

28. Zimmermann R, Konig V, Bauditz J, Hopf U. Inferferon alfa in leukocytoclastic vasculitis, mixed cryoglobulinaemia and chronic hepatitis C. *Lancet* 1993 ; 341 : 561-2.

29. Pateron D, Fain O, Sehonnou J, Trinchet JC, Beaugrand M. Severe necrotizing vasculitis in a patient with hepatitis C virus infection treated by interferon. *Clin Exp Rheumatol* 1996 ; 14 : 79-81.

30. Gournay J, Ferrell LD, Roberts JP, Ascher NL, Wright TL, Lake JR. Cryoglobinemia presenting after liver transplantion. *Gastroenterology* 1996 ; 110 : 256-70.

31. Safadi R, Shouval D, E'id A, Ilan Y, Tur-Kaspa R, Jurim O. Hepatitis C associated cryoglobulinemia after liver transplantation. *Transpl Proc* 1997 ; 29 : 2684-6.

32. Hearth-Holmes M, Zahradka SL, Baethge BA, Wolf RE. Leukocytoclastic vasculitis associated with hepatitis C. *Am J Med* 1991 ; 90 : 765-6.

33. Deny P, Guillevin L, Bonacorsi S, Quint L. Association between hepatitis C virus and polyarteritis nodosa. *Clin Exp Rheumatol* 1992 ; 10 : 319.

34. Quint L, Deny P, Guillevin L, Granger B, Jarrousse B, Lhote F, Scavizzi M. Hepatitis C virus in patients with polyarteritis nodosa. Prevalence in 38 patients. *Clin Exp Rheumatol* 1991 ; 9 : 253-7.

35. Cacoub P, Lunel Fabian F, Le Thi Huong D. Polyarteritis nodosa and hepatitis C virus infection. *Ann Intern Med* 1992 ; 116 : 605-6.

36. Carson CW, Conn DL, Czaja AJ, Wright TL, Brecher ME. Frequency and significance of antibodies to hepatitis C virus in polyarteritis nodosa. *J Rheumatol* 1993 ; 20 : 304-9.

37. Theilman L, Gmelin K, Kallinowski B, Kommerel B, Koderisch J, Andrassy K. Prevalence of antibodies to hepatitis C virus in sera from patients with systemic necrotizing vasculitis. *Nephron* 1991 ; 57 : 482.

38. Cribier B. Porphyrie cutanée tardive : liens avec le virus de l'hépatite C. *Presse Med* 1997 ; 26 : 572-6.

39. Piperno A, D'Alba R, Roffi L, Pozzi M, Farina A, Vecchi L, Fiorelli G. Hepatitis C virus infection in patients with idiopathic hemochromatosis and porphyria cutanea tarda. *Arch Virol* 1992 ; 4 : 215-6.

40. Fargion S, Piperno A, Cappelini MD, Sampietro M, Fracanzani AL, Romano R, Caldarelli R, Marcelli R, Vecchi L, Fiorelli G. Hepatitis C virus and porphyria cutanea tarda: evidence of a strong associatation. *Hepatology* 1992 ; 16 : 1322-6.

41. De Castro M, Sanchez J, Herrera JF, Chaves A, Duran R, Garcia-Buey L, Garcia-Monzon C, Sequi J, Moreno-Otero R. Hepatitis C virus antibodies and liver disease in patients with porphyria cutanea tarda. *Hepatology* 1993 ; 17 : 551-7.

42. Herrero C, Vicente A, Bruguera M, Ercilla MG, Barrera JM, Vidal J, Teres J, Mascaro JM, Rodes J. Is hepatitis C virus infection a trigger of porphyria cutanea tarda? *Lancet* 1993 ; 341 : 788-9.

43. D'Alessandro-Gandolfo L, Biocalti G, Griso D, Macri A, Topi G. Frequency of viral hepatitis markers in porphyria cutanea tarda. *Eur J Dermatol* 1993 ; 3 : 180-2.

44. Lacour JP, Bodokh I, Castanet J, Bekri S, Ortonne JP. Porphyria cutanea tarda and antibodies to hepatitis C virus. *Br J Dermatol* 1993 ; 128 : 121-3.

45. Murphy A, Dooley S, Hillary IB, Murphy GM. HCV infection in porphyria cutanea tarda. *Lancet* 1993 ; 341 : 1534-5.

46. Ferri C, Baicchi U, Lacivita L, Greco F, Longrombardo G, Mazzoni A, Careccia G, Bombardieri S, Pasero G, Zigneco AL, Manns MP. Hepatitis C virus-related autoimmunity in patients with porphyria cutanea tarda. *Eur J Clin Invest* 1993 ; 23 : 851-5.

47. Hussain I, Hepburn NC, Jones A, Rorke KO, Hayes PC. The association of hepatitis C viral infection (HCV) with porphyria cutanea tarda (PCT) in the lothian region Scotland. *Gut* 1995 ; 35 : 40.

48. Stölzel U, Kostler E, Koska C, Stöffler-Meilicke M, Schuppan D, Somasundaram R, Doss MO, Nabermehl KO, Riecken EO. Low prevalence of hepatitis C virus infection in porphyria cutanea tarda in Germany. *Hepatology* 1995 ; 21 : 1500-3.

49. Navas S, Bosch O, Castillo I, Marriott E, Carreno V. Porphyria cutanea tarda and hepatitis C and B viruses infection: a retrospective study. *Hepatology* 1995 ; 21 : 279-84.

50. Lim HV, Harris HR, Fotiades J. Hepatitis C virus infection in patients with porphyria cutanea tarda evaluated in New-York. *Arch Dermatol* 1995 ; 131 : 849.

51. Cribier B, Petiau P, Keller F, Scmitt C, Vetter D, Heid E, Grosshans E. Porphyria cutanea tarda and hepatitis C viral infection. *Arch Dermatol* 1995 ; 131 : 801-4.

52. Salmon P, Oakley A, Rademaker M, Duffil M. Hepatitis C virus infection and porphyria cutanea tarda in Australasia. *Arch Dermatol* 1996 ; 132 : 91.

53. Malina L, Stransky J, Zdarsky E. Geographical differences in prevalence of hepatitis C virus infection in PCT (porphyria cutanea tarda). *Br J Dermatol* 1997 ; 136 : 287-8.

54. Kondo M, Horie Y, Okano JI, Kitamura A, Maeda N, Kawasaki H, Mishiro S, Yamamoto SI, Itou T, Saeki SI, Tanaka S, Okamoto H. High prevalence of hepatitis C virus infection in Japanese patients with porphyria cutanea tarda. *Hepatology* 1997 ; 26 : 246.

55. Rebora A, Patri PL, Rampini E. Erosive lichen planus and cirrhotic hepatitis. *Ital Gen Rev Dermatol* 1978 ; 15 : 123-7.

56. Mokni M, Rybojad M, Puppin D, Catala S, Veneza F, Djian R, Morel P. Lichen planus and hepatitis C virus. *J Am Acad Dermatol* 1991: 792.

57. Divano MC, Parodi A, Rebora A. Lichen planus, liver kidney microsomal (LKM1) antibodies and hepatitis C virus antibodies. *Dermatology* 1992 ; 185 : 132-3.

58. Cribier B, Garnier C, Laustriat D, Heid E. Lichen planus and hepatitis C virus infection: an epidemiologic study. *J Am Acad Dermatol* 1994 ; 31 : 1070-2.

59. Santander C, De Castro M, Garcia-Monzon C, Garcia-Bues L, Sanchez L, Herrera JF, Borque MJ, Moreno-Otero R. Prevalence of hepatitis C virus (HCV) infection and liver damage in patients with lichen planus. *Hepatology* 1994 ; 20 : 238 A.

60. Bellman B, Reddy RK, Falanga V. Lichen planus associated with hepatitis C. *Lancet* 1995 ; 346 : 1234.

61. Nagao Y, Sata M, Tanikawa K, Itoh K, Kameyama T. Lichen planus and hepatitis C virus in the northern Kyushu region of Japan. *Eur J Clin Invest* 1995 ; 25 : 910-4.

62. Sanchez-Perez J, De Castro M, Buezo GF, Hernandez-Herrera J, Borque MJ, Garcia-Diez A. Lichen planus and hepatitis C virus: prevalence and clinical presentation of patients with lichen planus and hepatitis C virus infection. *Br J Dermatol* 1996 ; 134 : 715-9.

63. Dupin N, Chosidow O, Lunel F, Fretz C, Szpirglas H., Frances C. Lichen buccal et hépatite C : une association fortuite ? *Rev Med Intern* 1996 ; 17 : 95 S.

64. Carrozzo M, Gandolfo S, Carbone M, Colombatto P, Broccoletti R, Garzino-Demo P, Ghisetti V. Hepatitis C virus infection in Italian patients with oral lichen planus: a prospective case-control study. *J Oral Pathol Med* 1996 ; 25 : 527-33.

65. Dupond AS, Lacour JP, Laffont C, Tramaloni S, Ortonne JP. Lichen érosif buccal et hépatite C : étude rétrospective réalisée chez 29 patients. *Ann Dermatol Venereol* 1997 ; 124 : 576-7.

66. Imhof M, Popal H, Lee JH, Zeuzen S, Milbradt R. Prevalence of hepatitis C virus antibodies and evaluation of hepatitis C virus genotypes in patients with lichen planus. *Dermatology* 1997 ; 195 : 1-5.

67. Pawlotsky JM, Bencaiki H, Pellet C. Lichen planus and hepatitis C virus (HCV) related chronic hepatitis: evaluation of HCV genotypes. *Br J Dermatol* 1995 ; 132 : 158-9.

68. Doutre MS, Couzigou P, Beylot-Barry M, Beylot C, Quinton A. Lichen plan et hépatite C. Hétérogénicité évolutive de 6 cas traités par l'Interféron alpha. *Gastroenterol Clin Biol* 1996 ; 20 : 709-10.

69. Bouloc A, Pawlotsky JM, Choukroun V, Norol F, Vernant JP, Revuz J, Bagot M. Cutaneous chromic graft-*versus*-host disease and hepatitis C virus. *Arch Dermatol* 1995 ; 131 : 853-5.

70. Reichel M, Mauro TM. Urticaria and hepatitis C. *Lancet* 1990 ; 336 : 823.

71. Raychaudhuri SP, Kaplan M. Chronic urticaria and hepatitis C. *Int J Dermatol* 1995 ; 34 : 823-4.

72. Kanazawa K, Yaoita H, Tsuda F, Okamoto H. Hepatitis C virus infection in patients with urticaria. *J Am Acad Dermatol* 1996 ; 35 : 195-8.

73. Smith R, Caul EO, Burton JL. Urticaria and hepatitis C. *Br J Dermatol* 1997; 136 : 980.

74. Doutre MS, Beylot-Barry M, Beylot C. Urticaria and hepatitis C infection. *Br J Dermatol* 1998 ; 138 :194-5.

75. Fisher AD, Wright TL. Pruritus as a symptom of hepatitis C. *J Am Acad Dermatol* 1994 ; 30 : 629-32.

76. Kanazawa K, Yaoita H, Tsuda F, Murata K, Okamoto H. Association of prurigo with hepatitis C virus infection. *Arch Dermatol* 1995 ; 131 : 852-3.

77. Antinori S, Esposito R, Aliprandi CA, Tadini G. Erythema multiform and hepatitis C. *Lancet* 1991 ; 337 : 428.

78. Berard F, Pincemaille B, Charhon A, Perrot H. Erythème polymorphe persistant associé à une infection chronique par le virus de l'hépatite C. Efficacité de l'interféron alpha. *Ann Dermatol Venereol* 1992; 124 : 329-31.

79. Dominogo P, Ris J, Martinez E, Casas F. Erythema nodosum and hepatitis C. *Lancet* 1990 ; 336 : 1377.

80. Patoux-Pibouin M, Le Gall F, Jouanolle H, Le Hir I, Deugnier Y, Chevran-Breton J. Dermohypodermite subintrante associée à une hépatite C chronique active due au virus C. *Ann Dermatol Venereol* 1991 ; 118 : 854-5.

81. El Darouti M, Abu El Ela M. Necrolytic acral erythema: a cutaneous marker of viral hepatitis C. *Int J Dermatol* 1996 ; 35 : 252-6.

82. Bodokh I, Lacour JP, Perrin C, Rainero C, Lebreton E, Grosshans E, Ortonne JP. Malakoplakie cutanée associée à une hépatite chronique due au virus de l'hépatite C. *Ann Dermatol Venereol* 1993 ; 20 : 808-10.

83. Nishika M, Miyairi M, Kosaka S. Dermatomyositis following infection with hepatitis C virus. *J Rheumatol* 1994 ; 21 : 1584-5.

9

The role of HHV8 in cutaneous tumours

Céleste LEBBÉ
Department of Dermatology, Laboratory of Pharmacology, Hôpital Saint-Louis, Paris, France.

HHV8: historical and molecular aspects

Several epidemiological characteristics of Kaposi's sarcoma (KS), such as a higher incidence in immunosuppressed patients, in developing countries, in homosexual or bisexual men and in HIV-infected female partners of bisexual men, have long suggested the role of an infectious agent. However all candidate infectious agents proposed until 1994 such as cytomegalovirus, human herpes virus 6, human papillomavirus 16 and 18 led to controversial results [1].

Kaposi's sarcoma-associated herpesvirus (KSHV) or human herpes virus 8 (HHV8) DNA sequences were first identified in 1994 using an original technique named « representational differential analysis » on KS and normal tissue from an HIV-positive patient [2]. This is a general method based upon subtractive hybridisation techniques to detect small differences between the sequences of two DNA populations [3]. Briefly, DNA extracted from a KS lesion and from normal skin of the same patient is cleaved with restriction endonucleases, ligated to oligonucleotide adaptors and amplified by PCR. These adaptors are then removed, KS fragments are ligated to new adaptors and then hybridised with DNA fragments amplified from normal tissue in excess. Taq polymerase is then added in order to fill in the ends of the hybrids. Three types of hybrids are obtained: homohybrids (two DNA strands from normal tissue), heterohybrids (hybridisation of one DNA strand from normal tissue and the homologous strand from the KS lesion) and a third type made of two DNA strands from KS lesion without homologous DNA from normal tissue. The latter hybrid is then amplified by another PCR using the adaptor oligonucleotides. Two DNA sequences of 330 and 631 base pairs were found using this technique. HHV8 was subsequently detected in primary effusion lymphoma (PEL)-

derived cell lines [4] (one of the three human diseases associated with HHV8) and in KS spindle cells from KS specimens [5] using electron microscopy. The 140.5 Kb genome of this γ herpes virus has been sequenced and 81 open reading frame (orf) or genes have been demonstrated [6] (*Graph 1*). Strong homologies with herpesvirus saimiri and, to a lesser extent, with Epstein-Barr virus (EBV) were shown. Some of the viral gene products are true oncogenes, such as viral interferon-regulatory factor (v-IRF) and viral G-protein coupled receptor (v-GPCR) [7, 8]. Some are related to cellular proteins implicated in the control of cell cycle (v-cyclin) [9] or in inhibition of apoptosis [10-12] (*Graph 2 and Graph 3*). Other viral proteins are homologous to cellular cytokines and potentially involved in cell proliferation or

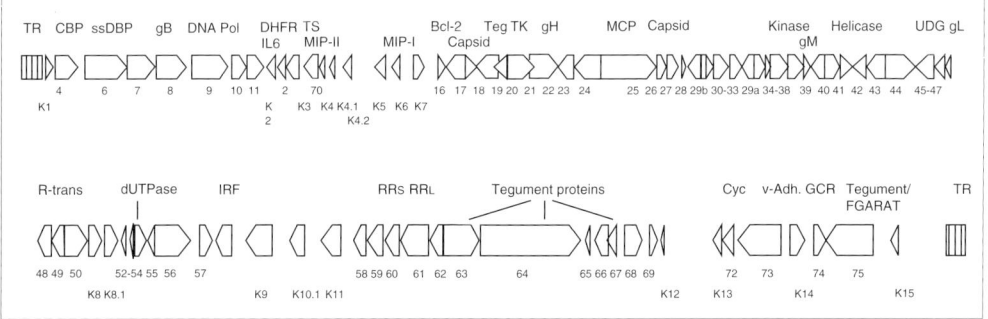

Graph 1. HHV8 genome. TR: terminal repeat; CBP: complement binding protein; gB: glycoprotein B; Pol: polymerase; IL6: interleukin 6; DHFR: dehydrofolate reductase; TS: thymidylate synthase; MIP: macrophage inflammatory protein; Teg: tegument protein; TK: thymidine kinase; MCP: major capsid protein; UDG: uracyl DNA glucosidase; IRF: interferon regulatory factor; RRs: ribonucleotide reductase, small; RRl: ribonucleotide reductase, large; FLIP: Flice inhibitory protein; Cyc: cyclin; LANA: latency associated nuclear antigen; Adh: adhesion molecule; GPCR: G protein coupled receptor; FGARAT: N-formylglycinamide ribotide amidotransferase. (From [6].)

Graph 2. Some elements of the G1/S checkpoint regulation. The eukaryotic cell cycle has 4 major phases in actively growing cells: G1 (gap 1 when the cell prepares itself for S phase), S (DNA replication) and G2 (gap 2) and M (mitosis) phases. These phases are coordinated in a complex fashion by changes in the activity of specific enzymes called cyclin dependant kinases (cdk) and cdk inhibitors (cdkI). In order to be activated, cdk associates with cell cycle-stage specific cyclins: cyclin D and cyclin E in G1, cyclin A in S and G2, and cyclin B in G2 and M. Driving the cell from G1 to phase S requires the phosphorylation of Rb (retinoblastoma) protein by cyclin/cdk complexes (G1/S checkpoint). This

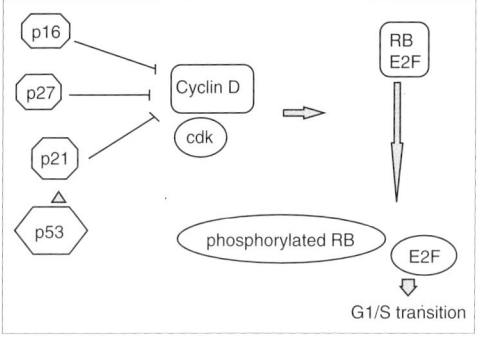

leads to the release of the transcription factor E2F proteins which can activate transcription of genes required to initiate or propagate the S phase of the cycle, when complexed with proteins of the DP family. Physiologically, cyclin-dependant kinases are down regulated by cdkI such as p21 (upregulated by p53), p16, p27 which therefore inhibit progression from G1 to S phase and lead to cell cycle arrest. By contrast HHV8 v-cyclin-cdk complexes could escape from down regulation by cdkI and drive infected cells to commitment in S phase.

chemotaxis, including v-IL6 and viral macrophage inflammatory proteins (v-MIP I and v-MIP II) [13, 14]. As for other γ herpesviruses, HHV8 can either remain episomal in infected cells without viral replication (latent infection), or it can replicate during a productive lytic phase (lytic infection). Despite the molecular piracy of this virus and although immortalised PEL-derived cell lines infected with HHV8 are available, *in vitro* immortalisation by HHV8 has not been described so far by only one team (*see* [74]). The biological role of this virus in human pathology is currently studied using PCR, reverse transcriptase PCR (RT-PCR) and *in situ* hybridisation.

Recently, serologic assays (mainly immunofluorescence assays, enzyme-linked immunosorbent assay-ELISA and Western blot assays) have been established recognising either latent or lytic antigens. The seroprevalence among blood donors seems to vary according to technical conditions and the geographic origin. It has been estimated to 0-5% in Great Britain and 0-3% in North America with studies using a latent immunofluorescence assay (IFA) recognising antibodies directed against the latency-associated nuclear antigen (LANA). By contrast, HHV8 seroprevalence was estimated around 20-25% in California using a lytic immunofluorescence assay on PEL-derived cells treated with agents allowing the virus to enter lytic replication [15-18]. The seroprevalence could be around 30% in Southern Italy [19] when latent IFA and ELISA confirmed by Western blot with recombinant orf 65 capsid protein were combined, and about 50% in Uganda using latent IFA [15]. Whether HHV8 is ubiquitous like most human herpes viruses or restricted to some individuals thus remains to be determined.

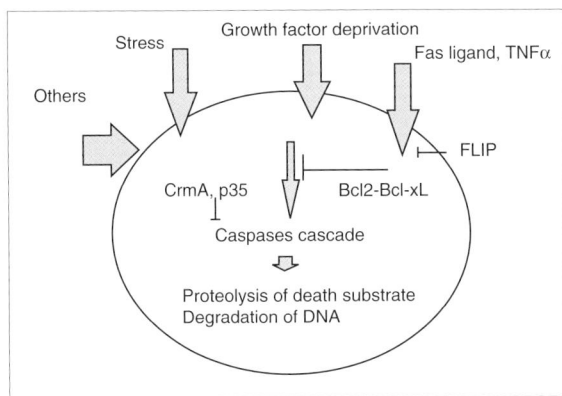

Graph 3. Factors involved in triggering, control and execution of apoptosis. Failure of control of cell cycle from mutations or rearrangements of various oncogenes or tumour repressor genes or viral infection play an important role in tumourigenesis. However, most normal cells respond to such alterations by apoptosis or programmed cell death, disclosing the importance of this phenomenon in cell homeostasis. The phases leading to apoptosis are summarised in this figure. Apoptosis triggering signals are multiple: growth factor deprivation, treatment with various cytotoxic agents, or gluco-corticoids, cellular stress (UV or X radiation) leading to DNA damage and therefore to p53 activation, hypoxia. Cell apoptosis can be induced by death factors such as Fas ligand and other molecules of the Tumor necrosis factor family (TNF) which includes TNF, CD30 ligand, CD40 ligand, CD27 ligand, and TRAIL (TNF-related apoptosis inducing ligand). Binding of Fas ligand to Fas or TNF to TNF receptor induces trimerization of the receptor which recruits an enzyme called caspase 8 or FLICE *via* an adaptor (FADD /MORT1). Activation of FLICE protease domain trigger the ICE protease cascade (interleukin 1β concerting enzyme) with subsequent proteolysis of death substrates. All apoptotic signals lead to the cascade activation of a family of cystein proteases called caspases which are the final executors of apoptosis. Negative or positive control of these phenomena include the mitochondrial Bcl2 family of proteins. For instance Bcl2 can influence the permeability transition of mitochondrial membranes upstream of caspases cascade, or interact with pro-domains of some caspases and inhibit apoptosis. Viral proteins can inhibit apoptotic signals. Some of them are homologous to Bcl2 (HHV8 Bcl2 or adenovirus Bcl2 for instance); baculovirus p35 and cowpox virus CrmA can inhibit the degradation phase of apoptosis by interacting with caspases; FLIP proteins inhibit the FLICE activation from death factors such as TNF.

HHV8 seroprevalence among HIV-positive homosexual patients without KS and among other patients sexually at risk suggests that HHV8 could be sexually transmitted, at least in Western countries [15, 17]. Up till now HHV8 has been associated to three human diseases, namely Kaposi's sarcoma, primary B cell lymphomas/primary effusion lymphoma (PEL) or body cavity based lymphomas [20] and 75% of multicentric Castleman's disease cases [21, 22]. Multicentric Castleman's disease is an uncommon polyclonal lymphoproliferative disorder occurring more frequently in association with KS, predominantly in HIV-infected patients [21, 22]. PEL is a rare clonal aggressive proliferation of large cells bearing an intermediate phenotype between anaplastic and immunoblastic cells and a B cell genotype. As for KS, it predominates in HIV-infected men and is frequently associated to KS. Co-infection with EBV of tumour cells is frequent but not constant. PEL *in vitro*-derived cell lines have been very useful tools to study the molecular biology of HHV8 [23].

Role of HHV8 in Kaposi's sarcoma

KS tissue

HHV8 sequences can be isolated from 90-100% of KS lesions using PCR, depending on the sensitivity of the technique and the nature of specimens (fresh-frozen or archival paraffin-embedded), irrespective of the clinicoepidemiological form (classic, endemic, epidemic, iatrogenic), the geographic origin and the nature of the tissue [2, 24, 25]. In KS lesions spindle cells, normal endothelial cells and monocytes are infected. Contrasting with PEL-derived cell lines, HHV8 sequences are rapidly lost from KS-derived spindle cells in culture [26]. *In situ*, most spindle cells harbour latent virus while replicative forms are found in some monocytes infiltrating the lesions [27, 28]. Expression of v-cyclin by most KS spindle cells and of v-GPCR, v-MIP-I and v-MIP-II by a few cells has been demonstrated using RT-PCR or *in situ* hybridisation [29-31]. GPCR induces the synthesis of VEGF (vascular endothelial growth factor), and v-MIP I and II appear to have potent angiogenic activity [8, 31]. v-cyclin activates cdk6 (*Graph 2*) but cellular inhibitors such as p16, p21 or p27 fail to inactivate the complex cyclin-kinase; this could lead to a defect of control of the cell cycle checkpoint G1/S and potentially to deregulated cell proliferation [9].

Normal tissues

HHV8 sequences have also been detected in normal skin in most patients [24, 32], and in peripheral blood mononuclear cells in about 50% of patients suffering from HIV-positive or -negative KS [24, 33, 34]. HHV8 viraemia, although fluctuating, could be related to tumour burden or progression of KS and was shown to be correlated with immunosuppression in HIV-infected patients [24, 34]. HHV8 sequences have also been variably isolated from the saliva, seminal liquid, prostate, lymph nodes, bone marrow and spleen from KS patients, a fact paralleling the multicentric pattern of KS [35, 36].

Serologic tests

HHV8 serologic tests recognising latent antigens are positive in 85-100% of classic KS and 71-81% of HIV-positive KS cases; combining lytic and latent assays increases sensitivity [15-18]. Recently, half of HIV-positive KS were found HHV8-seropositive 46 months before KS onset [15]. One case control HHV8 serological Italian study using latent IFA, an immunoperoxidase assay which is a technical modification of this test and two Western blot assays for LANA and recombinant orf 65 capsid protein, showed the presence of antibodies in

91% of 11 organ-graft recipients who developed posttransplantation KS before the graft, whereas only 12% of 17 control recipients who remained free of KS for at least two years after transplantation were positive. One patient who was seronegative at transplantation received an organ from a seropositive donor and developed KS three months later. Post-transplantation HHV8 seroconversion was demonstrated for another patient in this study who developed both KS and Castleman's disease. These results have been confirmed by others (D. Farge, submitted) and suggest that HHV8 infection is generally present before the onset of immunosuppression [37]. However HHV8 transmission by the graft is possible and further studies are awaited in order to assess this risk and to define monitoring of transplant patients.

Sensitivity of HHV8 to anti-herpetic drugs

Although *in vitro* data on PEL-derived cells have shown an antireplicative effect of antiherpetic drugs such as cidofovir, foscavir and ganciclovir, the clinical relevance of these studies remains to be better delineated [38]. Three retrospective analyses of unselected groups of patients with AIDS led to controversial conclusions concerning the risk of developing KS after receiving such drugs [39-41]. Among 6 HIV-positive patients with KS treated with foscavir, a small benefit was obtained since partial remission was demonstrated in one patient, while two patients remained stable and the remaining three had progressive disease [42].

Cutaneous disorders other than Kaposi's sarcoma

Various benign or malignant cutaneous proliferations have been investigated for the presence of HHV8 DNA sequences. Although controversial data have been published, most results were negative or only rarely positive.

Epithelial proliferations

Rady *et al.* [43] reported the detection of HHV8 sequences in 82% of 33 epithelial skin lesions (mainly squamous cell carcinomas and actinic keratoses but also basal cell carcinomas, *Verruca vulgaris*, atypical squamous proliferations and seborrheic keratoses) in four organ-transplant patients using PCR. Nishimoto *et al.* [44] detected HHV8 sequences in 13/21 Bowen's diseases, 3/11 actinic keratoses, 3/7 leukoplakias and 1/6 Paget's disease from non-immunosuppressed patients. However, nine other independent studies performed on a total of about 130 benign or malignant epithelial proliferations from immunocompetent or immunosuppressed hosts (AIDS, organ transplantation) using HHV8 single or nested PCR [45-53] failed to confirm such results.

Vascular proliferations

Vascular proliferations other than KS may exceptionally harbour HHV8 sequences [54]. Mc Donagh *et al.* [55] detected HHV8 DNA sequences in 7/24 (29%) angiosarcomas and 1/20 (5%) haemangiomas but not in 6 haemangiopericytomas. Gyulai *et al.* [56, 57] found viral sequences in 4/4 cases of angiolymphoid hyperplasia and one angiosarcoma. By contrast, 138 cases of non-KS vascular lesions (including 15 angiosarcomas, 75 haemangiomas, 3 haemangiopericytomas, 25 pyogenic granulomas, 15 lymphangiomas, 2 Kimura's disease) were negative [58]. The study of Tomita *et al.* [59] on 35 cases of angiosarcomas collected in Japan led to negative results; we obtained a similar negative result in 9 angiosarcomas, 4 cases of angiolymphoid hyperplasia and one case of Kimura's disease [60].

Lymphomas

Apart from one study [61] reporting the presence of HHV8 sequences in 7/48 non-epidermotropic cutaneous T cell lymphomas, 2/20 mycosis fungoides or Sézary syndrome and 2/6 parapsoriasis en plaques, four other studies which tested a total of about 90 cutaneous or peripheral blood cell specimens from cutaneous lymphomas yielded generally negative results [20, 62-64].

By contrast, controversial data were recently published concerning myeloma [65]. HHV8 sequences were detected in stromal dendritic cells from about 80% of bone marrow biopsies of myeloma patients in two independent studies [66, 67], whereas HHV8 serology was found negative in these patients [68-70].

Miscellaneous

Investigation of some other benign (such as dermatofibromas) or malignant cutaneous tumours (a small number of melanomas) also led to negative results [71, 72]. Positive results reported in 90% of sarcoid specimens by Di Alberti et al. [73] in one PCR study were disputed by others [71].

In conclusion, since the discovery of HHV8 in 1994, this virus has been definitely associated with three human diseases, i.e. Kaposi's sarcoma, primary effusion lymphomas and multicentric Castleman's disease. Although the large screening of most tumours, that has yielded negative results, and some sero-epidemiologic studies favour the hypothesis of a non-ubiquitous restricted virus, further studies are needed in order to better delineate the role of HHV8 and of potential infectious and non-infectious cofactors in associated diseases.

References

1. Lebbé C. Caractéristiques cellulaires et moléculaires du sarcome de Kaposi. *médecine/sciences* 1996 ; 10 : 1055-63.

2. Chang Y, Cesarman E, Pessin M, Lee F, Culpepper J, Knowles D, Moore P. Identification on a new human herpes virus-like DNA sequences in AIDS-associated Kaposi's sarcoma. *Science* 1994 ; 266 : 1865-9.

3. Lisitsyn N, Lisitsyn N, Wigler M. Cloning the difference between 2 complex genomes. *Science* 1993 ; 259 : 946-51.

4. Renne R, Zhong W, Herndier B, McGrath M, Abbey N, Kedes N, Ganem D. Lytic growth of Kaposi's sarcoma-associated herpesvirus (human herpesvirus 8) in culture. *Nature Med* 1996 ; 2 : 341-6.

5. Orenstein J, Alkan S, Blauvelt A, Jeang K, Weinstein M, Ganem D, Herndier B. Visualisation of human herpesvirus type 8 in Kaposi's sarcoma by light and transmission electron microscopy. *AIDS* 1997 ; 11 : F35-45.

6. Russo J, Bohenzky R, Chien M, Chen J, Yan M, Maddalena D, Parry J, Peruzzi D, Edelman I, Chang Y, Moore P. Nucleotide sequence of the Kaposi sarcoma-associated herpesvirus (HHV8). *Proc Natl Acad Sci USA* 1996 ; 93 : 14862-7.

7. Gao S, Boshoff C, Jayachandra S, Weiss R, Chang Y, Moore P. KSHV ORF K9 (vIRF) is an oncogene which inhibits the interferon signalling pathway. *Oncogene* 1997 ; 15 : 1979-85.

8. Bais C, Santomasso B, Coso O, Arvanitakis L, Geras Raaka E, Gutkind J, Ash A, Cesarman E, Gerhengorn M, Mesri E. G-protein-coupled receptor of KSHV isa viral oncogene and angiogenesis activator. *Nature* 1998 ; 391 : 86-9.

9. Swanton C, Mann D, Fleckenstein B, Neipel F, Peters G, Jones N. Herpes viral cyclin/Cdk6 complexes evade inhibition by CDK inhibitor proteins. *Nature* 1997 ; 390 : 184-7.

10. Thome M, Schneider P, Hofmann K, Fickenscher H, Meini E, Neipel F, Mattmann C, Burns K, Bodmer J, Schroter M, Scaffidi C, Krammer P, Peter M, Tschopp J. Viral FLICE-inhibitory proteins (FLIPs) prevent apoptosis induced by death receptors. *Nature* 1997 ; 386 : 517-21.

11. Sarid R, Sato T, Bohenzky R, Russo J, Chang Y. KSHV encodes a functional bcl-2 homologue. *Nature Med* 1997 ; 3 : 293-8.

12. Lewin B. *Cell cycle and growth regulation*. Genes, 6th ed. New York : Oxford University Press, 1997 : 1089-130.

13. Nicholas J, Ruvolo V, Burns W, Sandford G, Wan X, Ciufo D, Hendrickson S, Guo H, Hayward G, Reitz M. KSHV encodes homologues of macrophage inflammatory protein-1 and interleukin 6. *Nature Med* 1997 ; 3 : 287-92.

14. Moore P, Boshoff C, Weiss R, Chang Y. Molecular mimicry of human cytokine and cytokine response pathway genes by KSHV. *Science* 1996 ; 274 : 1739-44.

15. Gao S, Kingsley L, Li M, Zheng W, Parravicini C, Ziegler J, Newton R, Rinaldo C, Saah A, Phair J, Detels R, Chang Y, Moore P. KSHV antibodies among americans, italians and ugandans with and without Kaposi's sarcoma. *Nature Med* 1996 ; 2 : 925-8.

16. Lennette E, Blackbourn D, Levy J. Antibodies to HHV8 in the general population and in Kaposi's sarcoma patients. *Lancet* 1996 ; 348 : 858-61.

17. Kedes D, Operkalski E, Busch M, Kohn R, Flood J, Ganem D. The seropepidemiology of HHV8: distribution of infection in KS risk groups and evidence for sexual transmission. *Nature Med* 1996 ; 2 : 918-24.

18. Simpson G, Schulz T, Whitby D, Cook P, Boshoff C, Rainbow L, Howard M, Gao S, Bohenzky R, Simmonds P, Lee C, De Ruiter A, Hatzakis A, Tedder R, Weller I, Weiss R, Moore P. Prevalence of KSHV infection measured by antibodies to recombinant capsid protein and latent immunofluorescence antigen. *Lancet* 1996 ; 349 : 1133-8.

19. Calabro M, Sheldon J, Favero A, Simpson G, Fiore J, Gomes G, Angarano G, Chieco-Bianchi L, Schulz T. Seroprevalence of Kaposi's sarcoma associated herpesvirus/human herpesvirus 8 in several regions of Italy. *J Hum Virol* 1998 : in press.

20. Cesarman E, Chang Y, Moore P, Said J, Knowles D. Kaposi's sarcoma associated herpesvirus-like DNA sequences in AIDS-related body cavity based lymphoma. *N Engl J Med* 1995 ; 332 : 1186-91.

21. Soulier J. Herpès virus associé à la maladie de Kaposi KSHV/HHV8 : nouveaux résultats et nouvelles questions. *médecine/sciences* 1995 ; 11 : 1605-7.

22. Soulier J, Grollet L, Oksenhendler E, Cacoub P, Cazals-Hatem D, Babinet P, d'Agay M, Clauvel J, Raphael M, Degos L, Sigaux F. Kaposi's sarcoma-associated herpesvirus-like DNA sequences in multicentric Castleman's disease. *Blood* 1995 ; 86 : 1276-80.

23. Karcher D, Alkan S. HHV8 associated body cavity based lymphoma in human immunodeficiency virus-infected patients. *Hum Pathol* 1997 ; 28 : 801-8.

24. Lebbé C, Agbalika F, De Crémoux P, Deplanche M, Rybojad M, Masgrau E, Morel P, Calvo F. Detection of human herpesvirus 8 and human T-cell lymphotropic virus type 1 sequences in Kaposi's sarcoma. *Arch Dermatol* 1997 ; 133 : 25-30.

25. Alkan S, Karcher D, Ortiz A, Khalil S, Akhtar M, Ahraf Ali M. HHV8 in organ transplant patients with immunosuppression. *Br J Haematol* 1997 ; 96 : 412-4.

26. Lebbé C, De Crémoux P, Rybojad M, Costa da Cunha C, Morel P, Calvo F. Kaposi's sarcoma and new herpesvirus. *Lancet* 1995 ; 345 : 1180.

27. Boshoff C, Schulz T, Kennedy M, Graham A, Fisher C, Thomas A, McGee J, Weiss R, O'Leary J. Kaposi's sarcoma-associated herpesvirus infects endothelial and spindle cells. *Nature Med* 1995 ; 1 : 1274-8.

28. Blasig C, Zietz C, Haar B, Neipel F, Esser S, Brockmeyer N, Tschachler E, Colombini S, Ensoli B, Stürzl M. Monocytes in Kaposi's sarcoma lesions are productively infected by human herpes virus 8. *J Virol* 1997 ; 71 : 7963-8.

29. Davis M, Stürtzl M, Blasig C, Schreier A, Guo H, Reitz M, SR O, Browning P. Expression of HHV8-encoded cyclin D in Kaposi' sarcoma spindle cells. *J Natl Cancer Inst* 1997 ; 89 : 1868-74.

30. Cesarman E, Nador R, Bai F, Bohenzky R, Russo J, Moore P, Chang Y, Knowles Q. KSHV contains G protein coupled receptor and cyclin D homologs which are expressed in Kaposi's sarcoma and malignant lymphoma. *J Virol* 1996 ; 70 : 8218-23.

31. Boshoff C, Endo Y, Collins P, Takeuchi Y, Reeves J, Schweickart V, Siani M, Sasaki T, Williams T, Gray P, Moore P, Chang Y, Weiss R. Angiogenic and HIV inhibitory functions of KSHV encoded chemokines. *Science* 1997 ; 278 : 290-4.

32. Dupin N, Grandadam M, Calvez V, Gorin I, Aubin J, Havard S, Lamy F, Leibowitch M, Huraux J, Escande J, Agut H. Herpes virus-like DNA sequences in patients with mediterranean Kaposi's sarcoma. *Lancet* 1995 ; 345 : 761-2.

33. Moore P, Kingsley L, Holmberg S, Spira T, Gupta P, Hoover D, Parry J, Conley L, Jaffe H, Chang Y. Kaposi's sarcoma-associated herpesvirus infection prior to the onset of Kaposi's sarcoma. *AIDS* 1996 ; 10 : 175-80.

34. Whitby D, Howard M, Tenant-Flowers M, Brink N, Copas A, Boshoff C, Hatzioannou T, Suggett F, Aldam D, Denton A, Miller R, Weller I, Weiss R, Tedder R, Schulz T. Detection of Kaposi's sarcoma associated herpesvirus in peripheral blood of HIV-infected ndividuals and progression to Kaposi's sarcoma. *Lancet* 1995 ; 346 : 799-802.

35. Corbellino M, Poirel L, Bestetti G, Pizzuto M, Aubin J, Capra M, Bifulco C, Berti E, Agut H, Rizzardini G, Galli M, Parravicini C. Restricted tissue distribution of extralesional KSHV sequences in AIDS patients with Kaposi's sarcoma. *AIDS Res* 1996 ; 12 : 651-7.

36. Vieira J, Huang M, Koelle D, Corey L. Transmissible KSHV in saliva of men with a history of Kaposi's sarcoma. *J Virol* 1997 ; 71 : 7083-7.

37. Parravicini C, Olsen S, Capra M, Poli F, Sirchia G, Gao S, Berti E, Nocera A, Rossi E, Besttetti G, Pizzuto M, Galli M, Moroni M, Moore P, Corbellino M. Risk of KSHV transmission from italian post-transplant Kaposi'sarcoma patients. *Blood* 1997 ; 90 : 2826-9.

38. Kedes D, Ganem D. Sensitivity of KSHV replication to antiviral drugs. *J Clin Invest* 1997 ; 99 : 2082-6.

39. Jones J, Hanson D, Chu S. AIDS associated Kaposi's sarcoma. *Science* 1995 ; 267 : 1078-9.

40. Costagliola D, Mary-Kraus M. Can antiviral agents decrease the occurrence of Kaposi' sarcoma? *Lancet* 1995 ; 346 : 578.

41. Mocroft A, Youle M, Gazzard B, Morcinek J, Halai R, Phillips A. Anti-herpesvirus treatment and risk of Kaposi' sarcoma in HIV infection. *AIDS* 1996 ; 10 : 1101-5.

42. Cordero E, Lopez-Cortes L, Viciana P, Alarcon A, Pachon J. Foscarnet and AIDS-associated Kaposi's sarcoma. *AIDS* 1997 ; 11 : 1787-8.

43. Rady P, Yen A, Rollefson J, Orengo I, Bruce S, TK H, Tyring S. Herpesvirus-like DNA sequences in non-Kaposi's sarcoma skin lesions of transplant patients. *Lancet* 1995 ; 345 : 1339-40.

44. Nishimoto S, Inagi R, Yamanishi K, Hosokawa K, Kabibushi M, Yoshikawa K. Prevalence of human herpesvirus-8 in skin lesions. *Br J Dermatol* 1997 ; 137 : 179-84.

45. Wolf P, Pütz B, Tilz G, Kerl H. Rare presence of HHV8 in skin tumors from patients with psoriasis treated with oral psoralen plus UV-A. *Arch Dermatol* 1997 ; 133 : 538.

46. Boshoff C, Talbot S, Kennedy M, O'Leary J, Schulz T, Chang Y. HHV8 and skin cancers in immunosuppressed patients. *Lancet* 1996 ; 347 : 338-9.

47. Cathomas G, Tamm M, McGandy C, Itin P, Gudat F, Thiel G, Mihatsch M. Absence of KSHV in transplantation related tumors other than Kaposi's sarcoma. *Transplant Proc* 1997 ; 29 : 836-7.

48. Dictor M, Rambech E, Way D, Witte M, Bendsöe N. HHV8 DNA in Kaposi's sarcoma lesions, AIDS Kaposi's sarcoma cell lines, endothelial Kaposi's sarcoma simulators, and the skin of immunosuppressed patients. *Am J Pathol* 1996 ; 148 : 2009-16.

49. Lebbé C, Tatoud R, Morel P, Calvo F, Euvrard S, Kanitakis J, Faure M, Claudy A. HHV8 sequences are not detected in epithelial tumors from patients receiving transplants. *Arch Dermatol* 1997 ; 133 : 111.

50. Dupin N, Gorin I, Escande J, Calvez V, Grandadam M, Hureaux J, Agut H. Lack of evidence of any association btween HHV8 and various skin tumors from both immunocompetent and immunosuppressed patients. *Arch Dermatol* 1997 ; 133 : 139.

51. Noël J, P H, Andre J, Simonart T, Verhest A, Haot J, Burny A. Herpesvirus-like DNA sequences and Kaposi's sarcoma. *Cancer* 1996 ; 77 : 2132-6.
52. Mitsuishi T, Sata T, Matsukura T, Kawashima M. HHV8 DNA is rarely found in Bowen's disease of non-immunosuppressed patients. *Br J Dermatol* 1997 ; 136 : 803-4.
53. Uthman A, Brna C, Weninger W, Tschachler E. No HHV8 in non Kaposi's sarcoma mucocutaneous lesions from immunodeficient HIV positive patient. *Lancet* 1996 ; 347 : 1700-1.
54. Koizumi H, Ohkawaba A, Itakura O, Kikuta H. Herpesvirus-like DNA sequences in classic Kaposi's sarcoma and angiosarcoma in Japan. *Br J Dermatol* 1996 ; 135 : 1009-10.
55. McDonagh D, Liu J, Gaffey M, Layfield L, Azumi N, Traweek T. Detection of Kaposi's sarcoma-associated herpesvirus-like DNA sequences in angiosarcoma. *Am J Pathol* 1996 ; 149 : 1363-8.
56. Gyulai R, Kemeny L, Adam E, Nagy F, Dobozy A. HHV8 DNA in angiolymphoid hyperplasia of the skin. *Lancet* 1996 ; 347 : 1837-8.
57. Gyulai R, Kemény L, Kiss M, Adal E, Nagy F, Dobozy A. Herpesvirus-like DNA sequences in angiosarcoma in a patient without HIV infection. *N Engl J Med* 1996 ; 334 : 540-1.
58. Jin Y, Tsai S, Yan J, Hsiao J, Lee Y, Su I. Detection of Kaposi's sarcoma associated herpesvirus like DNA sequence in vascular lesions. *J Clin Pathol* 1996 ; 105 : 360-3.
59. Tomita Y, Naka N, Aozasa K, Cesarman E, Knowles D. Absence of Kaposi's sarcoma associated herpesvirus-like DNA sequences in angiosarcomas developing in body-cavity and other sites. *Int J Cancer* 1996 ; 66 : 141-2.
60. Lebbé C, Pellet C, Flageul B, Sastre X, Avril M, Bonvalet D, Morel P, Calvo F. Sequences of HHV8 are not detected in various non Kaposi's sarcoma vascular lesions. *Arch Dermatol* 1997 ; 133 : 919-20.
61. Sander C, Simon M, Puchta U, Raffeld M, Kind P. HHV8 in lymphoproliferative lesions in the skin. *Lancet* 1996 ; 348 : 475-6.
62. Pastore C, Gloghini A, Volpe G, Nomdedeu J, Leonardo E, Mazza U, Saglio G, Carbone A, Gaidano G. Distribution of KSHV sequences among lymphoid malignacies in Italy and Spain. *Br J Haematol* 1995 ; 91 : 918-20.
63. Dupin N, Franck N, Calvez V, Gorin I, Grandadam M, Hureaux J, Leibowitch M, Agut H, Escande J. Lack of HHV8 DNA sequences in HIV-negative patients with various lymphoproliferative disorders of the skin. *Br J Dermatol* 1997 ; 136 : 827-30.
64. Pawson R, Catovsky D, Schulz T. Lack of evidence of HHV8 in mature T-cell lymphoproliferative disorders. *Lancet* 1996 ; 348 : 1450-1.
65. Rettig M, Ma H, Vescio R, Pold M, Schiller G, Belson D, Savage A, Nishikubo C, Wu C, Fraser J, Said J, Berenson J. KSHV infection of bone marrow dendritic cells from multiple myeloma patients. *Science* 1997 ; 276 : 1851-4.
66. Said J, Rettig M, Heppner K, Vescio R, Schiller G, Ma H, Belson D, Savage A, Shintaku I, Koeffler H, Asou H, Pinkus G, Pinkus J, Schrage M, Green E, Berenson J. Localization of KSHV in bone marrow biopsy samples from patients with multiple myeloma. *Blood* 1997 ; 90 : 4278-82.
67. Brousset P, Meggetto F, Attal M, Delsol G. Kaposi's sarcoma associated herpesvirus infection and multiple myeloma. *Science* 1997 ; 278 : 1972.
68. Masood T, Tulpule A, Arora NLC, Whitman J. Kaposi's sarcoma associated herpesvirus infection and multiple myeloma. *Science* 1997 ; 278 : 1970-1.
69. Marcelin A, Dupin B, Bouscary D, Bossi P, Cacoub P, Ravaud P, Calvez V. HHV8 and multiple myeloma in France. *Lancet* 1997 ; 350 : 1144.
70. MacKenzie J, Sheldon J, Morgan G, Cook G, Schulz T, Jarrett R. HHV-8 and multiple myeloma in the UK. *Lancet* 1997 ; 350 : 1144-5.
71. Regamey N, Erb P, Tamm M, Cathomas G. Human herpesvirus 8 variants. *Lancet* 1998 ; 351 : 680.
72. Foreman K, Bonish B, Nickoloff B. Absence of HHV8 DNA sequences in patients with immunosuppression-associated dermatofibromas. *Arch Dermatol* 1997 ; 133 : 108-9.
73. Di Alberti L, Piattelli A, Artese L, Favia G, Patel S, Saunders N, Porter S, Scully C, Ngui S, Teo C. HHV8 variants in sarcoid tissues. *Lancet* 1997 ; 350 : 1655-61.
74. Flore O, Rafii S, O'Leary JJ, Hyjek EM, Cesarman E. Transformation of primary human endothelial cells by Kaposi's sarcoma-associated herpesvirus. *Nature* 1998 ; 394 : 588-92.

10

Influence of organ transplantation on preexisting dermatoses

Alain CLAUDY
Department of Dermatology, Edouard-Herriot Hospital, Lyon, France.

Cutaneous lesions can be a significant problem in transplant recipients. Factors such as skin type, climate and level of immunosuppression have been implicated as modifiers of these clinical manifestations. With the advent of effective immunosuppression, organ transplantation has become an established and successful mode of treating end-stage organ disease. The graft-preserving immunosuppression predisposes recipients to complications, namely malignant tumors and infections [1]. The impact of organ transplantation on the evolution of common preexisting dermatosis has been so far poorly evaluated.

Skin lesions of hemodialyzed patients

Several dermatologic conditions are associated with chronic renal failure, such as pruritus, xerosis, easy bruising, increased pigmentation, yellow or yellow-brown color superimposed upon pallor in anemic patients, decreased sweating, keratosis pilaris, half-and-half nails, calciphylaxis, perforating collagenosis and β2 microglobulin-associated amyloidosis [2]. All these signs tend to subside within weeks after transplantation. A dermatological examination has been performed on 49 patients (30 males, 19 females aged 24-64 years) 3.1 years after successful kidney transplantation [3]. When sufficient renal function is restored, the alterations of uremic skin disappear. The decrease in sweat secretion, a common symptom in uremic patients, is no more observed after renal transplantation. The ichtyosiform aspect of uremic skin and the increased fragility of the skin is observed in only a minority of transplanted patients. The generalized pruritus and Raynaud's phenomenon that are frequent in uremic patients disappear completely. However, severe actinic elastosis and Dupuytren's contractures usually persist after transplantation.

Successful renal transplantation can also reverse cutaneous microangiopathy in normal-appearing skin of patients on hemodialysis. Cardiovascular disease is a major cause of morbidity and mortality among patients on maintenance hemodialysis. Hyperlipidemia associated with dialysis is not corrected by renal transplantation [4].

Specific skin lesions may appear during hemodialysis. They include local complications at the site of insertion of the cannula into the arteriovenous fistula (extravasation, phlebitis, bacterial colonization of the cannula, blood or peritoneal cavity), allergic dermatitis resulting from the adhesive tape used to secure the dialysis cannula. All these local complications disappear after successful kidney transplantation.

Bullous dermatosis of hemodialysis is often encountered. It may be due to a specific skin reaction that occurs during hemodialysis, or to porphyria cutanea tarda (PCT) that develops while on hemodialysis, or to a phototoxic drug reaction [5]. Bullous dermatosis of hemodialysis consists of subepidermal bullae on the dorsum of the hands that are clinically and histologically similar to PCT. Porphyrin levels may be normal or elevated. Iron overload is a possible precipitating factor. Uroporphyrin is normally moderately dialysable, suggesting that protein binding of the uroporphyrin may occur. There is no known effective treatment for bullous dermatosis of hemodialysis except from kidney transplantation which allows a progressive disappearance of the cutaneous signs.

Cutaneous lesions in patients with cirrhosis

Boldys et al. [6] monitored 11 patients with liver cirrhosis. Etiology of the disease was alcohol abuse in 5 cases, post-inflammatory in 4 cases and primary biliary cirrhosis in 2 cases. One month after liver transplantation a reduction of spider telangiectasias, erythema palmare and nail changes was observed. During the next few months, leg discoloration, gynecomastia and hippocratic fingers disappeared but Dupuytren's contractures remained unchanged. There was no correlation between sex hormone levels and skin changes, except from a decrease of the total testosterone level and an increase of the ratio free/total testosterone in women and a decrease in estradiol level in men after transplantation. Skin changes typical for liver cirrhosis can be reversible after liver transplantation.

Infectious diseases

The prevalence of cutaneous infections is higher in transplant recipients than in control groups. Preexisting infections such as onychomycosis, dermatophytosis, candidiasis, human papilloma virus (HPV) infections, paronychia and *Herpes simplex* usually worsen after grafting and their prevalence increases with the duration of immunosuppression. *Tinea versicolor* may be present in 5-10% of patients pretransplantation and develops in 15-20% of patients posttransplantation, mainly in those who tan easily [1]. Repeated topical treatments are useful to prevent frequent recurrences. *Tinea versicolor* is the only condition that decreases with the duration of immunosuppression if correctly treated [1].

Herpes simplex virus infections

Herpes simplex virus (HSV) is a common cause of infection in transplant patients. Over 60% of them have circulating anti-HSV antibodies indicating previous exposure to the virus. The majority of posttransplant infections result from reactivation of the latent virus. Forty percent of the patients with pretransplant HSV antibody titers develop clinical posttransplantation infection [7]. Some studies have reported higher infection rates based on asymptomatic viral shedding rather than clinical disease. Rejection of the graft with higher doses of immunosuppression is more frequent among patients who develop HSV infection. Therefore, the incidence of HSV infection in transplant patients is relatively low in those sero-positive prior to transplant. Even though acyclovir is capable of preventing reactivation of the latent virus, prophylactic therapy must be undertaken with caution because of the risk of emergence of drug- resistant strains. Restricting the drug to therapeutic use reduces the cost and diminishes the risk for acyclovir resistance [7].

If HSV infection is known to reactivate in previously seropositive transplant recipients, it is generally thought that the infection is not transmissible by the transplant itself. However two cases of disseminated HSV infection occurring in a heart and a pancreatic transplant recipient implicated the allografts as the source of the virus [8]. Both recipients were seronegative pretransplant and developed an antibody response with temporal antigenic specificity and complement-enhanced neutralization consistent with primary infection. These findings suggest that HSV transplanted in donor tissues may cause severe infection in seronegative and immunosuppressed transplant recipients.

HPV infections

HPVs are the causative agents of condylomata acuminata, common warts and other epithelial proliferative lesions. Keratinocytes infected by HPV are stimulated to proliferate; specific types of HPV, namely types 16 and 18, have an increased tendency to induce dysplastic lesions and play an essential role in the genesis of cervical and anal carcinomas in transplanted patients [9].

Immunocompromised individuals have an increased prevalence of HPV-associated lesions and neoplasia, a higher number of invasive carcinomas and a higher rate of recurrences than immunocompetent individuals. HPV lesions preexisting to the graft are more likely to undergo rapid progression as much as the presence of viral DNA, extent of disease and potential for malignant transformation appear to correlate with the degree of immunosuppression [9]. Treatment options for transplanted patients remain similar to those for normal individuals. Cutaneous and mucosal warts can be treated by usual methods; however in the setting of deep immunosuppression, lesions tend to become numerous and extensive and therefore refractory to local treatments. A reduction of the immunosuppressive treatment may be useful, especially for genital lesions which usually progress toward malignancy. Better antiviral drugs, frequent monitoring for disease progression and better education to reduce spread of HPV infection are highly needed in organ transplantation.

Acne

Steroid acne is common in organ transplant patients; it affected 42% of patients in one series of heart transplant recipients. Steroid acne usually appears within two weeks of systemic steroid therapy or even earlier if acne is active before transplantation and regresses upon drug discontinuation [10]. Adults are more commonly affected, but cases in children and infants have been reported. This type of acne differs from adolescent acne. The lesions are monomorphous with papules and papulo-pustules scattered on the face, upper trunk and upper limbs. On the contrary, when present before transplantation, acne is often exacerbated by steroids and shows the same polymorphic appearance as adolescent acne. Topical therapy is usually inefficient. Progressive improvement is noticed only when steroids are notably diminished. Moderate dose isotretinoin (0.3 to 0.5 mg/k/day) may be added to the tapering of steroids for 3 to 6 months.

Skin cancers

The immunosuppressive therapy significantly increases the incidence of certain malignancies that arise *de novo* after transplantation. The main question is whether immunosuppressive therapy affects the growth of preexisting tumors, either those untreated or those with residual cells at the time of transplantation. In a study of 913 renal transplant recipients, Penn [11] provided conflicting results regarding the effect of immunosuppression on existing cancer cells. There was a high incidence of new tumors or recurrences in patients with non-melanoma skin cancers (basal and squamous cell carcinomas) and a higher incidence of multiple skin cancers occurring *de novo* after transplantation. Penn hypothesized that imidazole breakdown products of azathioprine sensitize the skin to ultraviolet light and may enhance the predisposition to cancer in persons who already have had one or more skin cancers [11]. The conclusion drawn from this study is that heavy immunosuppression, given early after transplantation, is responsible for recurrences of tumors within the first two years after transplantation, whereas chronic immunosuppression may foster the development of late recurrences. There is now a bulk of evidence suggesting that immunosuppression favors the growth of existing malignant cells [12].

Renal transplantation exposes patients with preexisting Kaposi's sarcoma (KS) in apparent remission to a high risk of recurrences [13]. KS regresses only when all immunosuppression is discontinued after transplant removal. The outcome of recurrent KS is similar to that of a first episode in transplant recipients. Cyclosporin A (CsA), steroids and azathioprine have long been recognized to promote KS. Tapering of immunosuppressive drugs is often done at the cost of graft loss. Optimal HLA matching in order to minimize the risk of rejection and decrease the need for immunosuppression is highly desirable in patients with preexisting KS to be grafted.

Nevi and malignant melanoma

Melanocyte proliferation, both benign and malignant, may follow organ transplantation as a result of immunosuppression. Melanocytic nevi show considerable variation in different age groups. They are uncommon in infancy but increase in number through childhood and adolescence. The case of a child who developed numerous benign melanocytic nevi following renal transplantation has been reported, whereas his identical non-immunosuppressed sibling did not develop excess nevi [14]. This phenomenon is common in children undergoing renal transplantation, but is not seen in children on dialysis for renal disease. An inverse association of chronic sun exposure and age with numbers of nevi has been found in a cohort of adult renal transplant recipients [15]. It may comprise patients who may have had in the past clinically atypical nevi, which may have disappeared at the time of examination. It has been suggested that accumulating solar effects may contribute to the natural maturation and elimination of common acquired nevi in late adulthood [16]. The possibility that immunosuppression *per se* is associated with an increased incidence of clinically atypical nevi or excess numbers of clinically normal nevi is not excluded [17]. In a cohort of 38 children with a renal allograft and in 38 individually age and sex-matched healthy controls, a significant increase in the total number of nevi in the renal transplant group compared with the control group ($p < .05$) was noted with most marked increases occurring on the back and acral sites. A strong positive correlation between nevi count and duration of immunosuppression independant of age was also found ($p < .005$) [18].

Organ allograft recipients are also prone to malignant melanoma (MM). MM may be transmitted from the donors. In a study of Penn [19], eleven donors (kidney, liver, heart) who had occult MM provided organs to 20 recipients; in these, three never had evidence of MM, one showed local spread of tumor beyond the allograft and 16 developed metastases. Within the last group, 11 patients died from MM and 4 of them experienced complete remission following transplant nephrectomy and discontinuation of immunosuppressive therapy. MM treated pretransplantation recur posttransplantation in 20% of the cases [19], notwithstanding the duration of the MM before transplantation. MM may also occur *de novo*. MM constitute 5.2% of posttransplant skin cancers compared with 2.7% in the general population. 27% of patients with cutaneous MM also have other skin cancers. Penn suggests that the risk of MM may be reduced by stringent selection of donors, by waiting at least 5 years between treatment of MM and transplantation, by reducing sunlight exposure and by early excision of suspicious dysplastic nevi [19].

Autoimmune diseases

Autoimmune disease are diverse and may involve most organs to various degrees. Immunosuppressive treatments have been attempted successfully but the risk of side-effects is a major concern in diseases that are not usually life-threatening. The objective of immunosuppression in autoimmune diseases is to improve the clinical status by slowing the autoimmune response, without exposing the patients to unacceptable risks with regard to disease prognosis. The immunosuppressive agents routinely used comprise five drugs or drug classes (steroids, azathioprine, cyclophosphamide, CsA and methotrexate), three of which are used in transplanted patients. Autoimmune diseases should therefore improve in grafted patients. In some cases the transplanted organs may be involved by the autoimmune process [20]. Recurrence of systemic lupus erythematosus may affect the transplanted kidneys, necessitating increased immunosuppressive therapy. In dialysed patients with systemic sclerosis, there is also a possibility of recurrence of the disease, raising the difficulty of distinguishing this situation from chronic vascular kidney rejection. Furthermore, the use of CsA after transplantation in systemic scleroderma aggravates alterations of vascular endothelium and adds a risk of kidney viability [21].

Linear IgA bullous dermatosis

This rare condition has been reported in association with coeliac disease, lymphoproliferative disorders, systemic lupus erythematosus, immune nephritis and drugs. One case of adult linear IgA bullous dermatosis has been observed after heart transplantation; the striking feature was that the eruption appeared while the patient was receiving immunosuppressive treatment. A potential side-effect of CsA was not ruled out. Dapsone (100 mg/day) resulted in clearing of the lesions [22].

Alopecia areata

CsA is now a widely used immunosuppressive agent in organ transplantation. One of the most common dermatological side effects of the drug is dose-dependant hypertrichosis, which affects more than 80% of patients with variable degrees of hirsutoid hair growth on different areas of the face and body. Hypertrichosis is usually noted 8 weeks after initiation of therapy. The development of hypertrichosis is not hormone-induced, but is probably due to a direct effect of the drug on hair growth.

Several authors have proposed that alopecia areata (AA) has an autoimmune pathogenesis based on autoreactivity of T lymphocytes against an unknown antigen of the hair bulb. Support for this hypothesis came from reports of a case of AA that improved by CsA.

The mechanism of action of CsA in AA is unknown. The infiltrate around the hair bulbs consists predominantly of CD4+ cells and the decrease in the mean number of CD4+ and CD8+ cells per hair follicle significantly correlates with terminal hair regrowth [23].

Topically applied CsA is ineffective due to its poor penetration through the epidermis. Systemically administered CsA has been thought to be effective in AA but the results of the literature are controversial. In 1990, Gupta et al. [23] reported 6 patients in which 6 mg/kg/day of CsA for 12 weeks induced hair regrowth on the scalp of all patients within the second and fourth week of therapy. However, hair loss occurred in all patients within 3 months of CsA discontinuation. Similar results were obtained in human allograft recipients during the late eighties [24]. Then appeared reports of patients in whom AA developed during the course of CsA therapy following kidney, liver or heart transplantation [25, 26]. Two explanations were brought upon. Firstly, the immunosuppressive dosage taken by the patients was inadequate to prevent T-cell activation. The second, not mutually exclusive explanation would be that the immunopathology of AA does not primarily depend on the activation of CD4+ T lymphocytes [27]. IL1 has been recently suggested as a crucial mediator inducing cessation of hair growth. It has been demonstrated that CsA enhances IL1β mRNA expression while inhibiting IL2, IL3, IFNγ, GM-CSF and TNFα. This fact could therefore explain why CsA may be a failure in AA occurring in allograft recipients [28].

In conclusion, CsA does not have a therapeutic effect in grafted patients with AA, especially those with alopecia universalis. This may be due to the fact that the doses of CsA sufficient to protect from rejection of the transplanted organ are insufficient to protect against AA [29]. A newly discovered macrolide antibiotic immunosuppressant, FK 506, effective against graft rejection at much lower doses compared to CsA, has proven to induce stimulation of hair growth by topical (but not oral) administration in mice. Use of topical application of FK 506 in humans is under investigation.

Psoriasis

The relationship between psoriasis, dialysis and transplantation remains unclear. Psoriasis may be exacerbated, appear *de novo* or improve during dialysis and after transplantation. Steroids and immunosuppressive drugs are known to be active on psoriasis. Psoriatic patients receiving kidney transplants should therefore theoretically be improved by immunosuppressive treatments. However, exacerbation of psoriasis may occur in these patients. Stress experienced by transplanted patients is more likely to be associated with psoriasis, even though there is considerable individual variation in the ability to cope. Stress can affect the immune system directly through neuroendocrine changes or indirectly.

Several transplanted patients are infected with hepatitis C virus (HCV) from transfusions or from the donor organ. HCV is known to induce psoriasis or to exacerbate long-lasting psoriasis [30, 31]. In non-transplanted patients HCV-induced psoriasis may benefit from interferon therapy; in transplanted patients, this treatment should be ruled out because of the risk of immunological rejection.

A rapid steroid withdrawal after renal transplantation may transform psoriatic plaques into generalized pustular psoriasis. Meinardi et al. [32] reported the successful use of CsA in a patient with generalized pustular psoriasis. The oral dose of CsA was 12 mg/kg/day. A reduction of CsA dosage to 5 mg/kg/day resulted in relapse of pustulation. Coulson et al. [33] failed to suppress generalized pustular psoriasis with CsA in a renal-transplanted patient, although they did not achieve whole blood levels of CsA as high as in the case of Meinardi et al. [32].

Bland emollients may be sufficient to control the disease. When psoriasis is generalized, erythrodermic or pustular, systemic therapy may be required. Early after renal transplantation, particularly if evidence of graft rejection exists, etretinate should be used with caution. Methotrexate is the agent most frequently used. It has immunosuppressant activity, which may be of benefit if graft rejection is evident after organ transplantation. Although methotrexate is excreted via the kidney, use of small doses (2.5 to 5 mg per week) may be highly effective [33].

Atopic dermatitis

Atopic individuals exhibit a « late phase T cell reaction » when exposed to relevant allergens and are at increased risk for developing autoimmune disorders such as alopecia areata, vitiligo and lichen planus.

CsA is known to improve patients with severe refractory atopic dermatitis suggesting that inhibition of T cell functions may be important for the control of disease. Immunosuppressive treatments given to organ-transplant recipients with atopic dermatitis should therefore improve their status.

It has been hypothesized that atopic patients might also exhibit an increased incidence of cellular hypersensitivity to allografts. Seung and Lorincz [34] conducted a 6-month retrospective study comparing episodes of acute renal transplant rejection in nine atopic patients versus nine non-atopic ones. The conclusion of the study was that atopic individuals exhibit an increased incidence and severity of rejection of renal transplants when compared with non-atopic individuals with renal allografts.

Lichen planus

The cause of lichen planus (LP) is unknown. The most common hypotheses incriminate a viral cause, immunologic abnormalities, neurologic changes and emotional stress. A possible autoimmune basis for LP has been suggested, based on evidence of a cell-mediated immune response directed against basal epidermal keratinocytes. Recent studies have demonstrated that hepatitis C virus could be the cause of some cases of LP [35]. It is conceivable that the higher the prevalence of HCV in the transplanted population, the higher the prevalence of HCV as a cause of LP will be. These observations provided the basis for trials of LP with immunosuppressive drugs such as high dose steroids, azathioprine or topical CsA, i.e. treatments used in grafted patients. Therefore, the incidence of LP in patients receiving allografted organs is potentially high due to the prevalence of HCV infection, but the immunosuppressive treatments given to these patients should prevent its occurence or diminish its duration.

The association of LP and primary biliary cirrhosis (PBC) is probably more than coincidental and may be due to the fact that both conditions are based on alterations of cell-mediated immune responses. One patient presenting with generalized LP associated with PBC unrelated to D-penicillamine and unresponsive to usual treatments was reported to have cleared his skin lesions after liver transplantation and immunosuppressive therapy with CsA [36].

Porphyrias

Liver transplantation can be successfully performed in patients with erythropoietic protoporphyria who have severe liver disease [37]. Skin photosensitivity progressively improves after transplantation and disappears in one to four years even though the erythrocyte and serum protoporphyrin levels may remain elevated [38]. However, the transplanted liver remains susceptible to protoporphyrin-induced damage [38]. The rationale for transplantation is that the new liver would reduce the metabolic disturbance and thus abrogate the porphyric symptoms. More relevant patients with protoporphyria and longer follow-up is necessary in order to determine the ultimate outcome and validity of this technique.

References

1. Lugo-Janer G, Sanchez JL, Santiago-Delpin E. Prevalence and clinical spectrum of skin diseases in kidney transplant recipients. *J Am Acad Dermatol* 1991 ; 24 : 410-4.
2. Gupta AK, Gupta MA, Cardella CJ, Haberman HF. Cutaneous associations of chronic renal failure and dialysis. *Int J Dermatol* 1986 ; 25 : 498-504.
3. Altmeyer P, Kachel HG, Schäfer G, Bassbinder W. Normalisierung der urämischen Hautveränderungen nach Nierentransplantation. *Hautarzt* 1986 ; 37 : 217-21.
4. Gilchrest BA, Rowe JW, Mihm MC. Clinical and histological skin changes in chronic renal failure: evidence for a dialysis-resistant, transplant-response microangiopathy. *Lancet* 1980 ; II : 1271-5.
5. Stevens BR, Fleischer AB, Piering F, Crosby DL. Porphyria cutanea tarda in the setting of renal failure. *Arch Dermatol* 1993 ; 129 : 337-9.
6. Boldys H, Pageaux GP, Larrey D, Michel H. Evolution of cutaneous changes observed in cirrhosis patients before and after liver transplantation. *Pol Arch Med Wewn* 1993 ; 89 : 151-8.
7. Tomlanovich SJ, Sabatte-Caspillo J, Melzer J, Amend W, Vincenti F, Feduska N, Salvatierra O. The incidence and impact of *Herpes simplex* virus infections in the first month following renal transplantation. *Transplant Proc* 1989 ; 21 : 2091-2.
8. Goodman JL. Possible transmission of *Herpes simplex* virus by organ transplantation. *Transplantation* 1989 ; 47 : 609-13.
9. Euvrard S, Kanitakis J, Claudy A. Skin cancers in immunocompromised patients. In : Grob JJ, Stern RS, MacKie RM, Weinstock WA, eds. *Epidemiology, causes and prevention of skin diseases*. Blackwell Science, 1997 : 189-97.
10. Hurwitz RM. Steroid acne. *J Am Acad Dermatol* 1989 ; 21 : 1179-81.
11. Penn I. The effect of immunosuppression on pre-existing cancers. *Transplantation* 1993 ; 55 : 742-7.
12. Penn I. Effect of immunosuppression on pre-existing cancers. *Transplant Proc* 1993 ; 25 : 1380-2.
13. Doutrelepont JM, De Pauw L, Gruber SA, Dunn DL, Qunibi W, Kinnaert P, Vereerstraeten P, Penn I, Abramowicz D. Renal transplantation exposes patients with previous Kaposi's sarcoma to a high risk of recurrence. *Transplantation* 1996 ; 62 : 463-6.
14. McGregor JM, Barker JNWN, Macdonald DM. The developement of excess numbers of melanocytic nevi in an immunosuppressed identical twin. *Clin Exp Dermatol* 1991 ; 16 : 131-2.
15. Bouwes Bavinck JN, Crijns M, Vermeer BJ, van der Wouds F, Claas FHJ, Pfister H, Green A, Bergman W. Chronic sun exposure and age are inversely associated with nevi in adult renal transplant recipients. *J Invest Dermatol* 1996 ; 106 : 1036-41.
16. Harth Y, Friedman-Birnbaum R, Linn S. Influence of cumulative sun exposure on the prevalence of common acquired nevi. *J Am Acad Dermatol* 1992 ; 27 : 21-4.
17. Barker JNWN, Macdonald DM. Eruptive dysplastic nevi following renal transplantation. *Clin Exp Dermatol* 1988 ; 13 : 123-5.
18. Smith CH, McGregor JM, Barker JNWN, Morris RW, Rigden SPA, MacDonald DM. Excess melanocytic nevi in children with renal allografts. *J Am Acad Dermatol* 1993 ; 28 : 51-5.

19. Penn I. Malignant melanoma in organ allograft recipients. *Transplantation* 1996 ; 61 : 274-8.

20. Nyberg G, Blohmé I, Persson H, Olausson M, Svalander C. Recurrence of systemic lupus erythematosus in transplanted kidneys: a follow-up transplant biopsy study. *Nephrol Dial Transplant* 1992 ; 7 : 1116-23.

21. Ruiz JC, Val F, de Francisco ALM, de Bonis E, Zubimendi JA, Prieto M, Arias M. Progressive systemic sclerosis and renal transplantation: a contra-indication to cyclosporin. *Nephron* 1991 ; 59 : 330-2.

22. Petit D, Borradori L, Rybojad M, Morel P. Linear IgA bullous dermatosis after heart transplantation. *J Am Acad Dermatol* 1990 ; 22 : 851.

23. Gupta AK, Ellis CN, Cooper KD, Nickoloff BJ, Ho VC, Chan LS, Hamilton TA, Tellner DC, Griffiths CEM, Voorhees JJ. Oral cyclosporin for the treatment of alopecia areata. *J Am Acad Dermatol* 1990 ; 22 : 242-50.

24. Gebhart W, Schmidt JB, Schemper M, Spona J, Kopsa H, Zazgornik J. Cyclosporin-A-induced hair growth in human renal allograft recipients and alopecia areata. *Arch Dermatol Res* 1986 ; 278 : 238-40.

25. Misciali C, Peluso AM, Cameli N, Tosti A. Occurence of alopecia areata in a patient receiving systemic cyclosporin A. *Arch Dermatol* 1996 ; 132 : 843-4.

26. Roger D, Charmes JP, Bonnetblanc JM. Alopecia areata occurring in a patient receiving cyclosporin A. *Acta Derm Venereol (Stockh)* 1994 ; 74 : 154.

27. Davies MG, Bowers PW. Alopecia areata arising in patients receiving cyclosporin immunosuppression. *Br J Dermatol* 1995 ; 132 : 835-6.

28. Parodi A, Micalizzi C, Basile GC, Rebora A. Alopecia universalis and cyclosporin A. *Br J Dermatol* 1996 ; 135 : 657.

29. Monti M, Barbareschi M, Caputo R. Alopecia universalis in liver transplant patients treated with cyclosporin. *Br J Dermatol* 1995 ; 133 : 663.

30. Kanazawa K, Aikawa T, Tsuda F, Okamoto H. Hepatitis C virus infection in patients with psoriasis. *Arch Dermatol* 1996 ; 132 : 1391-2.

31. Yamamoto T, Katayama I, Nishioka K. Psoriasis and hepatitis C virus. *Acta Derm Venereol (Stockh)* 1995 ; 75 : 482-3.

32. Meinardi MMHM, Westerhof W, Bos JD. Generalized pustular psoriasis (von Zumbusch) responding to cyclosporin A. *Br J Dermatol* 1987 ; 16 : 269-70.

33. Coulson IH, Evans CD, Holden CA. Generalized pustular psoriasis after renal transplantation: failure to suppress with cyclosporin A. *Clin Exp Dermatol* 1988 ; 13 : 416-7.

34. Seung LM, Lorincz AL. Incidence of acute renal transplant rejection in atopic individuals. *Arch Dermatol* 1994 ; 130 : 584-8.

35. Pawlotsky JM, Dhumeaux D, Bagot M. Hepatitis C virus in dermatology. *Arch Dermatol* 1995 ; 131 : 1185-93.

36. Oleaga JM, Gardeazabal J, de Galdeano S, Diaz PJL. Generalized lichen planus associated with primary biliary cirrhosis which resolved after liver transplantation. *Acta Derm Venereol. (Stockh)* 1995 ; 75 : 87.

37. Steinmuller T, Doss MO, Steffen R, Blumhardt G, Bechstein WO, Frank M, Sieg I, Kretschmar R, Neuhaus P. Liver transplantation in erythropoietic protoporphyria. *Dtsch Med Wochenschr* 1992 ; 117 : 1097-102.

38. Bloomer JR, Weimer MK, Bossenmaier IC, Snover DC, Payne WD, Ascher NL. Liver transplantation in a patient with protoporphyria. *Gastroenterology* 1989 ; 97 : 188-94.

11

Herpes virus infections and prophylaxis

Gérard GUILLET
Department of Dermatology, University of Brest, France.

Immunosuppression is a necessary condition for allograft transplantation. The induced immunosuppression occurs after any kind of graft (kidney, heart, lung, liver and bone marrow). It is of major importance in the early post-transplantation period since the treatment is intensive. The deep immunosuppression will last for a variable time depending on the treatment requested for the specific organ grafted and on the threat of rejection. Herpes virus infections are expected to occur during severe immunosuppression. Viral infection causes morbidity to the patient and also occasionally to the graft itself. Bone marrow allograft recipients are especially concerned because 75% of them may develop viral infections due to the type and dose of administered drugs: more than cyclosporine and steroids, anti-lymphocyte serum and OKT3 monoclonal antibody induce a high risk for herpes virus infections.

Herpes simplex virus infections

Herpes simplex virus (HSV) infections occur shortly after bone marrow transplantation. Primary infection is a very rare event as compared with the reactivation of orolabial, ocular and genital infections, representing 98% of all HSV infections in bone marrow graft recipients. They manifest usually with extensive mucocutaneous ulcerations (*Figures 12 and 13, page 219*), but uncommon clinical presentations may be observed, such as hyperkeratotic papules, nodules of the tongue or chronic mouth ulcers. These mucocutaneous lesions may last for weeks before healing occurs. Before acyclovir became available, HSV infections were a primary cause of death in 3% of all bone marrow transplant recipients [1, 2] due to pneumonia or meningitis. In this respect, confusion between pulmonary herpetic infection and rejection of the grafted lung was a major problem [3]. Some criteria have been evaluated to predict the risk of HSV infection with respect to HSV serology prior to transplantation [4]. This risk is of utmost importance in seropositive HSV patients; it is more severe in bone marrow transplant recipients and very frequent in kidney recipients since 30% of them develop infection in the first 10 days after transplantation. For this reason, therapeutic guidelines were established for HSV prophylaxis, based on the serological status of grafted patients and on the expected time of HSV onset after transplantation [5-7].

Statistical data allow to predict a high risk of infection for seropositive bone marrow transplant recipients; 50-80% of them will develop HSV infections in the first two weeks post-graft. The risk is also important but lower after heart, lung or kidney transplantation: 50% of seropositive patients will develop HSV infection in the early two months after transplantation with moderate to severe manifestations. The risk is lower for liver transplant recipients (31% of patients in the first two weeks). Therefore protection against active HSV infection through prophylactic treatment merits consideration. Oral intake of acyclovir (200 mg every 8 hours daily for 30 days) [6] was shown to decrease the incidence of HSV infections down to 5% in kidney, heart and lung allograft recipients. In bone marrow grafted patients, a dramatic decrease from 80% to 15% is obtained with acyclovir given at the dose of 5 mg/kg three times daily for 4 weeks followed by oral intake of 800 mg four times daily during 6 months. However, the risk of HSV infection outset remains identical once acyclovir has been withdrawn.

Varicella zoster virus infections

Infection with the varicella zoster virus (VZV) is another expected complication in immunocompromised patients [4, 8-11]. The clinical expression of VZV infection may be especially severe, manifesting as generalized zoster or complicated necrotic varicella with possibilities of pulmonary infection, severe hepatitis and Reye's syndrom. The high morbidity of VZV infection is correlated with the immune status of the patient. The risk of VZV infection is higher in bone marrow than in kidney graft recipients, but clinical manifestations may be very severe in both. In the event of loss of specific anti-VZV immunity, patients may develop an unusual varicella characterized by an extensive non-inflammatory vesicular eruption that may be associated with specific hepatitis, pneumonia or encephalomeningitis [12]. Patients who maintain a specific VZV immunity will develop common manifestations of zoster or a generalized eruption combining zoster and varicella: zoster-varicella is defined by the outbreak of at least 20 vesicles outside the plaque of zoster. In order to decrease this risk in kidney recipients, acyclovir should be administered at a dose of 200 mg four times daily for 6 weeks. The benefit is major since VZV infections are abrogated. For bone marrow recipients, intravenous acyclovir is recommended at a dose of 250 mg/m^2 twice daily from day 5 to day 28, followed by oral intake for 6 months. The incidence of VZV decreases from 36% to 0% but there is no significant difference after acyclovir is withdrawn after 6 months of treatment. In any case, graft recipients not receiving the treatment are advised to consult if an infectant contact or a possible outbreak are suspected.

Cytomegalovirus infections

Among HSV infections, cytomegalovirus (CMV) is associated with significant morbidity and mortality in immunocompromised patients [5, 13-18]. Immunosuppression allows for unusual cutaneous presentation of CMV infections with a maculopapular rash spreading down from the trunk to the limbs but sparing the palms and soles, and periorificial ulcers of the anal, genital or mammary area, with mucous membrane involvement [19, 20].

Cutaneous manifestations are benign and non-specific, and the diagnosis relies on histocytologic findings. However, dermatologists should be aware of the fact that a cutaneous eruption may suggest CMV infection if fever, leukopenia and severe visceral involvement (hepatitis, pancreatitis, oesophagitis) are present. The predictable period of outset for CMV infection in bone marrow transplant recipients is 3 months following transplantation, with expected complications such as aplasia, pneumonia, retinitis or myocarditis. In renal allograft recipients the morbidity is increased due to the risk of kidney rejection in the first month posttransplantation; it should be suspected in the presence of renal dysfunction resulting from tubulointerstitial nephritis or vasculitis. For this reason, protection against active CMV infection is recommendable during the four first months following transplantation, according to the predictable risk evaluated on the basis of serological anti-CMV status [21].

In seronegative kidney allograft recipients, the incidence of CMV infection ranges from 70% to 80% when the renal graft is provided by a seropositive donor, but is as low as 1.1% if the donor and the recipient are both seronegative. Prophylaxis with acyclovir 800 to 3,200 mg daily for 3 months decreases these rates to 16% and 0%, respectively. When the donor and the recipient are both CMV-seropositive prior to transplantation, the incidence of CMV infection ranges from 15% to 30%, and acyclovir treatment decreases this rate to 11%. Seventy five percent of liver graft recipients develop CMV viraemia but only 25% of them develop visceral infection. Prophylactic treatment with acyclovir at a daily dose of 3,200 mg from day 1 up to 3 months reduces the rate of viraemia (from 75% to 14%) and of infection (from 25% to 4.5%) [17].

CMV infection occurs in 38% of bone marrow allograft recipients within 3 months after transplantation [22]. Intravenous administration of acyclovir at a dose of 500 mg/m^2 from day 5 to day 30 decreases the incidence of CMV infection from 38% down to 22%.

Epstein-Barr virus infections

Epstein-Barr virus (EBV) infection is not uncommon in allograft recipients [1] but the precise risk is poorly evaluated. Infected patients may develop oral hairy leukoplakia and lymphoproliferative diseases. Lymphomas occur 2 to 4 years after transplantation depending on the degree of immunosuppression; this risk seems to increase with the use of OKT3 treatment that shortens the delay of lymphomas to 6 months after transplantation. Such lymphomas are located in the central nervous system, the liver and gut; the graft itself was reportedly involved in 20 cases. However, data regarding the benefit of prophylaxis against EBV infection are lacking since this is generally considered a benign and rare infection of late onset.

Human herpes virus 8 infections

Human herpes virus 8 (HHV8) or Kaposi's sarcoma herpes virus (KSHV) may be responsible for three diseases in the setting of immunosuppression, namely Kaposi's sarcoma [22], primary effusion lymphomas, and Castleman disease. Rady et al. [23] reported the detection of nucleotide sequences of HHV8 in epithelial skin tumours of transplant recipients but this finding was not confirmed by subsequent studies [24]. So far no prospective data on the efficacy of antiherpetic drugs in the prophylaxis of HHV8 infection are available.

Specific considerations according to the grafted organ

Since the risks and severity of HSV infections correlate with the type of immunosuppression (*i.e.* with the type of grafted organs), prophylaxis differs according to the speciality.

Nephrologists consider that an anti-HSV1 treatment should not be invariably administered: common labial herpes as well as recurrent herpes is expected within 5 to 10 days after transplantation but may be treated with a classical therapy, rather than prophylaxis. Nephrologists are more concerned with CMV or VZV infection: a past history of possible contacts or suspicion of CMV infection requires immediate prophylactic treatment. The risk is high in patients treated with thymoglobulin or OKT3, and intravenous ganciclovir is given for 3 weeks if CMV infection is predictable. For renal transplant recipients, oral acyclovir is recommended at the dose of 200 mg four times daily for 2 months to prevent HSV and VZV infection, or at the dose of 3,200 mg daily for 3 months against CMV. Prophylactic treatment with high doses of ganciclovir and acyclovir may decrease the incidence of viraemia in seronegative patients but the decrease of CMV infection and graft rejection is not significant [25].

For heart and lung transplant recipients there is presently no consensus on prophylaxis, but it is suggested that HSV antibody-positive patients should receive prophylactic acyclovir for the first two months after surgery, and at any time of increased immunosuppression [3].

Hepatologists are concerned with the risk of cytolysis and CMV viraemia in the early months after liver transplantation; however antiviral prophylaxis is not systematically given. Prophylaxis in this group of patients is still controversial [18]. It is namely a matter of discussion in the event of tritherapy (cyclosporine, steroids and OKT3). Prophylaxis mainly relies upon a careful evaluation of the possibility of CMV and VZV infection. For liver transplant recipients, low doses of acyclovir for 4 weeks may delay the onset of HSV infection. The prevention of CMV infection necessitates higher doses.

Haematologists administer prophylactic treatment depending on the intensity and length of immunosuppression; this is prescribed for a variable period (8 months to 2 years) and may be protracted in the event of graft-*versus*-host reaction. This approach is highly efficient concerning CMV and HSV infection, and prevents from clinical misdiagnosis between chemotherapy-induced mucitis and herpes infection.

Considering VZV, 10-15% of grafted patients develop herpes zoster one year post-graft. Therefore rational prophylaxis relies on the balance between predictable risk and morbidity, and toxicity or resistance to the drug. If prophylaxis is not given, a short treatment is prescribed in any case of risk or in the case of patent infection. For bone marrow allograft recipients, a prophylactic treatment with acyclovir 250 mg/m^2 three times daily from day 3 to day 18 is required against HSV infection. A dose of 250 mg/m^2 twice daily from day 5 to day 32 followed by oral intake of 400 mg three times daily for 6 months is required for VZV infection. CMV infection prophylaxis necessitates a dose of 3,200 mg daily for 3 months.

The main concern is the uncertainty regarding the long-term efficacy of such treatments; however there is a consensus for systematic prophylaxis in any case of major risk such as bone marrow allograft recipients or recent history of suspected infection in other types of graft recipients.

The interest of other antiviral drugs such as ganciclovir or foscarnet still needs evaluation. Protocols have been carried out to compare high dose oral acyclovir or valacyclovir, the valine ester of acyclovir [24] and regimens with ganciclovir, hyperimmune globulin, foscarnet, newer antiviral agents or even CMV vaccine [15]. Presently, however, most studies on prophylaxis concern HIV-infected patients rather than transplant recipients. A review of human trials suggests that acyclovir offers the best favourable combination of safety and efficacy [26] although the optimal dose of intravenous *versus* oral acyclovir is not clearly established for some types of transplant recipients [14]. Valaciclovir should be given to prevent HSV infections in bone marrow and in other graft recipients as well as to treat severe infections so as to avoid administration of high intravenous acyclovir doses [27]. Valaciclovir, however, is not indicated for the treatment of CMV infection and/or prophylaxis.

References

1. Saral R, Burns W, Prentice H. Herpes virus infections: clinical manifestations and therapeutic strategies in immunocompromised patients. *Clin Haematol* 1984 ; 13 : 645-60.
2. Taylor C, Sviland L, Pearson A, Dobb M, Reid M, Craft A, Hamilton P, Protor S. Virus infections in bone marrow transplant recipients: a three-year prospective study. *J Clin Pathol* 1990 ; 43 : 633-7.
3. Smyth R, Higen-Bottam T, Scott J, Wreghitt T, Stewart S, Clelland C, MC Goldrick J, Wallork J. *Herpes simplex* virus infection in heart lung tansplant recipients. *Transplantation* 1990 ; 49 : 735-9.
4. Lundgren G, Wilczek H, Lönnqvist B, Lindholm A, Wahren B, Ringden O. Acyclovir prophylaxis in bone marrow transplant recipients. *Scand J Infect Dis* 1985 ; 47 : 137-44.
5. Griffin P, Colbert J, Williamson E, Fiddian A, Hickmoyt E, Sells R, Salaman J. Oral acyclovir prophylaxis of herpes infections in renal transplant recipients. *Transplant Proc* 1985 ; 178 : 84-5.
6. Seale L, Jones C, Kathpalia S, Jackson G, Mozes M, Madoux M, Packham D. Prevention of herpes virus infections in renal allograft recipients by low dose oral acyclovir. *JAMA* 1985 ; 254 : 3435-48.
7. Selby P, Powles R, Easton D, Perren T, Stolle K, Jameson B, Piddian A, Tryhorn Y, Stern H. The prophylactic role of intravenous and long-term oral acyclovir after allogenic bone marrow transplantation. *Br J Cancer* 1989 ; 59 : 434-8.
8. Ljungman P, Lönnqvist B, Gahrton G, Ringden O, Sundquist V, Wahren B. Clinical and subclinical reactivation of varicella-zoster virus in immunocompromised patients. *J Infect Dis* 1986 ; 153 : 840-7.
9. Haagsma E, Klompmaker I, Grond J, Bijleveld C, The T, Schirm J, Gibs C, Sloof M. Herpes virus infections after orthotopic liver transplantation. *Transplant Proc* 1987 ; 19 : 4054-6.
10. Stoffel M, Squifflet J, Pirson Y, Lamy M, Alexandre G. Effectiveness of oral acyclovir prophylaxis in renal transplant recipients. *Transplant Proc* 1987 ; 19 : 2190-3.
11. Wacker P, Hartmann O, Benhamou E, Salloum E, Lemerle J. Varicella-zoster virus infections after autologous bone marrow transplantation in children. *Bone Marrow Transplant* 1989 ; 4 : 191-4.
12. Sassolas B, Moal C, Schollhammer M, Bourbigot B, Guillet G. Varicelle d'évolution fulminante chez un transplanté rénal. *Nouv Dermatol* 1995 ; 14 : 11.
13. Prentice H, Gluckman E, Powles R, Ljungman P, Milpied N, Ranada J, Mandelli F, Kho P, Kennedy L, Bell A. Impact of long term acyclovir on cytomegalovirus infection and survival after allogenic bone marrow transplantation. *Lancet* 1994 ; 343 : 749-54.
14. Sturgill M, Hatton J. Use of intravenous acyclovir for prophylaxis of cytomegalovirus infection in renal transplant recipients. *J Pharm Technol* 1993 ; 9 : 150-9.
15. Balfour H. Prevention of cytomegalovirus disease in renal allograft recipients. *Scand J Infect* 1991 ; 78 : 88-93.
16. Mollison L, Richards M, Johnson P, Hayes K, Munckhof W, Jones R, Dabkowski P, Angus P. High dose oral acyclovir reduces the incidence of cytomegalovirus infection in liver transplant recipients. *J Infect Dis* 1993 ; 168 : 721-4.
17. Stratta R, Shaefer M, Cushing K, Markin R, Wood R, Langnas A, Reed E, Woods G, Donovan J, Pillen T, Li S, Duckworth R, Shaw B. Successful prophylaxis of cytomegalovirus disease after primary CMV exposure in liver transplant recipients. *Transplantation* 1991 ; 51 : 90-7.
18. Saliba F, Eyraud D, Samuel D, David J, Arulnaden J, Dussaix E, Mathieu D, Bismuth H. Randomized controlled trial of acyclovir for the prevention of cytomegalovirus infection and disease in liver transplant recipients. *Transplant Proc* 1993 ; 25 : 1444-5.

19. Bournerias I, Boisnil S, Patey O, Deny P, Gharakmanian S, Duflo B, Gentilini M. Unusual cutaneous cytomegalovirus involvement in patients with acquired immunodeficiency syndrome. *Arch Dermatol* 1989 ; 125 : 1243-6.

20. Lesher JL. Cytomegalovirus infection and the skin. *J Am Acad Dermatol* 1988 ; 18 : 1333-8.

21. Kurtz J. Prevention and treatment of cytomegalovirus infection. *Curr Opin Infect Dis* 1988 ; 1 : 595-8.

22. Guillet G, Chouvet B, Thivolet J, Perrot H. Traitements immunosuppresseurs et maladie de Kaposi. *Ann Dermatol Venereol* 1980 ; 107 : 907-10.

23. Rady P, Yen A, Rollefson J. Herpes virus like DNA sequences in non-Kaposi's sarcoma lesions of transplant patients. *Lancet* 1995 ; 345 : 133-40.

24. Lebbé C, Tatoud R, Morel P, Calvo F, Euvrard S, Kanitakis J, Faure M, Claudy A. Human herpes virus 8 sequences are not detected in epithelial tumors from patients receiving transplants. *Arch Dermatol* 1997 ; 133 : 111.

25. Pouteil-Noble C. Infection à cytomégalovirus après transplantation rénale. *Presse Med* 1997 ; 26 : 7-9.

26. Raffi F. Perspectives d'avenir du valaciclovir dans le traitement et la prévention des infections à *Herpes viridae* chez le patient immunodéprimé. *Presse Med* 1997 ; 26 (suppl 1) : 19-23.

27. Milpied N. Infections à herpès virus et à virus varicelle-zona après greffes de moëlle. *Presse Med* 1997 ; 26 (suppl 1) : 4-6.

12

Oral hairy leukoplakia in immunocompromised patients

Peter H. ITIN
Department of Dermatology, University of Basel,
and Department of Dermatology, Kantonsspital Aarau, Switzerland.

In recent years stomatologic markers for severe immunosuppression in organ transplant patients have been increasingly appreciated. King et al. [1] investigated the rising prevalence of dysplastic and malignant lip lesions in renal transplant recipients and confirmed this tendency suggested by several earlier case reports. New oral disorders have been described in organ transplant patients during the last years. Benign gingival hyperplasia for example is quite a common undesired effect of cyclosporin therapy. Two patients with cyclosporin-associated posttransplant lymphoproliferative disorders presenting as gingival hyperplasia were reported [2]. Menni et al. [3] discussed the cutaneous and oral findings in 32 children after renal transplantation and described lingual fungiform papillae hypertrophy which was subsequently confirmed in patients under cyclosporin treatment [4].

In 1988 the first HIV-negative but otherwise severely immunosuppressed patients with oral hairy leukoplakia (OHL) were documented [5, 6]. OHL was initially described in 1981 by Greenspan et al. [7]. At the beginning, OHL was seen only in homosexual men with HIV infection, although in 1986 the risk group for HIV-infected patients who may develop OHL was expanded. OHL is rare in HIV-infected children and has been reported in only seven cases so far [8]. The only infectious agent consistently found in lesional tissue of OHL was Epstein-Barr virus (EBV). In 1989, EBV-receptors on oral keratinocyte plasma membranes were detected. This fact explained the predilection site of OHL on the lateral border of the tongue. EBV has been shown to replicate in lesional tissue of OHL.

Clinical features

OHL may appear unilaterally or bilaterally including the ventral surface of the tongue and rarely the buccal mucosa. The lesion is whitish and unremovable (*Figure 14, page 219*). OHL lesions are corrugated and shaggy with several keratin projections that give it a hairy appearance [9]. As a rule OHL is painless but burning sensations may occur. It seems likely that these subjective complaints may result from coinfection with *Candida* that is found in about half of the cases.

Histological examination

Histology shows parakeratosis and acanthosis, hair-like projections and ballooning of cells with inclusion bodies (*Figure 15, page 219*). Hyperkeratosis, acanthosis, hair-like projections and koilocyte-like features are found in 100%, 80%, 80%, and 98% of cases, respectively [10]. Intranuclear inclusions were considered as the histological hallmark of OHL [11]. Three types of nuclear inclusions were separated by light microscopy: eosinophilic central Cowdry type A inclusions with a halo; eosinophilic or basophilic variants with homogenous nuclear surface and marginal clumping of the chromatin; in the third inclusion type, the nuclei had a light steel-gray or ground-glass appearance with peripheral margination and clumping of chromatin. The absence of Langerhans cells in lesional tissue might be an important factor in the pathogenesis of OHL [12]. In up to 50% of OHL lesions *Candida albicans* coinfection may be found by PAS staining. *In situ* hybridization for EBV correlates well with cytopathic changes seen in OHL under light microscopy. Transmission electron microscopy of lesional tissue shows herpes-type virus, typical for EBV (*Figure 16*). Immunohistochemical studies in OHL show expression of keratins 6 and 16, which are markers for high turnover epithelia. Non-cornifying keratins are reduced compared with controls. The absence of suprabasal expression of keratin 19, which has been associated with premalignant changes, may explain why malignant transformation does not occur in OHL.

Virological studies

In situ hybridization demonstrates the presence of EBV-DNA in the upper part of the mucosal epithelium [13]. The topographic distribution of EBV-DNA infected cells in OHL supports the view that active viral replication is correlated with epithelial cell differentiation. Recent data document that OHL is maintained by repeated direct infection of the upper epithelial cells with virus from saliva or other infected cells from oral mucosa and not by reactivation of latent EBV. The absence of demonstrable EBV latency in the basal and suprabasal cells of OHL upholds this hypothesis [14-16]. The fact that continuous reinfection is necessary to maintain the lesion may contribute to the highly variable course of OHL. The

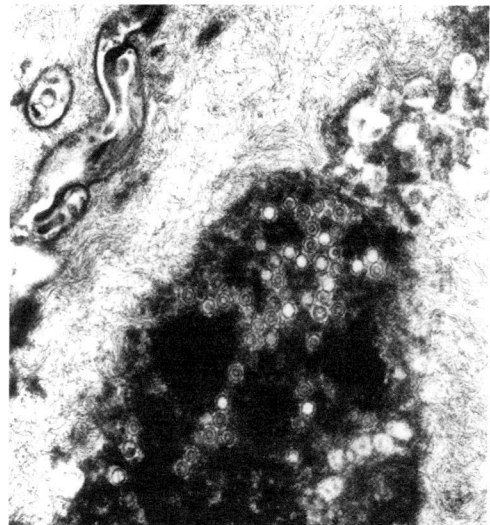

Figure 16. Electronmicroscopic aspect of lesional tissue in OHL. Typical herpes particles are visible.

clinical appearance of OHL may disappear or change dramatically within only few days. The necessity of continuous EBV-shedding for maintenance of OHL may explain why clinical OHL is almost restricted to HIV-infected or otherwise severely immunosuppressed persons as this population sheds continuously EBV in the throat and supplies the tongue epithelium with replicative EBV [17, 18]. In OHL co-infection with multiple strains of replicating EBV has been documented [19, 20]. Documentation of EBV is necessary to distinguish OHL from pseudo-oral hairy leukoplakia. Confirmation of the diagnosis of OHL by exfoliative cytologic methods is reliable and increasingly replaces biopsies [8]. EBV was found in 20% of heart transplant patients by negative staining electron microscopy in scrape material of the lateral border of the tongue [21]. Documentation of EBV-DNA by *in situ* hybridization and the polymerase chain reaction in the analysis of biopsies and exfoliative cytology specimens for the definitive diagnosis of OHL was extremely helpful in the study of Mabruk *et al.* [22]. Growing evidence exists that OHL involves coinfection with more than one strain of replicating EBV, some of which have mutations of the EBV nuclear antigen [19, 23]. It has been shown that HIV-negative patients with OHL have indeed coinfection with multiple EBV-strains and interstrain recombination [20]. No expression of EBNA-1, EBNA-2, EBNA-3 RNA (markers for latency) were detected in OHL cDNA library [24]. However the latent membrane protein-1 is expressed in OHL. Therefore EBV virions in OHL are infectious and able to infect and transform lymphocytes [25]. This fact may further explain why true OHL is more prevalent in immunosuppressed patients. It seems that continuous oral shedding of EBV with one strain is not sufficient to produce OHL. Multiple different EBV strains are necessary for the production of clinically manifest OHL. Coinfection with several strains and homologous recombination during viral replication generates virus variations [20].

Differential diagnosis

In 1989 Green *et al.* [26] coined the term « pseudo-hairy leukoplakia » for oral lesions mimicking hairy leukoplakia. The clinical and histologic features are identical as in true OHL. Only few reports on pseudo-oral hairy leukoplakia exist. In pseudo-oral hairy leukoplakia, no lesional EBV can be detected and HIV infection is absent [27].

Although the clinical appearance of OHL is characteristic, several entities have to be ruled out. A variety of intraoral diseases may clinically mimic OHL [28]. The differential diagnosis includes candidiasis (chronic hyperplastic, pseudomembranous and atrophic). Furthermore, lichen planus, graft-*versus*-host reaction, idiopathic leukoplakia, white sponge nevus, leucokeratosis nicotinica, geographic tongue, uremic stomatitis, marked edema, occlusal trauma, and chronic tongue chewing expand the spectrum of differential diagnosis.

Treatment

Although in most cases no treatment is required, several options for the management of OHL have been described, such as topical or systemic antifungals, topical retinoids, acyclovir, azidothymidine, podophyllin or surgical excision.

Table I. Oral hairy leukoplakia in HIV-seronegative patients

Author	Nb	Predisposing condition	T-helper cell count	EBV-DNA demonstration
Itin [5] 1988	1	Renal transplant	540	Yes
Epstein [6] 1988	2	Bone-marrow transplantation	Not done	Not done
Greenspan [35] 1989	1	Renal transplant	Not done	Yes
Syrjänen [36] 1989	1	Leukemia	Not done	Yes
Schmidt-Westhausen [37] 1990	1	Heart transplant	Helper/suppressor 0.2	Yes (immuno-histo-chemistry)
MacLeod [38] 1990	1	Renal transplant	Not done	Yes
Reggiani [39] 1990	1	Liver transplant	Not done	Not done
Kanitakis [40] 1991	1	Renal transplant	Not done	Yes
Ficarra [41] 1991	1	Myelodysplastic syndrome	547	Yes
Epstein [34] 1991	8	Bone marrow transplant	Not done	2/8
Itin [30] 1991	7	Renal transplant	37-1715	1/1
Schmidt-Westhausen [24] 1991	2	Heart transplant	Helper/suppressor 2.0	2/2
Marcoux [42] 1991	1	Renal transplant	Not done	Yes (electron-microscopy-
Eisenberg [43] 1992	2	No immuno-suppression	Not done	2/2
Felix [44] 1992	1	No immuno-suppression	365	Yes
Epstein [45] 1993	10	Bone marrow transplant	not done	3/10
Schmidt-Westhausen [46]	3	Liver transplant	Helper/suppressor 1.04/1.54/1.68	Yes (electron-microscopy)
Konzelberg 1993	1	Osler disease	251	Yes (electron-microscopy)
Lozada-Nur [47] 1994	4	No immuno-suppression	Not done	4/4
Flückiger [48] 1994	1	Ulcerative colitis	170	Yes (electron-microscopy)
King [32] 1994	18	Renal transplant	Not done	Not done
Schiodt [49] 1995	1	Behcet's disease	595	Yes
Kaminsky [50] 1995	1	Fabry's disease	449	Not done
Miranda [51] 1996	1	Systemic lupus erythematosus	–	–
Zakrzweska [52] 1995	1	Bronchial asthma	Normal	Yes
Blomgren [53] 1996	1	Multiple myeloma	Not done	Yes

OHL in organ transplant or otherwise severely immunosuppressed patients without HIV-infection: prevalence and own experience

In 1988 the first cases of OHL-like lesions in organ transplant patients without HIV-infection appeared in the literature [5, 6]. Further severely immunosuppressed patients have been reported with the same constellation (Table I). Nowadays, it is concluded that OHL is not restricted to HIV-infected persons but that it is a marker for severe immunosuppression [29]. The fact that EBV can be found in oropharyngeal excretions in immunosuppressed and even healthy people provides a clue as to why OHL is not restricted to HIV-infection [17]. The marked decrease of Langerhans cells in OHL indicates a dysfunction of the immune system. During the last few years we have observed more than 10 renal transplant patients with OHL, one of which had been infected with HIV from the renal graft. In 6 out of 7 patients of on early study no HIV-infection was present [30]. In a prospective study on 50 renal transplant patients (28 men, 22 women), 4 patients (2 men, 2 women) (8%) with OHL were found [31]; in addition, a bone-marrow transplanted patient with OHL was documented. King et al. [32] found a 11.3% prevalence of OHL in renal transplant recipients versus 0% in controls. In another study, no OHL cases were found among 100 HIV-negative immunocompromised patients with haematologic or other malignancies [33]. Epstein et al. [34] reported on eight out of 50 patients that had undergone bone marrow transplantation with suspicious lesions of OHL. In two patients of his series histology was compatible with OHL and EBV-DNA was found in the lesional tissue. Another patient showed clinically and histologically typical features of OHL, but EBV could not be demonstrated. This patient seems to have pseudo-oral hairy leukoplakia.

In conclusion, OHL is not restricted to HIV infection and may serve as marker for severe immunosuppression as found in organ transplanted patients.

References

1. King GN, Healy CM, Glover MT, et al. Increased prevalence of dysplastic and malignant lip lesions in renal-transplant recipients. N Engl J Med 1995 ; 332 : 1052-7.

2. Oda D, Persson GR, Haigh WG, Sabath DE, Penn I, Aziz S. Oral presentation of posttransplantation lymphoproliferative disorders. An unusual manifestation. Transplantation 1996 ; 61 : 435-40.

3. Menni S, Beretta D, Piccinno R, Ghio L. Cutaneous and oral lesions in 32 children after renal transplantation. Pediatr Dermatol 1991 ; 8 : 194-8.

4. Silverberg NB, Singh A, Echt AF, Laude TA. Lingual fungiform papillae hypertrophy with cyclosporin A. Lancet 1996 ; 348 : 967.

5. Itin P, Rufli T, Rüdlinger R, et al. Oral hairy leukoplakia in a HIV-negative renal transplant patient: a marker for immunosuppression? Dermatologica 1988 ; 177 : 126-8.

6. Epstein JB, Priddy RW, Sherlock CH. Hairy leukoplakia-like lesions in immunosuppressed patients following bone marrow transplantation. Transplantation 1988 ; 46 : 462-4.

7. Itin PH. Oral hairy leukoplakia. 10 years on. Dermatology 1993 ; 187 : 159-63.

8. Itin PH, Bircher AJ, Litzisdorf Y, Rudin C. Oral hairy leukoplakia in a child: confirmation of the clinical diagnosis by ultrastructural examination of exfoliative cytologic specimens. Dermatology 1994 ; 189 : 167-9.

9. Mabruk M, Flint SR, Coleman DC, Toner M, Atkins GJ. Diagnosis and treatment of oral hairy leukoplakia. J Eur Acad Dermatol 1996 ; 6 : 127-34.

10. Schiodt M, Greenspan D, Daniels TE, Greenspan JS. Clinical and histologic spectrum of oral hairy leukoplakia. *Oral Surg Oral Med Oral Pathol* 1987 ; 64 : 716-20.

11. Fernández JF, Benito C, Lizaldez EB, Montañés MA. Oral hairy leukoplakia: a histopathologic study of 32 cases. *Am J Dermatopathol* 1990 ; 12 : 571-8.

12. Daniels TE, Greenspan D, Greenspan JS, *et al*. Absence of Langerhans cells in oral hairy leukoplakia, an AIDS-associated lesion. *J Invest Dermatol* 1987 ; 89 : 178-82.

13. Talacko AA, Teo CG, Griffin BE, Johnson NW. Epstein-Barr virus receptors but not viral DNA are present in normal and malignant oral epithelium. *J Oral Pathol Med* 1991 ; 20 : 20-5.

14. Thomas JA, Felix DH, Wray D, Southam JC, Cubie HA, Crawford DH. Epstein-Barr virus gene expression and epithelial cell differentiation in oral hairy leukoplakia. *Am J Pathol* 1991 ; 139 : 1369-80.

15. Niedobitek G, Young LS, Lau R, *et al*. Epstein-Barr virus infection in oral hairy leukoplakia: virus replication in the absence of a detectable latent phase. *J Gen Virol* 1991 ; 72 : 3035-46.

16. Sandvej K, Krenacs L, Hamilton-Dutoit SJ, Rindum JL, Pindborg JJ, Pallesen G. Epstein-Barr virus latent and replicative gene expression in oral hairy leukoplakia. *Histopathology* 1992 ; 20 : 387-95.

17. Diaz-Mitoma F, Preiksaitis JK, Leung WC, Tyrrell DLJ. DNA-DNA dot hybridization to detect Epstein-Barr virus in throat washings. *J Infect Dis* 1987 ; 155 : 297-303.

18. Ferbas J, Rahman MA, Kingsley LA, *et al*. Frequent oropharyngeal shedding of Epstein-Barr virus in homosexual men during early HIV infection. *AIDS* 1992 ; 6 : 1273-8.

19. Walling DM, Edmiston SN, Sixbey JW, Abdel-Hamid M, Resnick L, Raab-Traub N. Coinfection with multiple strains of the Epstein-Barr virus in human immunodeficiency virus-associated hairy leukoplakia. *Proc Natl Acad Sci USA* 1992 ; 89 : 6560-4.

20. Walling DM, Clark NM, Markovitz DM, et al. Epstein-Barr virus coinfection and recombination in non-human immunodeficiency virus-associated oral hairy leukoplakia. *J Infect Dis* 1995 ; 171 : 1122-30.

21. Schmidt-Westhausen A, Gelderblom HR, Hetzer R, Reichart PA. Demonstration of Epstein-Barr virus in scrape material of lateral border of tongue in heart transplant patients by negative staining electron microscopy. *J Oral Pathol Med* 1991 ; 20 : 215-7.

22. Mabruk MJEMF, Flint SR, Toner M, *et al*. In situ hybridization and the polymerase chain reaction (PCR) in the analysis of biopsies and exfoliative cytology specimens for definitive diagnosis of oral hairy leukoplakia. *J Oral Pathol Med* 1994 ; 23 : 302-8.

23. Webster-Cyriaque J, Edwards RH, Quinlivan EB, Patton L, Wohl D, Raab-Traub N. Epstein-Barr virus and human herpesvirus 8 prevalence in human immunodeficiency virus-associated oral mucosal lesions. *J Infect Dis* 1997 ; 175 : 1324-32.

24. Lau R, Middeldorp J, Farrell PJ. Epstein-Barr virus gene expression in oral hairy leukoplakia. *Virology* 1993 ; 195 : 463-74.

25. Palefsky JM, Berline J, Penaranda ME, Lennette ET, Greenspan D, Greenspan JS. Sequence variation of latent membrane protein-1 of Epstein-Barr virus strains associated with hairy leukoplakia. *J Infect Dis* 1996 ; 173 : 710-4.

26. Green TL, Greenspan JS, Greenspan D, De Souza YG. Oral lesions mimicking hairy leukoplakia: a diagnostic dilemma. *Oral Surg Oral Med Oral Pathol* 1989 ; 67 : 422-6.

27. Itin PH, Rufli T. Oral hairy leukoplakia. *Int J Dermatol* 1992 ; 31 : 301-6.

28. Conklin RJ, Blasberg B. Common inflammatory diseases of the mouth. *Int J Dermatol* 1991 ; 30 : 323-35.

29. Cathomas G. Oral hairy leukoplakia. *Acta Derm Venereol (Stockh)* 1990 ; 70 : 362-3.

30. Itin P, Rufli T, Huser B, Rüdlinger R. Orale Haarleukoplakie bei nierentransplantierten Patienten. *Hautarzt* 1991 ; 42 : 487-91.

31. Itin PH, Grimm R, Huser B. Enoral complications in renal transplant recipients. *Dermatology* 1992 ; 185 : 227-8.

32. King GN, Healy CM, Glover MT, *et al*. Prevalence and risk factors associated with leukoplakia, hairy leukoplakia, erythematous candidiasis, and gingival hyperplasia in renal transplant recipients. *Oral Surg Oral Med Oral Pathol* 1994 ; 78 : 718-26.

33. Ramael M, Colebunders R, Colpaert C, et al. The prevalence of hairy leukoplakia in HIV seropositive and HIV seronegative immunocompromised patients. *Int JSTD AIDS* 1992 ; 3 : 251-4.

34. Epstein JB, Sherlock CH, Greenspan JS. Hairy leukoplakia-like lesions following bone-marrow transplantation. *AIDS* 1991 ; 5 : 101-2.

35. Greenspan D, Greenspan JS, De Souza YG, Ungar AM. Oral hairy leukoplakia in an HIV-negative renal transplant recipient. *J Oral Pathol Med* 1989 ; 18 : 32-4.

36. Syrjänen S, Laine P, Happonen RP, Niemelä M. Oral hairy leukoplakia is not a specific sign of HIV-infection but related to immunosuppression in general. *J Oral Pathol Med* 1989 ; 18 : 28-31.

37. Schmidt-Westhausen A, Gelderblom HR, Reichart PA. Oral hairy leukoplakia in an HIV-seronegative heart transplant patient. *J Oral Pathol Med* 1990 ; 19 : 192-4.

38. MacLeod RI, Long LQ, Soames JV, Ward MK. Oral hairy leukoplakia in an HIV-negative renal transplant patient. *Br Dent J* 1990 ; 169 : 208-9.

39. Reggiani M, Pauluzzi P. Hairy leucoplakia in liver transplant patient. *Acta Derm Venereol (Stockh)* 1990 ; 70 : 87-8.

40. Kanitakis J, Euvrard S, Lefrancois N, Hermier C, Thivolet J. Oral hairy leukoplakia in a HIV-negative renal graft recipient. *Br J Dermatol* 1991 ; 124 : 483-6.

41. Ficarra G, Miliani A, Adler-Storthz K, et al. Recurrent oral condylomata acuminata and hairy leukoplakia: an early sign of myelodysplastic syndrome in an HIV-seronegative patient. *J Oral Pathol Med* 1991 ; 20 : 398-402.

42. Marcoux C, Bourlond A, Malfait Y, Kwembeke F. Leucoplasie orale et immunodépression. *Ann Dermatol Venereol* 1991 ; 118 : 457-60.

43. Eisenberg E, Krutchkoff D, Yamase H. Incidental oral hairy leukoplakia in immunocompetent persons. A report of two cases. *Oral Surg Oral Med Oral Pathol* 1992 ; 74 : 332-3.

44. Felix DH, Watret K, Wray D, Southam JC. Hairy leukoplakia in an HIV-negative, nonimmunosuppressed patient. *Oral Surg Oral Med Oral Pathol* 1992 ; 74 : 563-6.

45. Epstein JB, Sherlock CH, Wolber RA. Hairy leukoplakia after bone marrow transplantation. *Oral Surg Oral Med Oral Pathol* 1993 ; 75 : 690-5.

46. Schmidt-Westhausen A, Gelderblom HR, Neuhaus P, Reichart PA. Epstein-Barr virus in lingual epithelium of liver transplant patients. *J Oral Pathol Med* 1993 ; 22 : 274-6.

47. Lozada-Nur F, Robinson J, Regezi JA. Oral hairy leukoplakia in nonimmunosuppressed patients. Report of four cases. *Oral Surg Oral Med Oral Pathol* 1994 ; 78 : 599-602.

48. Flückiger R, Laifer G, Itin P, Meyer B, Lang C. Oral hairy leukoplakia in a patient with ulcerative colitis. *Gastroenterology* 1994 ; 106 : 506-8.

49. Schiodt M, Norgaard T, Greenspan JS. Oral hairy leukoplakia in an HIV-negative woman with Behcet's syndrome. *Oral Surg Oral Med Oral Pathol Oral Radiol Endod* 1995 ; 79 : 53-6.

50. De Kaminsky AR, Kaminsky C, Fernandez Blanco G, et al. Hairy leukoplakia in an HIV-seronegative patient. *Int J Dermatol* 1995 ; 34 : 420-4.

51. Miranda C, Lozada-Nur F. Oral hairy leukoplakia of an HIV-negative patient with systemic lupus erythematosus. *Compend Contin Educ Dent* 1996 ; 17 : 408-10.

52. Zakrzewska JM, Speight PM. Oral hairy leukoplakia in a HIV-negative asthmatic patient on systemic steroids. *J Oral Pathol Med* 1995 ; 24 : 282-4.

53. Blomgren J, Bäck H. Oral hairy leukoplakia in a patient with multiple myeloma. *Oral Surg Oral Med Oral Pathol Oral Radiol Endod* 1996 ; 82 : 408-10.

13

Cutaneous manifestations of opportunistic infections (excluding viral and parasitic ones)

Jacqueline CHEVRANT-BRETON
*Deparment of Dermatology, Centre Hospitalier Régional
et Universitaire de Rennes-Pontchaillou, Rennes, France.*

Along with graft rejection, infections are the main complications developing in organ transplant recipients [1-5].

Opportunistic infections can be defined as infections due to agents which are not usually pathogenic unless they develop in an immunosuppressed host, or as those due to regular pathogens when they cause unusually extensive or aggressive disease.

Etiopathogenic factors of opportunistic infections

The skin and mucosae are the first barrier against infections from the external environment. Any alteration of this barrier (be it accidental, iatrogenic or even nosocomial), a change of skin flora or moistening of the skin under occlusive dressings contribute to skin infection. The blood supply of the skin can favour a metastatic spread from viscera, gut or the respiratory tract to the skin, or from a primary skin site to blood and viscera. The immune status of the patient is mainly determined by the immunosuppressive drugs but also by the viral status (especially cytomegalovirus) [5, 6] which aggravates immunosuppression. On the other hand, the nature of organ transplantation influences the course of infections; these are more severe in liver and heart than in kidney transplant recipients.

Chronology of infections

Almost the same pattern is observed in all types of organ transplantation. During the first month post-transplant, three types of infections can develop:
– those present in the allograft recipient prior to transplantation (mostly bacterial);
– those transmitted by the allograft,
– those due to surgery, usually caused by bacteria and candida.

Between the first and the sixth post-transplant month, infections are due to immuno-modulating viruses (mainly CMV) and opportunistic pathogens (*Pneumo-cystis carinii*, *Listeria monocytogenes* and fungi). In the late period (after 6 months) chronic viral infections are observed. Patients with a poor allograft function with some degree of rejection are at higher risk for opportunistic infections; reduction of the immunosuppressive treatment or even retransplantation may be necessary.

Clinical aspects of opportunistic infections

Skin lesions are usually atypical or non-specific (*Table I*). Acute, diffuse or rash lesions suggest an invasive systemic dissemination whereas a unique, chronic lesion suggests a primary localized disease. An epidemic outbreak of infection is usually the result of nosocomial contamination. Some infections are restricted to limited geographic areas. They all must be differentiated from other skin lesions, especially of iatrogenic origin.

The diagnosis of opportunistic infection must be confirmed by strict identification of the presumed pathogen, if possible within two or more lesions, by direct examination and cultures. Multiple infections with bacteria, viruses, fungi and/or parasites may develop in the same patient, even within the same lesion. The diagnosis of systemic fungal infection is often difficult since the symptoms are unreliable and often absent (except from fever). Laboratory tests should be carried out when no biopsy can be obtained; however blood cultures can be negative and serological tests are of limited value. *In vitro* assessment of fungi sensitivity to drugs is not as reliable as with bacteria.

Processing of the skin should be performed as summarized in *Table II*, so as to cover the full spectrum of bacteria, fungi, parasites and viruses. A new application of an anti-BCG antibody for rapid detection of various tissue micro-organisms, namely bacteria and fungi (but not spirochetes, viruses and protozoa) has recently been proposed [7].

Bacterial infections

Ecthyma gangrenosum

Ecthyma gangrenosum and/or necrotic cellulitis are caused by *Pseudomonas aeruginosa*, but also *Pseudomonas maltophilia* [8], other gram-negative bacteria and staphylococci. Septicaemia should be suspected when multiple petechial, ecchymotic or necrotic lesions appear suddenly. The diagnosis must be confirmed by biopsy and/or blood cultures so as to eliminate aspergillosis, mycobacteriosis and deep fungal infections.

Atypical bacteria

Other new atypical bacteria such as *Leuconostoc*, *Bacillus subtilis* and *Rhodococcus equi* are new candidates for skin infection.

Table I. Dermatological symptoms of opportunistic infections and their etiologic agents in organ grafted patients (modified from [1] and [2]).

Abscesses	*Aspergillus spp, Chaetoconidium, Cryptococcus neoformans, Fusarium solani, Mucoraceae, Mycobacterium avium-intracellulare, M. fortuitum, M. kansasii, Nocardia spp, Pseudomonas aeruginosa, T. Rubrum, M. canis*
Cellulitis	*Aspergillus spp, Candida spp, C. neoformans, Histoplasma capsulatum, Mucoraceae, M. kansasii, Nocardia spp, Paecilomyces, Pseudomonas aeruginosa, Prototheca spp*
Ecthyma gangrenosum	*Candida spp, Mucoraceae, Pseudomonas aeruginosa,* other gram-negative bacteria, *Scedosporium*
Erythematous macules	*Alternaria alternata, Aspergillus spp, Mucoraceae, H. capsulatum,* HIV primoinfection
Haemorrhagic lesions	*A. alternata, Aspergillus spp, Candida spp, C. neoformans, H. capsulatum, Trichosporon beigelii*
Papules, nodules	*Aspergillus spp, Candida spp, C. neoformans, Fusarium spp., H. capsulatum, Mucoraceae, M. tuberculosis* (miliary), *M. chelonei, M. fortuitum, M. kansasii, M. marinum, M. szulgai, Prototheca spp, T. beigelii, T. rubrum, Pneumocystis carinii, Rochalimea*
Plaques	*A. alternata, Aspergillus spp, Candida spp, C. neoformans, M. kansasii, M. tuberculosis, Prototheca spp, Coccidioides immitis, H. capsulatum.*
Pustules	*Aspergillus spp, C. neoformans, Fusarium spp, H. capsulatum, Mucoraceae, M. kansasii, Prototheca spp*
Subcutaneous nodules, panniculitis	*Candida spp, Chaetoconidium, H. capsulatum, Mucoraceae, M. fortuitum, M. intracellulare, M. kansasii, M. marinum, M. tuberculosis, M. chelonei, M. malmoense, Nocardia spp, Scytalidium hyalinum, Fusarium solani, Pseudomonas aeruginosa*
Cysts	*Exophiala janselmei, Scedosporium*
Blisters, vesicles	*Aspergillus spp, Alternaria spp, Candida spp, C. neoformans,* Herpes simplex, herpes zoster, *Mucoraceae, Prototheca spp, Pseudomonas aeruginosa*
Ulcers	*Candida spp, Rhizopus spp, H. capsulatum,* cytomegalovirus
Verrucous and keratotic lesions	*Alternaria spp, C. immitis, Blastomyces dermatitidis, Exophiala spp,* Papilloma virus, scabies
Pseudo-molluscum contagiosum	*Cryptococcus, Penicillium marneffei*
Angiomatoid lesions	*Bartonella (Rochalimea)*
Sporotrichoid dissemination	Sporotrichosis, mycobacteriosis, fusariosis, histoplasmosis, coccidioidomycosis, nocardiosis, blastomycosis, leishmaniasis

Atypical mycobacterial infections

Atypical mycobacterial infections are not uncommon [9]: about 100 cases have been reported, two thirds of which after kidney transplantation. Non-tuberculous mycobacterial infections (NTM) appear late in the post-transplantation period and the diagnosis is usually delayed. NTM are often the cause of chronic infection of the skin and soft tissue of extremities, manifesting with violaceous painful nodules, progressing to abscesses with occasionally a sporotrichoid diffusion [10]. Tenosynovitis and osteoarthritis can occur. General symptoms are usually absent; however, pulmonary involvement is present in about 1/3 of cases and dissemination in about 50% of cases. The diagnosis relies on the identification of the type of NTM (*M. kansasii, fortuitum chelonei, marinum, avium, scrofulaceum*...) in abscess fluid or in biopsy specimens by histochemical stains and cultures. Management usually associates surgery, reduction of immunosuppressive treatment and antibiotics.

Table II. Processing of skin for the diagnosis of opportunistic infections

Material
- Skin scraping - puncture wound drainage, curettage, skin biopsy, hair, nails...

Transport
- Saline solution (fungi)
- Sterile water (bacteria)
- Special medium for viruses
- Formaldehyde (for histological examination)

Direct preparations
- Wet mount for fungal elements
  - Potassium hydroxide
  - Saline solution
  - India ink
- Stained smears
  - Gram's stain
  - Acid-fast stain
- Immunofluorescence (herpes virus)

Histologic examination
- Haematoxylin-eosin stain
  - PAS stain
  - Silver methenamine (Gomori-Grocott)
  - Acid-fast stain
  - BCG immunostain [7]
  - Special techniques - PCR

Cultures
- Aerobic and anaerobic bacteria
  - Thioglycollate broth
  - Sheep blood agar
- Atypical mycobacteria (25°-37°C)
  - Löwenstein-Jensen medium
  - Middle brook 7.H. 10 agar
- Fungi
  - Sabouraud's dextrose agar
  - Mycosal agar
  - Special media (e.g. for dematiae)

Nocardiosis

Nocardiosis [11] is caused by a soil-borne, ubiquitous aerobic actinomycetes; this is usually introduced through the respiratory tract and may then progress to an acute or chronic infection, or even disseminate through the blood to the skeleton, soft tissues and the nervous system. Four types of nocardiosis have been described, *i.e.* mycetoma, lymphocutaneous infection, superficial skin infection (abscess, cellulitis...), and disseminated disease. In the USA, cutaneous nocardiosis [12] is infrequent in organ transplant recipients (less than 0.2% after renal transplantation), especially after the introduction of cyclosporin [13]. Multiple risk factors are known, including (among others) early rejection, major immunosuppressive therapy, neutropenia, uraemia, and age below 10 or over 40 years.

The diagnosis is made by skin or organ biopsy and culture of skin, sputum or tracheal washing so as to determine the primary or metastatic nature of the infection, the responsible species of Nocardia (*N. asteroides* or more rarely *N. brasiliensis*) and the mode of contamination. Treatment usually associates antibiotics (sulfonamides, tetracyclines, amikacin, amoxicillin associated with clavulanic acid...) and surgery.

Actinomycosis

Actinomycosis of the face has been described in a renal transplant patient [14]. It is due to *Actinomyces israeli*, a gram-positive, anaerobic non-acid fast bacterium, a common saprophyte of the oral, respiratory and digestive tract, and is promoted by traumatisms and tooth caries. It displays the characteristic histological aspect of a gram-positive actinomycotic granule. Oral or i.v. penicillin in high doses is the treatment of choice.

Other atypical bacterial infections

Botryomycosis

Botryomycosis is a rare chronic suppurative disease caused by various bacteria; it is often misdiagnosed as a fungal infection because of its histological aspect (bacteria in clusters surrounded by an amorphous eosinophilic coat). It is usually resistant to antibiotic therapy. One fatal case of mural endocarditis with cutaneous botryomycosis has been described in a heart transplant patient [15].

Malakoplakia

Malakoplakia [16] is an inflammatory disorder (33 cases reported until 1996) caused by several gram-negative rods and gram-positive cocci, and is characterised by accumulation of phagocytic macrophages filled with round, concentric, lamellar, von Kossa-positive inclusion bodies. It has been reported in nine renal transplant [16] and one heart transplant recipient [17] and usually manifests with perineal, inguinal, abdominal or facial nodules and abscess-like lesions.

Bartonellosis

Bartonellosis or bacillary angiomatosis [18], due to *Rochalimea quintana* or *Rochalimea henselae*, presents as solitary or multiple angiomatoid nodules of the skin sometimes accompanied by peliosis, hepatitis and fever. One case of abscess of the sternum has been described in a renal transplant recipient [19]. The diagnosis is confirmed by histochemical stains (Whartin-Starry) and ultrastructural demonstration of the responsible pathogen within the lesions. Macrolides are usually successful.

Opportunistic fungi

General comments

Opportunistic fungal infections occur mostly between the first and sixth months after organ transplantation [1, 20]. The incidence and severity of invasive fungal infections depend on the nature of the grafted organ. They occur in about 5% of renal, 10% of heart and over 20% of liver transplant recipients [21]. New fungal opportunists are continually appearing [22]; some of them (such as *Candida species*, *Aspergillus* or *Fusarium*) are invasive, cause fungaemia and are responsible for a high mortality rate. Several other fungi are rare and usually unknown. The diagnosis can be very difficult; it necessitates the use of special culture media devoid of cyclohexamide (which inhibits saprophytes) and prolonged incubation for up to 4-6 weeks to permit identification of slow-growing organisms. Furthermore, some fungi can change their morphology in different tissues and may thus lead to a false diagnosis of species [22]. The less pathogenic the fungus is the more strict the criteria should be: concordance of two or three direct examinations and cultures, histologic demonstration of the fungus in the epidermis and/or the dermis. Some of these fungi have not (yet) been observed after solid organ transplantation, but are known to occur after bone marrow transplantation or in the course of other immunodeficiency conditions [23]. The symptoms may vary depending on the route of entry. The skin and intestine are the main ones. Nasal or sinus infection extends sometimes to the face and the palate as facial granuloma. The treatment of these infections is not well codified [24, 25].

Classification of fungi

Fungi can be classified on the basis of their morphology [20].

- Yeasts are unicellular organisms; they multiply asexually by budding (*Candida, Cryptococcus, Trichosporon, Malassezia, Saccharomyces*).
- Molds have hyphae; they multiply asexually by spore production or fragmentation of hyphae and are of 2 types:
    - Septate hyphae with cross walls include:
        - Hyaline fungi, comprising:
            1) *Aspergillus* and other hyalohyphomycoses (*Fusarium scedosporium, Acremonium, Paecilomyces, Scopulariopsis...*),
            2) Dermatophytes (*Trichophyton-Microsporum-Epidermophyton* genera)
            3) Dimorphic fungi (*Histoplasma capsulatum, Penicillium marneffei, Coccidioides immitis, Sporothrix schenckii*),
        - Dematiaceous fungi (*Alternaria, Exophiala, Wangiella sp...*);
    - Aseptate hyphae characterize the Zygomycete class – zygomycosis or mucormycosis (obsolete term of phycomycosis) of different genera (*rhizopus* and *Mucor* species).

Yeasts

Candida

Candida (especially *Candida albicans*) [20-21] is the most common cause of systemic fungal infection, but other species are also involved, such as *C. tropicalis, C. parapsilosis, C. glabrata, C. lusitaniae, C. pseudotropicalis, C. guillermondi*. The mortality rate is high (70-75%) except for *C. parapsilosis* (30%), frequently showing skin lesions (23%). The classical triad of disseminated candidiasis associates fever, myalgias and discrete, painless, erythematous papulonodules with a pale centre, or occasionally purpuric or pustular-necrotic lesions. The diagnosis is made by culture of skin biopsy or blood (positive in only half of cases), stools, urine, sputum, even if correlation with an invasive disease is not always clearly established. Amphotericin B remains the treatment of choice. When possible, catheters should be removed. 5 fluorocytosin (5 FC) can be added if *C. tropicalis* is suspected.

Cryptococcus

Cryptococcus neoformans [26-28] is found in the soil, in pigeon droppings and nesting places. Inhalation of *C. neoformans* can be silent until dissemination occurs *via* the bloodstream, mostly to the central nervous system and the skin (10-20%). Cutaneous lesions can be isolated for months before the infection becomes overt; they can be exceptionally primary. Various non-specific lesions have been described, such as papules occasionally umbilicated mimicking molluscum contagiosum, vesicles or pustules, ulcers, subcutaneous masses, purpura, cellulitis, vegetating plaques and oral ulcers [26]. The diagnosis is readily made with India ink stain of yeast capsules in skin touch, smear or biopsy and late agglutination for cryptococcal antigen, but culture of blood and/or cerebrospinal fluid must confirm this test. Amphotericin B and 5 FC are the main treatments and should be given for at least 4 to 6 weeks; azoles have been successful on some occasions.

Trichosporon beigelii

Trichosporon beigelii (or *cutaneum*) is a yeast of the soil occasionally found as part of the normal flora of the skin and mouth; it causes white piedra of terminal hair and occasionally nail disease. Immunosuppressed neutropenic patients can present disseminated trichosporonosis of the lungs, kidneys, liver, spleen and heart. Skin lesions are found in 30% of patients; they manifest as purpuric papules or nodules with central necrosis (trunk, arms and face) or as cellulitis of the leg. Dermal invasion with vasculitis has been observed histologically. Cultures are positive in 90% of cases [29]. The prognosis is poor, partly because the yeast is resistant to amphotericin B. Only three cases of cutaneous infection in organ transplant recipients have been reported [30-31].

Molds

Septate molds

Hyaline hyphae
Aspergillus [20, 32, 33]
Aspergillosis is the second major fungal complication in organ transplant patients. It is mostly due to *Aspergillus fumigatus*, rarely to *A. flavus*, *A. niger*, *A. terreus*, *A. nidulans* or *A. ustus*. Cutaneous aspergillosis is usually secondary to systemic dissemination and manifests with a maculopapular eruption progressing to pustular and necrotic lesions, abscess or granulomas. A primary infection can occur associated with adhesive tape, armboards, indwelling catheters or even with air contamination (sometimes during hospital renovations). Cutaneous lesions include erythematous-violaceous, haemorrhagic necrotic lesions, cellulitis, abscesses, ulcers and disseminated papulonodules. The diagnosis should be made rapidly in a patient with unremitting fever, pulmonary distress and shock, by direct examination of skin lesions and cultures (cultures of sputum, blood and cerebrospinal fluid are often negative). Vascular thromboses are frequent with *Aspergillus* (as well as with zygomycosis). In case of systemic infection the prognosis is poor. Treatment with amphotericin B and/or 5 FC is urging; itraconazole may be used.

Other hyalohyphomycoses
They are rare but emerging:
– *Fusarium* [34] is a serious pathogen. *F. solani*, a ubiquitous soil saprophyte, may contaminate wounds, burns or the eyes; it can also disseminate mainly from the skin or from the gut, especially in neutropenic patients. Skin lesions are present in over 80% of cases. One of the earliest signs is an eruption of erythematous, papulopustular and necrotic nodules of the skin and oral mucosa, sometimes with a sporotrichoid spreading. Histology is similar to aspergillosis. The mortality rate is high (over 70%); neutrophil recovery is necessary because of a frequent resistance to amphotericin B and 5 FC.
– *Paecilomyces* [20]. *P. lilacinus* may cause cellulitis in renal transplant recipients.
– *Scedosporium* (*S. apiospermum*) or *Monosporium* or *pseudo-Allescheria boydii* is a frequent cause of mycetoma in the USA, disseminating exclusively in neutropenic or organ transplant recipients [35]. Skin lesions present as ecthymatous nodules in 30% of cases and CNS involvement is present in 40% of cases. *S. apiospermum* and *S. prolificans* are often resistant to amphotericin B, 5 FC and azoles, therefore surgical resection of localized lesions may be necessary.
– *Acremonium* (*cephalosporium*) is mainly responsible for mycetoma in renal transplant recipients. Surgery is required but the course may be lethal [36].

Dermatophytes
Extensive atypical tinea of the face or the scalp may occur. Exceptionally, dermal invasion of *T. rubrum* [37] or *M. canis* [38] may cause granulomas, abscesses or cellulitis.

Dimorphic fungi
These fungi have two aspects, a mold phase at 25° C and a yeast phase at 37° C. They are infrequent in Europe but frequent in the USA and South America. They include *H. capsulatum, B. dermatitidis, Coccidioides immitis, P. brasiliensis* and *Sporothrix Schenckii* which are true pathogens, disseminating aggressively, often reactivating ancient disease in immunosuppressed patients.
• Histoplasmosis [20]. Oral ulcerative, nodular or vegetating lesions are frequent (about 20% of cases). Dissemination to the skin manifests with a painful erythematous rash, cellulitis or pseudo-erythema nodosum. Skin biopsy is the best method for a timely diagnosis, showing characteristic pseudo-encapsulated yeasts (2-4 µm) within macrophages. High dose amphotericin B is required.
• Coccidioidomycosis [20, 39] is a systemic mycosis encountered in the South-west part of the USA and in Central and South America. Skin lesions appear when the disease disseminates, manifesting with multiple papulonodules, plaques or suppurative verrucous granulomas that are often misdiagnosed. Amphotericin B and/or fluconazole or itraconazole is the best treatment.
• *Penicillium marneffei* [23] is found in South East Asia. The presence of papular molluscum contagiosum-like lesions in a patient with fever, anaemia, hepatomegaly and lymph-node enlargement should raise the diagnosis in an immunosuppressed patient.

Dematiaceous fungi
Dematiaceous fungi [20, 30, 40-48] are emerging pathogens in the 1980s. They are characteristic by virtue of their brown melanin pigment, readily visible in haematoxylin-eosin stained sections. Three types of diseases, probably representing different forms of a continuum, are caused by these fungi, including phaeohyphomycosis, chromoblastomycosis and mycetoma.

Phaeohyphomycosis
Phaeohyphomycosis is due to the interaction between the fungus and its host. It affects any organ including the skin. It can get various aspects in tissues, such as yeast-like cells, pseudo-hyphal elements, septate hyphae or all of them; staining for melanin may therefore be necessary. Cutaneous and especially subcutaneous localized skin lesions are frequent in kidney transplant recipients. Systemic forms may occur; they often start in the lung with dissemination to other organs such as the brain.

Chromoblastomycosis
Chromoblastomycosis, which represents a special form of phaeohyphomycosis, is a post-traumatic chronic localized infection of the skin manifesting with nodular, tumoural, verrucous, cicatricial lesions or plaques; muriform sclerotic bodies within a dermal inflammatory infiltrate and abscess are characteristic. Management includes surgery, associated with amphotericin B, 5 FC or azoles.

Mycetoma
Mycetoma is a tumour-like nodule containing granules.
• *Alternaria* [43-44] are ubiquitous molds of the soil acting as plant pathogens and airborne laboratory contaminants. They are involved in asthma and rarely in osteomyelitis, sinusitis and keratitis. More than 80 cases of dermal alternariosis have been reported, mostly in immunosuppressed patients. Lesions are promoted by local trauma; they manifest with unique or multiple ulcerative, vegetating or keratotic papulo-nodules on the limbs or the cephalic extremity (*Figures 17 and 18, page 219 and Figure 19, page 220*). They can be chronic, extensive or relapsing but systemic disease does not occur. Strict criteria of pathogenicity should be met. Cultures on special media are necessary to identify the genera, mostly *Alternaria alternata* or *A. stemphyloïdes, A. tenuissima* and *A. chartarum*. Spore-like bodies and hyphae are present in granulomatous or abscess-like lesions (*Figure 20, page 220*), sometimes causing vascular

damage. No codified treatment exists. Topical antifungals, oral azoles and surgery are required; tapering of immunosuppressive treatment is helpful.
• *Exophiala* [45, 46]. *E. janselmei* (the most frequent) but also *E. pisciphila*, *E. moniliae*, *E. spinifera*, are as ubiquitous in the environment as *Alternaria* sp. Following traumatic inoculation usually located on the distal limbs, they cause different types of phaeohyphomycotic lesions, including verrucous-keratotic (*Figure 21, page 220*), ulcerative or cystic lesions (*Figure 22, page 220*). Systemic fatal dissemination (often from the lung) is very unusual. Surgical resection of the cysts is necessary along with treatment with azoles (*e.g.* itraconazole).
• *Bipolaris* and *Exserohilum* [47] were first reported with *Drechsclera genera*. *B. spicifera* and *E. rostratum* are the main ones responsible for cutaneous nodular or ulcerative lesions, sinusitis and osteomyelitis. In heart transplant recipients they may disseminate through the blood (fungaemia) mainly to the CNS.
• *Wangiella dermatitis* [20] (*Fonsecae* or *Phialophora*) infection has mostly been described in Japan. Infection is usually post-traumatic and located to the skin, mucosae and lymph nodes but may disseminate to the brain and viscera. Most antifungals are ineffective and surgical treatment is usually necessary.
• *Cladophialophora bantiana* [48] has caused a recalcitrant ulcerated tumoural lesion in a renal transplant recipient and was cured with itraconazole.

Aseptate molds

Zygomycetes

Zygomycoses or mucormycosis [49] includes the genera *Rhizopus, Mucor, Rhizomucor* and *Absidia*. Four percent of them have been described in organ transplant patients, usually as skin ecthyma gangrenosum or deep cellulitis, frequently at the site of adhesive tape or skin trauma. Visceral dissemination is rare. Histologically, a dermal granulomatous infiltrate containing non-septate, thick-walled hyphae with right angle branching is typical. This angioinvasive fungus resembles *Aspergillus*. Contrasting with visceral involvement (lung, brain and gut), the prognosis of purely cutaneous mucormycosis is rather good, especially in acral (limb) localisations; however, long-term morbidity is substantial. Surgery with grafting plus amphotericin B are usually successful. In rare cases dissemination occurs to rhino-cerebral sites, skin, intestine and lungs.

Prototheca

Prototheca infection, mostly with *Prototheca wickerhamii*, is due to unicellular algae sometimes classified as fungi and growing on standard mycological media. It has been described in kidney transplant recipients [1, 50] and manifests with slowly enlarging eczematous plaques, herpetiform lesions, ulcers and cellulitis. The lesions develop on the head, the neck and the elbow, causing bursitis. Systemic dissemination is exceptional. Histologically it induces pseudoepitheliomatous changes and a dermal suppurative granulomatous infiltrate with often typical forms of morula that usually stain positively for fungal stains. The treatment is not codified. Surgery, when possible associated with amphotericin B and/or tetracyclines, is recommended; azoles such as itraconazole have been successful [50].

References

1. Wolfson JS, Sober AJ, Rubin RH. Dermatologic manifestations of infections in immunocompromised patients. *Medicine* 1985 ; 64 : 115-33.

2. Kaye E, Johnson A, Wolfson JS, Sober AJ. Dermatologic manifestations of infection in the compromised host. In : Rubin RH, Young LS, eds. *Clinical approach to infection in the compromised host*, third edition. London : Plenum Medical Book, 1994.

3. Gentry LO, Zeluff B, Kielhofner MA. Dermatologic manifestations of infectious diseases in cardiac transplant patients. *Infect Dis Clin North Am* 1994 ; 8 : 637-53.

4. Waser M, Maggiorini M, Lüthy A, Laske A, Von Segesser L, Mohacs P, Opravil M, Turina M, Follath F, Gallino A. Infectious complications in 100 consecutive heart transplant recipients. *Eur J Clin Microbiol Infect Dis* 1994 ; 13 : 12-8.

5. Castaldo P, Stratta RJ, Wood RP, Markin RS, Patil KD, Shaefer MS, Langnas AN, Reed EC, Li S, Pilen TJ, Shaw BW. Fungal disease in liver transplant recipients: a multivariate analysis of risk factors. *Transplant Proc* 1991 ; 23 : 1517-9.

6. Georges MJ, Snydman DR, Werner BG, Griffith J, Falagas ME, Dougherty NN, Rubin RH. The independant role of cytomegalovirus as a risk factor for invasive fungal disease in orthotopic liver transplant recipients. *Am J Med* 1997 ; 103 : 106-13.

7. Kutzner H, Argenyi BZ, Requena L, Rütten A, Hügel H. A new application of BCG antibody for rapid screening of various tissue microorganisms. *J Am Acad Dermatol* 1998 ; 38 : 56-60.

8. Burns RL, Lowe L. *Xanthomonas maltophilia* infection presenting as erythematous nodules. *J Am Acad Dermatol* 1997 ; 37 : 836-8.

9. Patel R, Roberts GD, Keating MR, Paya CV. Infections due to nontuberculous myco-bacteria in kidney, heart, and liver transplant recipients. *Clin Infect Dis* 1994 ; 19 : 263-73.

10. Dalovisio JR, Pankey GA. Dermatologic manifestations of nontuberculous mycobacterial diseases. *Infect Dis Clin North Am* 1994 ; 8, 3 : 677-88.

11. Lerner PI. Nocardiosis. *Clin Infect Dis* 1996 ; 22 : 891-905.

12. Kalb RE, Kaplan MH, Grossman ME. Cutaneous nocardiosis. *J Am Acad Dermatol* 1985 ; 13 : 125-33.

13. Arduino RC, Johnson PC, Miranda AG. Nocardiosis in renal transplant recipients undergoing immunosuppression with cyclosporin. *Clin Infect Dis* 1993 ; 16 : 505-12.

14. Rivera M, Marcen R, Aguilera A, Fernandez-Lucas M, Quereda C, Carrillo R, Ortuno J. Facial actinomycosis in a renal transplant patient. *Nephron* 1994 ; 68 : 149-50.

15. Defraigne JO, Demoulin JC, Piérard GE, Detry O, Limet R. Fatal mural endocarditis and cutaneous botryomycosis after heart transplantation. *Am J Dermatopathol* 1997 ; 19 : 602-5.

16. Lowitt MH, Kariniemi AL, Niemi KM, Kao GF. Cutaneous malakoplakia: a report of two cases and review of the literature. *J Am Acad Dermatol* 1996 ; 34 : 325-32.

17. Rémond B, Dompmartin A, De Pontville M, Moreau A, Mandard JC, Leroy D. Mala-koplakie cutanée chez un transplanté cardiaque. *Ann Dermatol Venereol* 1993 ; 120 : 805-8.

18. Adal KA, Cockerell CJ, Petri WA. Cat scratch disease bacillary angiomatosis and other infections due to Rochalimaea. *N Engl J Med* 1994 ; 330 : 1509-15.

19. Bruckert F, de Kerviler E, Zagdanski AM, Molina J, et al. Sternal abscess due to bartonella (*Rochalimae henselae*) in a renal transplant patient. *Skeletal Radiol* 1997 ; 26 : 431-3.

20. Radentz WH. Opportunistic fungal infections in immunocompromised hosts. *J Am Acad Dermatol* 1989 ; 20 : 989-1003.

21. Hibberd PL, Rubin RH. Clinical aspects of fungal infection in organ transplant recipients. *Clin Infect Dis* 1994 ; 19 : S33-40.

22. Perfect JR, Schell WA. The new fungal opportunists are coming. *Clin Infect Dis* 1996 ; 22 : S112-8.

23. Vartivarian SE, Anaissie EJ, Bodey GP. Emerging fungal pathogens in immunocom-promised patients: classification, diagnosis, and management. *Clin Infect Dis* 1993 ; 17 : 487-91.

24. Armstrong D. Treatment of opportunistic fungal infections. *Clin Infect Dis* 1993 ; 16 : 1-9.

25. Sanchez JL, Noskin GA. Recent advances in the management of opportunistic fungal infections. *Comp Ther* 1996 ; 22 : 703-12.

26. Haight DO, Esperanza LE, Greene JN, Sandin RL, DeGregorio MSR, Spiers ASD. Case report: cutaneous manifestations of cryptococcosis. *Am J Med Sci* 1994 ; 308 : 192-5.

27. Barfield L, Iacobelli D, Hasmimoto K. Secondary cutaneous cryptococcosis: case report and review of 22 cases. *J Cutan Pathol* 1988 ; 15 : 385-92.

28. Dupond A, Humbert P, Faivre B, Hory B, Barale T, Laurent R, Agache P. Localisations cutanées septicémiques d'une cryptococcose chez une greffée rénale. *Ann Dermatol Venereol* 1993 ; 120 : 612-5.

29. Piérard GE, Read D, Piérard-Franchimont C, Lother Y, Rurangirwa A, Arrese Estrada J. Cutaneous manifestations in systemic trichosporonosis. *Clin Exp Dermatol* 1992 ; 17 : 79-82.

30. Nahass GT, Rosenberg ST, Leonardi CL, Penneys SN. Disseminated infection with *Trichosporon beigelii*. Report of a case and review of the cutaneous and histological manifestations. *Arch Dermatol* 1993 ; 129 : 1020-3.

31. Mirza SH. Disseminated *Trichosporon beigelii* infection causing skin lesions in a renal transplant patient. *J Infect* 1993 ; 27 : 67-70.

32. Weitzman I. Saprophytic molds as agents of cutaneous and subcutaneous infection in the immunocompromised host. *Arch Dermatol* 1986 ; 122 : 1161-8.

33. Melda I. Cutaneous aspergillosis. *Dermatol Clin* 1996 ; 14 : 137-40.

34. Martino P, Gastaldi R, Raccah R, Girmenia C. Clinical patterns of Fusarium infections in immunocompromised patients. *J Infect* 1994 ; 28 : 7-15.

35. Lopes JO, Alves SH, Benevenga JP, Salla A, Khmohan C, Sylva CB. Subcutaneous pseudoallescheriasis in a renal transplant recipient. *Mycopathologia* 1994 ; 125 : 153-6.

36. Fincher RM, Fisher JF, Lovell RD, Newman CL, Espinel-Ingroff A. Infection due to the fungus acremonium (cephalosporium). *Medicine* 1991 ; 70, 6 : 398-409.

37. Novick NL, Tapia L, Bottone EJ. Invasive *Trichophyton rubrum* infection in an immunocompromised host. Case report and review of the literature. *Am J Med* 1987 ; 82 : 321-5.

38. Demidovich CW, Kornfeld BW, Gentry RH, Fitzpatrick JE. Deep dermatophyte infection with chronic draining nodules in an immunocompromised patient. *Cutis* 1995 ; 55 : 237-9.

39. Quimby SR, Connolly SM, Winkelmann RK, Smilack JD. Clinicopathologic spectrum of specific cutaneous lesions of disseminated coccidioidomycosis. *J Am Acad Dermatol* 1992 ; 26 : 79-85.

40. Fader RC, MacGinnis MR. Infections caused by dematiaceous fungi: chromoblastomycosis and phaeohyphomycosis. *Infect Dis Clin North Am* 1988 ; 2 : 925-38.

41. Singh N, Chang FY, Gayowski T, Marino IR. Infections due to dematiaceous fungi in organ transplant recipients: case report and review. *Clin Infect Dis* 1997 ; 24 : 369-74.

42. Rossmann SN, Cernoch PL, Davis JR. Dematiaceous fungi are an increasing cause of human disease. *Clin Infect Dis* 1996 ; 22 : 73-80.

43. Chevrant-Breton J, Boisseau-Lebreuil M, Freour E, Guiguen G, Launois B, Guelfi J. Les alternarioses cutanées humaines. À propos de 3 cas. Revue de la littérature. *Ann Dermatol Venereol* 1981 ; 108 : 653-62.

44. Chaidemenos G, Mourellou O, Karakatsanis G, Koussidou T, Panagiotidou D, Kapetis E. Cutaneous alternariosis in an immunocompromised patient. *Cutis* 1995 ; 56 : 145-50.

45. Sudduth EJ, Crumbley AJ, Farrar E. Phaeohyphomycosis due to *Exophiala species*: clinical spectrum of disease in humans. *Clin Infect Dis* 1992 ; 15 : 639-44.

46. Ronan SG, Uzoaru I, Nadimpalli V, Guitart J, Manaligod JR. Primary cutaneous phaeohyphomycosis: report of seven cases. *J Cutan Pathol* 1993 ; 20 : 223-8.

47. Adam RD, Paquin ML, Petersen EA, Saubolle MA, Rinaldi MG, Corgoran JG, Galgiani JN, Sobonya RE. Phaeohyphomycosis caused by the fungal genera *bipolaris* and *exserohilum*. A report of 9 cases and review of the literature. *Medicine* 1986, 65 : 203-17.

48. Jacyk WK, Du Bruyn JH, Holm N, Gryffenberg H, Karusseit VO. Cutaneous infection due to *Cladophialophora bantiana* in a patient receiving immunosuppressive therapy. *Br J Dermatol* 1997 ; 136 : 428-30.

49. Adam RD, Hunter G, Di Tomasso J, Comerci G. Mucormycosis: emerging prominence of cutaneous infections. *Clin Infect Dis* 1994 ; 19 : 67-76.

50. Boyd AS, Langley M, King LE. Cutaneous manifestations of Prototheca infections. *J Am Acad Dermatol* 1995; 32 : 758-64.

14

Extracutaneous tumors

Israel PENN

Department of Surgery, Transplantation Division, University of Cincinnati Medical Center, and Cincinnati Veterans Affairs Medical Center, Cincinnati, USA.

Physicians and, in particular, dermatologists should be aware of the complications of immunosuppressive therapy used to prevent and treat rejection of transplanted organs. A major problem is a wide variety of infections. In addition, each immunosuppressive drug has its own unique side effects. A third problem is an increased incidence of certain malignancies.

Overall there is a 3-4 fold increased risk of cancer compared with age-matched controls in the general population [1-8]. Prominent among the neoplasms are those arising in the skin. Overall the incidence of skin cancer is increased 4-21 fold, the highest rise being in areas of the world with high sunshine exposure. Apart from skin tumors, transplant patients do not exhibit an increased incidence of the neoplasms that are commonly seen in the general population (carcinomas of the lung, breast, prostate, colon, and invasive carcinomas of the uterine cervix). Instead, they are prone to develop a variety of mostly uncommon malignancies. Epidemiologic studies show increases of 28-49-fold of non-Hodgkin's lymphomas (NHL), 29-fold of lip carcinomas, 400-500-fold of Kaposi's sarcoma (KS), 100-fold of vulvar and anal carcinomas, 20 to 38-fold of hepatocellular carcinomas, 14-16-fold of *in situ* uterine cervical carcinomas, and small increases in sarcomas (excluding KS) and renal carcinomas [1-8]. This report is based on material collected by the Cincinnati transplant tumor registry (CTTR). The registry started collecting data in the fall of 1968 and gathers information from transplant centers throughout the world. Up till September 1997 the registry had data on 10,813 different types of cancer that occurred *de novo* after transplantation in 10,151 organ allograft recipients. In this report we shall mainly consider extracutaneous malignancies.

Types of malignancies

These are summarized in Table I.

Table I. 10,813 *de novo* cancers in organ allograft recipients

Type of neoplasm	N° of tumors*
Cancers of skin and lips	4,079
Lymphomas	1,801
Carcinomas of the lung	604
Kaposi's sarcoma	423
Carcinomas of uterus (cervix: 340, body: 64, unspecified: 4)	408
Carcinomas of the kidney (host kidney: 322, allograft kidney: 36, unspecified: 20)	378
Carcinomas of colon and rectum	365
Carcinomas of the breast	336
Carcinomas of the head and neck (excluding thyroid, parathyroid and eye)	302
Carcinomas of the vulva, perineum, penis, scrotum	267
Carcinomas of urinary bladder	240
Metastatic carcinoma (primary site unknown)	218
Carcinomas of prostate gland	200
Leukemias	192
Hepatobiliary carcinomas	161
Sarcomas (excluding Kaposi's sarcoma)	135
Carcinomas of thyroid gland	131
Cancers of stomach	126
Testicular carcinomas	82
Carcinomas of pancreas	79
Ovarian cancers	71
Miscellaneous tumors	215

*There were 10,151 patients of whom 621 (6%) had two or more distinct tumor types involving different organ systems. Of these, 39 patients each had 3 separate types of cancer and 1 had 4.

Time of appearance of cancers

The incidence of neoplasms increases with length of follow-up posttransplantation. An Australasian study of 6,596 patients showed that the percent probability of developing a malignancy following renal transplantation from cadaver donors 24 years postoperatively was 66% for skin tumors, 27% for non-skin neoplasms and 72% for any type of cancer [4]. These exceptional figures must be interpreted with caution as most malignancies were skin tumors (which are very common in Australia) and the number of 24 year survivors was small. Nevertheless, they emphasize the need to follow transplant patients indefinitely.

Review of the CTTR database showed that cancers occurred a relatively short time posttransplantation, with KS appearing at an average of 22 (median 13) months posttransplantation, lymphomas at an average of 34 (median 13) months, skin cancers at an average of 66 (median 51) months, and vulvar and perineal carcinomas appearing at the longest time posttransplantation, at an average of 115 (median 114) months [1-3]. If all tumors were considered the average time of their appearance was 64 (median 47) months.

Types of recipients

The 10,151 recipients comprised 8,312 who received kidney transplants, 1,041 heart, 464 liver, 173 bone marrow, 86 pancreas, 38 lung, 32 combined heart and lung, 4 upper-abdominal organ « cluster » transplants, and one small bowel transplant.

Age and gender of patients

The tumors occurred in a relatively young group of patients, whose average age at the time of transplantation was 43 years (range 8 days to 80 years). Forty percent were younger than 40 years at the time of transplantation. The average age of the patients at the time of diagnosis of their neoplasms was 48 years. Sixty-six percent of patients were male and 34% female, in keeping with the 2:1 ratio of male to female patients who undergo renal transplantation [1-3].

Organ-specific malignancies

Cancers of the skin and lips

These are discussed in detail elsewhere in this issue. A few facts from the CTTR are worth noting. They were the most common malignancies in the CTTR comprising 38% of all cancers. Of the 4,079 patients 3,592 (88%) had skin tumors, 239 (6%) had lip lesions, and 248 (6%) had cancers of the skin and lips.

In the general population most lymph node metastases and deaths from skin malignancies are caused by melanomas. In contrast squamous cell carcinomas (SCCs) were much more aggressive in transplant patients than the general population and accounted for the majority of lymph node metastases and deaths from skin cancer [1-3]. Thus, 5.7% of patients with skin or lip tumors in the CTTR had lymph node metastases. Of these 74% were from SCCs and only 17% from melanomas. Similarly 4.9% of patients died of skin or lip cancers, with 60% of deaths being from SCC and only 30% from melanomas [1-3]. Of 35 patients with Merkel cell tumors 20 (57%) had lymph node metastases and 17 (49%) died of their malignancies.

Lymphomas and lymphoproliferations

Only 52 (3%) of 1,801 lymphomas and lymphoproliferations (Table I) were cases of Hodgkin's disease whereas it comprises 10% of lymphomas in the general population. Similarly, myeloma and plasmacytoma comprised only 71 cases (4%) compared with a 19% incidence among lymphomas in the general population. The bulk of posttransplant lymphomas (1,678) were non-Hodgkin's lymphomas (NHLs) which made up 93.5% of lymphomas compared with only 71% in the general population [1-3].

Morphologically most NHLs were classified as immunoblastic sarcomas, reticulum cell sarcomas, microgliomas or large cell lymphomas [1-3]. As many lesions occupied the vague no-man's land between infection and neoplasia the term posttransplant lymphoproliferative disorder (PTLD) is now frequently used [9-10]. While most PTLDs represent Epstein-Barr virus (EBV)-induced lymphomas and lymphoproliferations some tumors showed no evidence of this virus despite a careful search for it [1-3].

Of PTLDs in the CTTR that were studied immunologically, 85% arose from B-lymphocytes, 14% were of T-cell origin and 0.3% were of null cell origin [1-3]. In 1,648 patients in whom the distribution of the lesions was known, 53% involved multiple organs or sites while 47% were confined to a single organ or site. While palpable lymph nodes were present in many patients PTLD differed from NHL in the general population in that extranodal disease was much more common affecting 1,157 (70%) of patients. Surprisingly, one of the most common extranodal sites was the central nervous system which was involved in 345 of 1,648 patients (21%) studied [1-3, 11]. The brain was usually involved whereas the spinal cord was rarely affected.

Another remarkable finding was the frequency of either macroscopic or microscopic allograft involvement which occurred in 23% patients with PTLD [1-3]. In some individuals with renal, cardiac or hepatic allografts the lymphomatous infiltrate was diagnosed as rejection when biopsies, done because of allograft dysfunction, were studied microscopically.

Skin lesions occurred in 51 of 1,648 patients (3%) of whom one had mycosis fungoides. Subcutaneous lesions were present in 12 patients (< 1%). Lesions of the oral cavity or pharynx, most commonly the tonsils in children, were found in 77 patients (5%).

The outcomes were studied in 1,217 patients with PTLD [1-3]. Of these 207 patients (17%) had no treatment, and the tumor was discovered at autopsy in 100 of them (48%). It is disturbing that so many patients died without treatment, either because the diagnosis was missed, or was made too late for effective therapy to be initiated. No data regarding therapy were available in 57 patients. Treatment was given to 953 patients of whom 368 (39%) had complete remissions. In 65 of these recipients (18%) the only treatment used was reduction or cessation of immunosuppressive therapy [1-3].

Kaposi's sarcoma

The frequent finding of Kaposi's sarcoma (KS) in the CTTR database (*Table 1*) stands in marked contrast with its incidence in the general population of the United States (before the acquired immunodeficiency syndrome – AIDS – epidemic started) where it comprised only 0.02% to 0.07% of all neoplasms [1-3, 12, 13]. The high incidence of KS in this worldwide collection of patients is comparable to that seen in tropical Africa where it occurs with greatest frequency, and comprises 3% to 9% of all cancers. It is remarkable that the number of transplant patients in the CTTR with KS (423) exceeded those with carcinomas of the colorectum (365), breast (336) or prostate (200) (*Table 1*). Apart from individuals with AIDS, who frequently have KS, there is probably no other large series, except possibly in tropical Africa, in which the number of patients with KS exceeds those who have these common malignancies.

KS affected males more than females in a 3:1 ratio, a figure far less than the 9:1 to 15:1 ratio seen with KS in the general population [1-3, 12]. Transplant-related KS was rare in children. Nine of 114 patients (8%) who were tested for the human immunodeficiency virus (HIV) were positive [12].

KS was most common in transplant patients who were Arab, black, Italian, Jewish or Greek [12]. Two studies reinforce these findings. KS occurred in 1.6% of 820 Italian renal transplant recipients [14] and was the most common cancer in renal allograft recipients in Saudi Arabia making up 76% of all cancers [15].

Fifty-eight percent of 419 patients, in whom the distribution of lesions is known, had nonvisceral KS confined to the skin, conjunctiva, or oropharyngolaryngeal mucosa and 41% had visceral disease, which involved mainly the gastrointestinal tract, lungs, and lymph nodes but also affected other organs [1-3, 12]. Of 242 patients with nonvisceral disease, the lesions were confined to the skin in 237 patients (98%) and to the mouth or oropharynx in 5 (2%). The 177 patients with visceral disease had no skin involvement in 42 instances (24%), but 6 of them (3%) had oral involvement, which provided a readily accessible site for biopsy and diagnosis of the disease. Of those with nonvisceral involvement, 130 (54%) had complete remissions after treatment. Interestingly, 45 (35%) of these remissions occurred when the only treatment was a drastic reduction of immunosuppressive therapy. In patients with visceral disease, only 51 of 177 patients (29%) had complete remissions. However, 30 of the 51 remissions (59%) occurred in response to reduction or cessation of immunosuppressive therapy only. Fifty-five percent of patients with visceral KS died. Of the deaths 72 of the 97 patients (74%) died of the neoplasm *per se*.

Of 39 kidney allograft recipients, in whom renal function was recorded following reduction or cessation of immunosuppressive therapy, 21 lost their allografts to rejection, 2 had impaired function, and 16 retained stable function [12].

Renal carcinomas

There were 378 patients with renal carcinomas (*Table 1*). This figure excludes 298 patients who had involvement of the native or allograft kidneys by lymphoma and 3 patients who had renal sarcomas. Of the tumors, 302 (80%) were renal cell carcinomas, hypernephromas, clear cell carcinomas or adenocarcinomas, 41 (11%) were transitional cell carcinomas or urothelial carcinomas, and 35 (9%) were miscellaneous carcinomas [1-3, 16].

A striking feature was that 91 of the 378 patients (24%) had incidentally discovered renal cancers, mostly renal cell carcinomas. These were discovered during workup for other disorders, at nephrectomy for hypertension or other reasons, during operation for some other disease, or at autopsy examination.

Unlike most other posttransplant neoplasms, that arose as complications of immunosuppressive therapy, many renal carcinomas were related to the underlying kidney disease in renal allograft recipients [1-3, 16], but no explanation is available for the 23 carcinomas that occurred in cardiac and 4 that occurred in liver allograft recipients. Most cancers in renal recipients developed in their own diseased kidneys, although 36 (10%) appeared in renal allografts, from 2 to 258 (average 77) months after transplantation [16]. Seven of the 36 tumors (19%) were diagnosed within 2 years of transplantation. It is possible that they may have been present in the allograft at the time of transplantation but were small enough to escape notice [16].

Two predisposing causes of renal carcinomas could be identified. Analgesic nephropathy was the underlying indication for transplantation in 29 of 315 (9%) transplant patients with carcinomas of their own diseased kidneys. This disorder is known to cause cancers, mostly transitional cell carcinomas, in various parts of the urinary tract. This is borne out in the CTTR series in which 17 of 29 (59%) patients with analgesia-related renal carcinomas had similar neoplasms elsewhere in the urinary tract [16].

Another predisposing cause of cancers in renal transplant recipients is acquired cystic disease (ACD) of the native kidneys. It occurs in 30-95% of patients receiving long-term hemodialysis, and is complicated by renal adenocarcinoma, which is increased 30-40 fold over its incidence in the general population [16]. With a successfully functioning transplant the ACD tends to regress, and theoretically the risk of developing carcinoma is reduced. However, cases of persistence of ACD and development of renal cell carcinoma have been reported in patients with successfully functioning renal allografts [16]. The precise incidence of ACD-related carcinomas in renal transplant recipients is not known.

Carcinomas of the vulva and perineum

This group of tumors includes carcinomas of the vulva, perineum, scrotum, penis, perianal skin or anus (*Table 1*) [1-3]. Females outnumbered males in a ratio of 2.5:1 in contrast with most other posttransplant malignancies where males outnumbered females by more than 2:1.

One-third of patients had *in situ* lesions [1-3]. A disturbing feature is that patients with invasive lesions were much younger (average age 42 years) than their counterparts in the general population, whose average age is usually between 50 and 70 years. Of 136 patients, in whom information was available, 78 (57%) had a history of condyloma acuminatum (genital warts) which must be regarded as a premalignant lesion. In women multicentric lesions were quite frequent not only involving several sites in the vulva, perianal area or anus, but sometimes the cervix and/or vagina as well [1-3]. While many patients with cancers of the vulva and perineum responded well to local or extensive excision of their lesions, 31 of 267 (12%) succumbed to the malignancy despite abdominoperineal resections or radical vulvectomies.

Carcinomas of the cervix

Carcinomas of the cervix occurred in 10% of women with posttransplant cancers (*Table 1*) [1-3]. At least 70% of patients had *in situ* lesions. The CTTR database showed a negligible increase in the incidence of *in situ* uterine cervical carcinoma compared with the general population. This is surprising in view of 2 epidemiologic studies that showed a 14- to 16-fold increased incidence in transplant patients. This suggests that many cases are being missed. In order to avoid this error every postadolescent female organ transplant recipient should have regular pelvic examinations and cervical smears [1-3].

Hepatobiliary tumors

Two epidemiologic studies showed a 20-38 fold increased incidence compared with controls [5, 8]. Most cases (115 of 161, 71%) in the CTTR (*Table 1*) were hepatomas and a substantial number of patients gave a preceding history of hepatitis B infection [8]. Since hepatitis C screening has become available, patients with a preceding history of this viral infection are being reported.

Sarcomas (excluding KS)

The majority involved the soft tissues or visceral organs whereas cartilage or bone involvement was uncommon [1-3, 12]. Of the 135 sarcomas, the major types were fibrous histiocytoma (24 cases), leiomyosarcoma (22), fibrosarcoma (12 including 2 cases of dermatofibrosarcoma), rhabdomyosarcoma (11), hemangiosarcoma (11), mesothelioma (9), liposarcoma (6), synovial sarcoma (5) and miscellaneous sarcomas (35).

Biological behavior of posttransplant cancers

Cancers in organ allograft recipients frequently demonstrated more aggressive behavior than did similar cancers in the general population [17].

Multiple tumors

Overall 621 of the 10,151 patients (6%) had two or more distinct tumor types that involved different organ systems. Of these 39 patients each had 3 separate types of malignancy and 1 had

4. The great majority of the patients with multiple tumors had some form of skin cancer. If patients with KS and carcinomas of the vulva and perineum are included with cancers of the skin and lips it was found that 497 patients with cutaneous tumors had 535 types of malignancy arising in other organs or sites. Of these 40 patients had carcinomas of the vulva and perineum associated with skin cancers in other locations.

The cutaneous cancers either preceded the other malignancies, or occurred at the same time, or appeared after the other neoplasms. The most frequent associations were skin cancer with a lymphoma: 74 patients (15%), uterine cervical carcinoma: 58 patients (12%) (of whom 36 patients had carcinomas of the vulva and 22 had cancers of other skin areas), lung cancer: 56 patients (11%), and head and neck cancer: 46 patients (9%). The frequent association of carcinomas of the vulva and uterine cervical carcinomas is not surprising as both are frequently related to infection by human papilloma virus, particularly types 16 and 18. The frequent association of skin cancers with malignancies located elsewhere emphasizes the need for the physician, treating a dermatological tumor, to do a thorough work up of any symptoms that might be caused by a neoplasm of one of the internal organs.

Treatment of posttransplant malignancies

The treatment of skin tumors is discussed elsewhere in this issue. Many cancers can be treated in the same way as in nontransplant patients [1-3]. For example, *in situ* carcinomas of the uterine cervix respond well to simple hysterectomy, cervical conization, or cryotherapy [1-3]. *In situ* carcinomas or small cancers of the vulva and perineum are treated by local excision. Large lesions required extensive operations such as total vulvectomy and inguinal node dissection, or abdominoperineal resection. Other neoplasms are treated by standard surgical, radiotherapeutic or chemotherapeutic modalities, but other treatments apply specifically to transplant-related malignancies. The antiviral agents acyclovir or ganciclovir may be used to treat EBV-related PTLD [1-3, 10]. Alpha-interferon has been used to treat some patients with KS or NHLs or other neoplasms [1-3]. Interferon is a potent immune modulator that increases membrane expression of class I antigens of the major histocompatibility complex, T-cell mediated cytotoxicity, and natural killer cell function. Thus it may stimulate rejection. However, conflicting findings have been reported in renal allograft recipients. A review of the literature suggests that small doses may be safe but large doses may precipitate rejection [18].

One option in treating posttransplant malignancies is reduction or cessation of immunosuppressive therapy [1-3, 19]. The value of this approach is borne out by experience with inadvertently transplanted malignancies, some of which regressed completely, following cessation of immunosuppressive therapy and removal of a renal allograft [2, 20]. As mentioned above, cessation or reduction of immunosuppressive therapy, when used by itself resulted in a substantial number of complete remissions of PTLD [1-3, 19] and KS [1-3, 12, 13]. However, such treatment has rarely caused regression of epithelial tumors. A drawback of this treatment is that it may precipitate allograft rejection with return of renal allograft recipients to dialysis therapy, but nonrenal allograft recipients may die of this complication. For example, this treatment caused impaired function or allograft loss from rejection in 21 of 39 renal recipients treated for KS [12]. Similarly, in a series of 14 renal recipients whose PTLD was treated (among other methods) by reduction or cessation of immunosuppression, 8 of 12 survivors lost their allografts [20, 21].

In patients requiring systemic cytotoxic therapy of widespread cancers we must remember that most agents depress the bone marrow [1-3]. It is, therefore, prudent to stop or reduce the administration of azathioprine, cyclophosphamide or mofetil mycophenolate dosage during such treatment to avoid severe bone marrow depression. As most cytotoxic drugs have immunosuppressive side effects, satisfactory allograft function may persist for prolonged periods. Treatment with prednisone may be continued as it is an important component of many cancer chemotherapy protocols. As many patients, particularly with PTLD, are already heavily immunosuppressed, chemotherapeutic agents should be used with caution as some patients have died of overwhelming infections following their use.

Acknowldegement

The author wishes to thank numerous colleagues, working in transplant centers throughout the world, who have generously contributed data concerning their patients to the Cincinnati transplant tumor registry.

Supported in part by a grant from Department of Veterans Affairs

References

1. Penn I. Why do immunosuppressed patients develop cancer? In : Pimentel E, ed. *Critical reviews in oncogenesis.* Boca Raton : CRC, 1989 ; 1 : 27-52.
2. Penn I. The problem of cancer in organ transplant recipients: an overview. *Transplant Sci* 1994 ; 4 : 23-32.
3. Penn I. Malignancy after immunosuppressive therapy: how can the risk be reduced? *Clin Immunother* 1995 ; 9 : 207-18.
4. Sheil AGR, Disney APS, Mathew TH, Amiss N. De novo malignancy emerges as a major cause of morbidity and late failure in renal transplantation. *Transplant Proc* 1993 ; 25 : 1383-4.
5. Kinlen LJ. Incidence of cancer in rheumatoid arthritis and other disorders after immunosuppressive treatment. *Am J Med* 1985 ; 78 (Suppl. 1A) : 44-9.
6. Blohme I, Brynger H. Malignant disease in renal transplant patients. *Transplantation* 1985 ; 39 : 23-35.
7. Harwood AR, Osoba D, Hofstader SL, Goldstein MB, Cardella CJ, Holecek MJ, Kunynetz R, Giammarco RA. Kaposi's sarcoma in recipients of renal transplants. *Am J Med* 1979 ; 67(5) : 759-65.
8. Schröter GPJ, Weil R III, Penn I, Speers WC, Waddell WR. Hepatocellular carcinoma associated with chronic hepatitis B virus infection after kidney transplantation. *Lancet* 1982 ; 2 : 381-2.
9. Nalesnik MA, Starzl TE. Epstein-Barr virus, infectious mononucleosis, and posttransplant lymphoproliferative disorders. *Transplant Sci* 1994 ; 4 : 61-79.
10. Hanto DW. Classification of Epstein-Barr virus-associated posttransplant lympho-proliferative diseases: implications for understanding their pathogenesis and developing rational treatment strategies. *Ann Rev Med* 1995 ; 46 : 381-94.
11. Penn I, Porat G. Central nervous system lymphomas in organ allograft recipients. *Transplantation* 1995 ; 59 : 240-4.
12. Penn I. Sarcomas in organ allograft recipients. *Transplantation* 1995 ; 60 : 1485-91.
13. Penn I. Kaposi's sarcoma in transplant recipients. *Transplantation* 1997 ; 64 : 669-73.
14. Montagnino G, Bencini PL, Tarantino A, Caputo R, Ponticelli C. Clinical features and course of Kaposi's sarcoma in kidney transplant patients: report of 13 cases. *Am J Nephrol* 1994 ; 14 : 121-6.
15. Al-Sulaiman MH, Al-Khader AA. Kaposi's sarcoma in renal transplant recipients. *Transplant Sci* 1994 ; 4 : 46-60.
16. Penn I. Primary kidney tumors before and after renal transplantation. *Transplantation* 1995 ; 59 : 480-5.
17. Barrett WL, First R, Aron BS, Penn I. Clinical course of malignancies in renal transplant recipients. *Cancer* 1993 ; 72 : 2186-9.
18. Min AD. Does interferon precipitate rejection of liver allografts? *Hepatology* 1995 ; 22 : 1333-5.

19. Starzl TE, Nalesnik MA, Porter KA, Ho M, Iwatsuki S, Griffith BP, Rosenthal JT, Hakala TR, Shaw BW Jr, Hardesty RL. Reversibility of lymphomas and lymphoproliferative lesions developing under cyclosporin-steroid therapy. *Lancet* 1984 ; 1 : 583-7.

20. Penn I. Neoplasia: an example of plasticity of the immune response. *Transplant Proc* 1996 ; 28 : 2089-93.

21. Hickey DP, Nalesnik MA, Vivas CA, Lopatin WB, Jordan ML, Starzl TE, Hakala TR. Renal retransplantation in patients who lost their allografts during management of previous post-transplant lymphoproliferative disease. *Clin Transplant* 1990 ; 4 : 187-90.

15

Cutaneous warts and carcinomas

Jan Nico BOUWES BAVINCK[1], Esther J. VAN ZUUREN[1], Jan TER SCHEGGET[2]
1. *Department of Dermatology, Leiden University Medical Centre, Leiden, The Netherlands.*
2. *Department of Virology, Academic Medical Centre, Amsterdam, The Netherlands.*

Transplant recipients are at an increased risk of developing keratotic skin lesions (*Figure 23, page 220*), and squamous and basal cell carcinomas (*Figure 24, page 220*) [1-6]. The cumulative incidence of skin cancer is steadily increasing in temperate climates from around 10%, ten years after the transplantation to 40%, twenty years after the transplantation [2, 7]: in Australia these figures at the same time periods are 40% and 70%, respectively (*Graph 4*) [5, 8]. In the general population basal cell carcinomas are more frequently seen than squamous cell carcinomas, but in the transplant population the ratio of squamous cell to basal cell carcinoma in renal transplant recipients is greater than 1 [1, 2, 5].

Human papillomavirus (HPV) infection can be considered as the most important cause for the development of keratotic skin lesions and may also play a role in the pathogenesis of skin cancer [6, 9]. Sooner or later most recipients will experience HPV infection. The number of viral warts is steadily rising after transplantation (*Graph 5*) [4]. The interval between the transplantation to the development of warts is clearly shorter than the interval from transplantation to the diagnosis of the first skin cancer [10].

Squamous cell carcinomas are almost exclusively localised on sun-exposed skin, whereas basal cell carcinomas also frequently develop on the trunk (*Figure 25*) [2]. The frequent occurrence of squamous cell carcinomas on the dorsum of the hands presents a specifically difficult therapeutical problem [11]. Transplant recipients often also experience leukoplakia, dysplasia and cancer of the lip (*Figure 26, page 221*) [12].

The problem of skin cancer is not limited to renal transplant recipients, but is also eminent in heart transplant recipients and recipients of other organs [13-16].

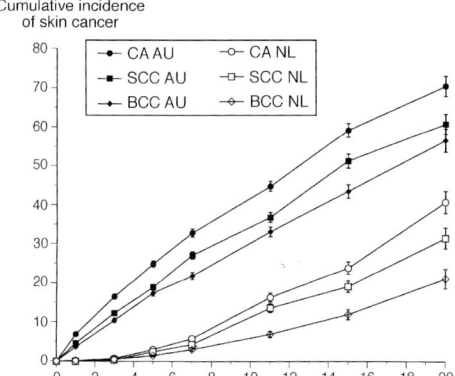

Graph 4. Cumulative incidence with 95% confidence interval of skin cancer in Australia and the Netherlands. CA denotes all skin cancers together; SCC: squamous cell carcinoma; BCC: basal cell carcinoma; AU: Australia; NL: the Netherlands (from [5]).

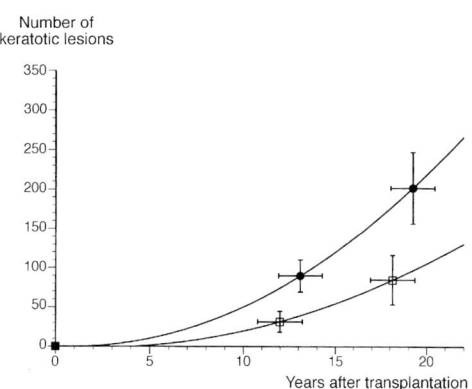

Graph 5. Increased number of keratotic skin lesions with increasing numbers of years since transplantation. Patients with skin cancer (n = 35) are indicated with solid circles and patients who did not develop skin cancer until 1995 (n = 31) with open squares. The horizontal and vertical bars represent 95% confidence intervals for years after transplantation and number of keratotic lesions, respectively. The curves are the result of second degree polynomial curve fitting with the point (0,0) as third point (unpublished observations).

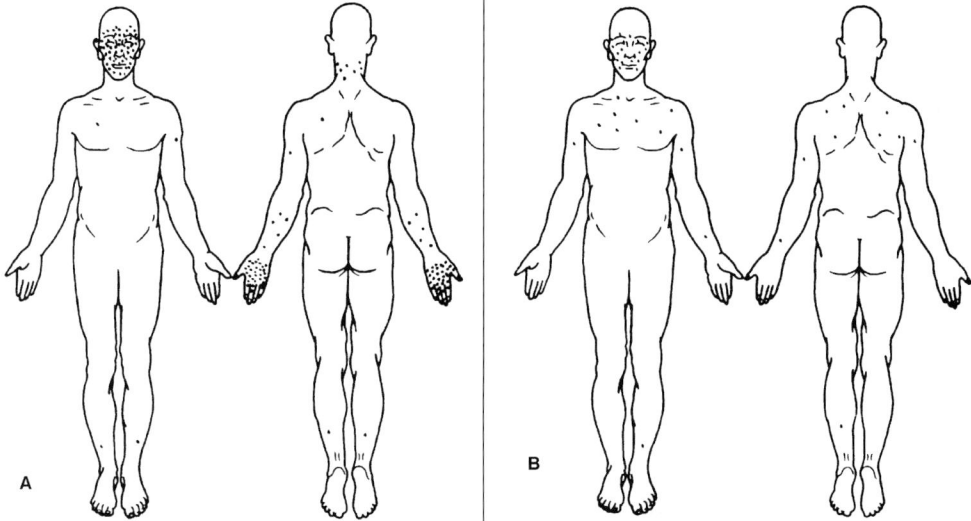

Figure 25. (A) Distribution of squamous cell carcinomas on sun-exposed sites and (B) of basal cell carcinomas on sun-exposed sites and the trunk (from [2]).

Clinicopathological aspects

The differentiation between squamous cell carcinomas and keratoacanthomas is often difficult to establish in transplant recipients, both on clinical and on histological grounds. Not infrequently, aggressive squamous cell carcinomas develop within a couple of weeks. Therefore, for therapeutical reasons, in this group of patients all keratoacanthomas should be regarded as squamous cell carcinomas. In addition, clinically benign appearing keratotic skin lesions sometimes show to be early squamous cell carcinomas by histological examination. Hence, frequent and early biopsy of such lesions is advocated, especially in inexperienced hands.

In renal transplant recipients, warts presenting on severely sun-damaged skin are difficult to distinguish clinically from other keratotic lesions. Keratotic skin lesions in this group of patients include actinic keratoses, *verrucae vulgares*, *verrucae planae*, seborrheic keratoses, EV-like lesions and hyperkeratotic papillomas. We biopsied a total of 155 keratotic skin lesions which were not clinically suspect for skin cancer. In 71 out of these 155 lesions there were no specific histological features to warrant diagnoses such as actinic keratoses, *verrucae planae*, *verrucae vulgares* or seborrheic keratoses (unpublished observation). These 71 histological slides did not show any signs of viral infection or cellular atypia, resulting in the *per exclusionem* diagnosis of hyperkeratotic papilloma. Therefore, a clear differentiation between all the different subtypes of keratotic skin lesions is not only difficult on clinical grounds, but also on histological grounds.

Environmental risk factors

Transplant recipients receive continuous immunosuppressive drugs, initially azathioprine and prednisone, and more recently cyclosporin A and FK506. The risk of skin cancer increases with time of immunosuppression [2, 5]. Several studies did not observe significant differences in the risk of developing skin cancer between recipients on cyclosporin and recipients who were treated with azathioprine [5, 17-19]. In light of these findings, it is difficult to maintain that skin cancer genesis in transplant recipients is largely due to enhanced carcinogenesis due to azathioprine metabolites, as proposed by Lennard *et al.* [20]. It is more likely that the increased risk of skin cancer following immunosuppression is independent of the agent(s) used, but is a result of the immunosuppression *per se*.

Exposure to sunlight is believed to be one of the most important risk factors for the development of both skin cancers and warts in transplant recipients [1, 3, 10]. Both exposure to the sun and smoking are risk factors for dysplastic and malignant lip lesions [12]. Except for its harmful effect by inducing DNA damage, ultraviolet light can also be harmful by inducing immunological unresponsiveness [21]. Ultraviolet light induced immunosuppression is discussed in Chapter 4.

HPV infection and skin cancer

The skin problems in transplant recipients mimic those seen in patients with epidermodysplasia verruciformis (EV). This rare syndrome is characterised by the presence of numerous flat warts, the occurrence of squamous cell carcinoma in 30% to 50% of patients, and possibly a defect in cell-mediated immunity [22, 23].

The number of keratotic skin lesions in transplant recipients is highly associated with skin cancer [1, 3, 10]. A wide diversity of HPV types can be detected in biopsies from premalignant lesions and skin cancers of transplant recipients [4, 9, 24-31]. The high prevalence of HPV

DNA detected in squamous cell carcinomas and basal cell carcinomas of these patients suggest a potential role for HPV infection in the aetiology of these lesions [32]. The types of HPVs that are possibly implicated are a matter of controversy [25, 33]. Mucosal HPVs (type 6, 11, 16, and 18) were detected by some groups [28, 31]. HPVs belonging to the EV-related subgroup (type 5, 8, 15, 19, 20, 22, 23, 24, 25, 36, 38 and at least 25 putative new EV-HPV types) were detected by other groups [24, 25, 33], and still another group detected non-EV HPVs such as HPV 41 or a HPV 29-related type [29], but also EV HPVs and mucosal HPVs [26]. This discrepancy is probably largely attributable to differences in the techniques used [25]. It is likely that more than one HPV types are present in the skin lesions, and dependent on the technique used, one or another type can be picked up. The existence of not yet established HPV types could be a second explanation for the controversies in the literature [24-26, 33].

The presence of HPV DNA (HPV 16) has been shown in 1 out of 25 carcinomas of the lip from non-immunosuppressed patients [34], but studies in renal transplant recipients are lacking. It is not unlikely that HPV DNA may be present in these lesions in a similar way as in squamous cell carcinomas of the skin.

Immunogenetic risk factors

There are several specific immunological and immunogenetic factors that may play a role in the development of skin cancer in transplant recipients [3, 35]. The non-specific immune surveillance against skin cancer is hampered in renal transplant recipients because of a depressed natural killer cell function [36-38]. Recent studies lay more strain upon the functioning of the specific cellular immune response through cytotoxic T lymphocytes. Specific immunological and immunogenetic factors may therefore play a role in the development of skin cancer in transplant recipients [3].

HLA antigens play a pivotal role in the cellular immune response to viral and tumour antigens [35, 39]. The HLA class II antigens are involved in recognition of foreign peptides by CD4 positive regulatory T lymphocytes [40], whereas the HLA class I antigens mainly serve as restriction elements for the reactivity of CD8 positive cytotoxic T lymphocytes [41].

An association between the occurrence of skin cancer and the class II antigen HLA-DR7 has been described [42]. We found the same trend, but in our study statistical significance was not reached [43].

Besides the induction phase of the immune response, the effector phase may be important since associations between the occurrence of skin cancer and class I antigens have also been found [44-46]. HLA-A11 was reported to be negatively associated with the development of skin cancer in renal transplant recipients [44]. The same trend of a negative association between HLA-A11 and non-melanoma skin cancers was found by others [42, 46, 47], although in most studies some HLA-A11 positive patients with skin cancers were found. However, recently, we found a positive association between HLA-A11 and skin cancer in an Australian population [48]. The reason of these apparently conflicting results is not clear yet.

HLA-B27 was reported to be positively associated with skin cancer, suggesting that susceptibility to skin cancer is associated with this class I antigen [42, 44]. This finding could be confirmed in the Australian population of transplant recipients [48].

Homozygosity for HLA antigens has been reported to be a risk factor for the development of several kinds of cancers [49, 50]. In homozygous individuals the number of different polymorphic class I and class II products is less than in heterozygous individuals. As a result, there are fewer possibilities for interaction with antigenic peptides and therefore fewer possibilities for recognition of foreign antigens [49]. Renal-transplant recipients who were homozygous for the HLA-DR antigen were also at an increased risk for skin cancer and keratotic skin lesions [3]. This finding provides additional, indirect evidence that an impaired response of CD4 positive regulatory T cells to HLA class II associated peptides might indeed be involved in the aetiology of skin cancer [45].

Immune response against HPV antigens

Patients without an apparent class switch from IgM to IgG to the fusion protein of the late antigen (L1) of human papillomavirus type 8 and β-galactosidase are at an increased risk of skin cancer as compared to the patients with a good humoral response to this fusion protein [51]. This indicates that the immune response against HPV antigens is relevant in these patients for the risk of developing skin cancer. The nature of this defect cannot be explained by factors that are related to transplantation, since the same association was also found when sera that were collected before the transplantation were considered [51]. The latter is a strong argument for a genetically determined predisposition for non-melanoma skin cancer in patients who have a poor antibody response to the HPV 8 L1 fusion protein. Moreover, this impaired antibody response is mainly found in patients who are HLA-DR7 positive, because a strong linkage between the absent class switch of antibody production to L1 of HPV 8 and HLA-DR7 was observed [51]. Since HLA-DR7 is also associated with the occurrence of non-melanoma skin cancer in renal transplant recipients [5, 42], this finding suggests that the development of non-melanoma skin cancer is also genetically controlled by genes in the class II region of the major histocompatibility complex.

Strategies for intervention and treatment

Regular surveillance of transplant recipients with skin problems and easy access of all patients to a dermatologist is advised, as well as early biopsy of suspicious lesions. This facilitates early removal of malignant and premalignant lesions to reduce the risk of skin cancer and metastasis in this patients population.

Because of the strong association with sun exposure, sun-protective measures are important to reduce the risk of skin cancer in transplant recipients. Particularly, the use of long sleeves, long trousers and a hat outdoors, especially in sunny climates, should be promoted. In addition, sunscreens can be prescribed, although its use can lead to a false feeling of safety, since protection by sunscreens is never complete.

Some controversy exists regarding the question whether tapering of the immunosuppressive drugs will reduce the risk for the development of additional skin cancers. Since there is no association between the cumulative doses of immunosuppressive drugs and the occurrence of skin cancer [3], reduction of the immunosuppressive therapy hypothetically will not decrease the risk of non-melanoma skin cancer, unless the dose is lowered to a level that may lead to an increased risk of graft rejection. However, other authors advocate that in patients with multiple skin cancers the immunosuppressive therapy should be reduced as much as possible, and, using this regimen, they observed an improvement of the skin condition in several patients [52, 53]. Controlled studies should be awaited to provide the final answer. However, changing the immunosuppressive regimen from azathioprine to cyclosporin A or *vice versa* does not seem to relieve the skin problems [5, 17-19].

Both oral and local retinoids may be of some help in the reduction of actinic keratoses and in the prevention of skin cancer in renal transplant recipients [54-59]. This subject is discussed in more detail in Chapters 22 and 23.

Resurfacing the dorsum of the hand can be a successful treatment for patients with multiple skin cancers on the back of the hand and can be used prophylactically in patients with severely actinically damaged skin [11, 60]. Nevertheless, this surgery should be reserved for carefully selected patients since it is an invasive procedure, recovery takes many months, and side effects are not negligible [11].

Acknowledgement

The authors are indebted to Drs. F.J. van der Woude, B.J. Vermeer, F.H.J. Claas, J.P. Vandenbroucke, R.G.J. Westendorp, H. Pfister, L. Gissmann, L.M. de Jong-Tieben, I.L.A. Boxman, and H.L. Smits for their contribution to important parts of the studies.

This work was supported by the Dutch Kidney Foundation and the Dutch Cancer Society. The research of Dr. Bouwes Bavinck has also been made possible by a fellowship of the Royal Netherlands Academy of Arts and Sciences.

References

1. Boyle J, MacKie RM, Briggs JD, Junor BJR, Aitchison TC. Cancer, warts, and sunshine in renal transplant recipients: a case-control study. *Lancet* 1984 ; 1 : 702-7.
2. Hartevelt MM, Bouwes Bavinck JN, Kootte AMM, Vermeer BJ, Vandenbroucke JP. Incidence of skin cancer after renal transplantation in the Netherlands. *Transplantation* 1990 ; 49 : 506-9.
3. Bouwes Bavinck JN, Vermeer BJ, van der Woude FJ, Vandenbroucke JP, Schreuder GMT, Thorogood J, Persijn GG, Claas FHJ. Relation between skin cancer and HLA antigens in renal-transplant recipients. *N Engl J Med* 1991 ; 325 : 843-8.
4. Barr BBB, Benton EC, McLaren K, Bunney MH, Smith IW, Blessing K, Hunter JAA. Human papillomavirus infection and skin cancer in renal allograft recipients. *Lancet* 1989 ; i : 124-9.
5. Bouwes Bavinck JN, Hardie DR, Green A, Cutmore S, Macnaught A, O'Sullivan B, Siskind V, van der Woude FJ, Hardie IR. The risk of skin cancer in renal transplant recipients in Queensland, Australia: a follow-up study. *Transplantation* 1996 ; 61 : 715-21.
6. Bouwes Bavinck JN, Berkhout RJM. HPV infections and immunosuppression. *Clin Dermatol* 1997 ; 15 : 427-37.
7. London NJ, Farmery SM, Will EJ, Davison AM, Lodge JPA. Risk of neoplasia in renal transplant patients. *Lancet* 1995 ; 346 : 403-6.
8. Hardie IR, Strong RW, Hartley LCJ, Woodruff PWH, Clunie CJA. Skin cancer in Caucasian renal allograft recipients living in a subtropical climate. *Surgery* 1980 ; 87 : 177-83.
9. Pfister H, ter Schegget J. Role of HPV in cutaneous premalignant and malignant tumors. *Clin Dermatol* 1997 ; 15 : 435-7.
10. Bouwes Bavinck JN, de Boer A, Vermeer BJ, Hartevelt MM, van der Woude FJ, Claas FHJ, Wolterbeek R, Vandenbroucke JP. Sunlight, keratotic skin lesions and skin cancer in renal transplant recipients. *Br J Dermatol* 1993 ; 129 : 242-9.
11. van Zuuren EJ, Posma AN, Scholtens REM, Vermeer BJ, van der Woude FJ, Bouwes Bavinck JN. Resurfacing of the hand as treatment and prevention of multiple skin cancers in renal transplant recipients. *J Am Acad Dermatol* 1994 ; 31 : 760-4.
12. King GN, Healy CM, Dent B, Glover MT, Kwan JTC, Williams DM, Leigh IM, Worthington HV. Increased prevalence of dysplastic and malignant lip lesions in renal-transplant recipients. *N Engl J Med* 1995 ; 332 : 1052-7.
13. Bouwes Bavinck JN, Robertson I, Wainwright RW, Green A. Excessive skin cancers and pre-malignant skin lesions in an Australian heart-transplant recipient. *Br Heart J* 1995 ; 74 : 468-70.
14. Euvrard S, Kanitakis J, Pouteil-Noble C, Dureau G, Touraine JL, Faure M, Claudy A, Thivolet J. Comparative epidemiologic study of premalignant and malignant epithelial cutaneous lesions developing after kidney and heart transplantation. *J Am Acad Dermatol* 1995 ; 33 : 222-9.

15. España A, Redondo P, Fernández AL, Zabala M, Herreros J, Llorens R, Quintanilla E. Skin cancer in heart transplant recipients. *J Am Acad Dermatol* 1995 ; 32 : 458-65.

16. Mihalow ML, Gattuso P, Abraham K, Holmes EW, Reddy V. Incidence of post-transplant malignancy among 674 solid-organ-transplant recipients at a single center. *Clin Transplant* 1996 ; 10 : 248-55.

17. Gruber SA, Gillingham K, Sothern RB, Stephanian E, Matas AJ, Dunn DL. *De novo* cancer in cyclosporin-treated and non-cyclosporin-treated adult primary renal allograft recipients. *Clin Transplant* 1994 ; 8 : 388-95.

18. Roeger LS, Sheil AGR, Disney APS, Mathew TH, Amiss N. Risk factors associated with the development of squamous cell carcinomas in immunosuppressed renal transplant recipients. *Clin Transplant* 1992 ; 6 : 202-11.

19. Shuttleworth D, Marks R, Griffin PJA, Salaman JR. Epidermal dysplasia and cyclosporin therapy in renal transplant recipients: a comparison with azathioprine. *Br J Dermatol* 1989 ; 120 : 551-4.

20. Lennard L, Thomas S, Harrington CI, Maddocks JL. Skin cancer in renal transplant recipients is associated with increased concentrations of 6-thioguanine nucleotide in red blood cells. *Br J Dermatol* 1985 ; 113 : 723-9.

21. Kripke ML. Ultraviolet radiation and immunology: something new under the sun-presidential address. *Cancer Res* 1994 ; 54 : 6102-5.

22. Orth G. Epidermodysplasia verruciformis. In : Salzman NP, Howley PM, eds. *The Papovaviridae, the papillomaviruses*. New York : Plenum Publishing Corp, 1987 : 199-243.

23. Cooper KD, Androphy EJ, Lowy D, Katz SI. Antigen presentation and T-cell activation in epidermodysplasia verruciformis. *J Invest Dermatol* 1990 ; 94 : 769-76.

24. Berkhout RJM, Tieben LM, Smits HL, Bouwes Bavinck JN, Vermeer BJ, ter Schegget J. Nested PCR approach for detection and typing of epidermodysplasia verruciformis-associated human papillomavirus types in cutaneous cancers from renal transplant recipients. *J Clin Microbiol* 1995 ; 33 : 690-5.

25. de Jong-Tieben LM, Berkhout RJM, Smits HL, Bouwes Bavinck JN, Vermeer BJ, van der Woude FJ, ter Schegget J. High frequency of detection of epidermodysplasia verruciformis-associated human papillomavirus DNA in biopsies from malignant and premalignant skin lesions from renal transplant recipients. *J Invest Dermatol* 1995 ; 105 : 367-71.

26. Shamanin V, zur Hausen H, Lavergne D, Proby CM, Leigh IM, Neumann C, Hamm H, Goos M, Haustein UF, Jung EG, Plewig G, Wolff H, de Villiers EM. Human papillomavirus infections in nonmelanoma skin cancers from renal transplant recipients and nonimmunosuppressed patients. *J Natl Cancer Inst* 1996 ; 88 : 802-11.

27. Euvrard S, Chardonnet Y, Pouteil-Noble CP, Kanitakis J, Thivolet J, Touraine JL. Skin malignancies and human papillomaviruses in renal transplant recipients. *Transplant Proc* 1993 ; 25 : 1392-3.

28. Euvrard S, Chardonnet Y, Pouteil-Noble C, Kanitakis J, Chignol MC, Thivolet J, Touraine JL. Association of skin malignancies with various and multiple carcinogenic and noncarcinogenic human papillomaviruses in renal transplant recipients. *Cancer* 1993 ; 72 : 2198-206.

29. Shamanin V, Glover M, Rausch C, Proby C, Leigh IM, zur Hausen H, de Villiers EM. Specific types of human papillomavirus found in benign proliferations and carcinomas of the skin in immunosuppressed patients. *Cancer Res* 1994 ; 54 : 4610-3.

30. Stark LA, Arends MJ, McLaren KM, Benton EC, Shahidullah H, Hunter JAA, Bird CC. Prevalence of human papillomavirus DNA in cutaneous neoplasms from renal allograft recipients supports a possible viral role in tumour promotion. *Br J Cancer* 1994 ; 69 : 222-9.

31. Soler C, Chardonnet Y, Allibert P, Euvrard S, Schmitt D, Mandrand B. Detection of mucosal human papillomavirus types 6/11 in cutaneous lesions from transplant recipients. *J Invest Dermatol* 1993 ; 101 : 286-91.

32. Burk RD, Kadish AS. Treasure hunt for human papillomaviruses in nonmelanoma skin cancers. *J Natl Cancer Inst* 1996 ; 88 : 781-2.

33. Höpfl R, Petter A, Pfister A. Human papillomavirus in nonmelanoma skin cancer? The phylogenetic tree of the papillomavirus family is not yet complete. *Arch Dermatol* 1996 ; 132 : 834.

34. Kawashima M, Favre M, Obalek S, Jablonska S, Orth G. Premalignant lesions and cancers of the skin in the general population: evaluation of the role of human papillomaviruses. *J Invest Dermatol* 1990 ; 95 : 537-42.

35. Streilein JW. Immunogenetic factors in skin cancer. *N Engl J Med* 1991 ; 325 : 884-7.

36. ten Berge RJM, Schellekens PTA, Surachno S, The TH, ten Veen JH, Wilmink JM. The influence of therapy with azathioprine and prednisone on the immune system of kidney transplant recipients. *Clin Immunol Immunopathol* 1981 ; 21 : 20-32.

37. Kelly GE, Sheil AGR, Taylor R. Nonspecific immunological studies in kidney transplant recipients with and without skin cancer. *Transplantation* 1984 ; 37 : 368-72.

38. Legendre CM, Guttmann RD, Yip GH. Natural killer cell subsets in long-term renal allograft recipients. A phenotypic and functional study. *Transplantation* 1986 ; 42 : 347-52.

39. Klitz W. Viruses, cancer and the MHC. *Nature* 1992 ; 356 : 17-8.

40. Neefjes JJ, Ploegh HL. Intracellular transport of MHC class II molecules. *Immunol Today* 1992 ; 13 : 179-84.

41. Monaco JJ. A molecular model of MHC class-I-restricted antigen processing. *Immunol Today* 1992 ; 13 : 173-9.

42. Czarnecki D, Zalcberg J, Nicholson I, Tait B. Skin cancer and HLA antigens. *N Engl J Med* 1992 ; 326 : 765.

43. Bouwes Bavinck JN, Vermeer BJ, van der Woude FJ, Vandenbroucke JP, Claas FHJ. Skin cancer and HLA antigens (reply). *N Engl J Med* 1992 ; 326 : 766.

44. Bouwes Bavinck JN, Kootte AMM, van der Woude FJ, Vandenbroucke JP, Vermeer BJ, Claas FHJ. On a possible protective effect of HLA-A11 against skin cancer and keratotic skin lesions in renal transplant recipients. *J Invest Dermatol* 1991 ; 97 : 269-72.

45. Bouwes Bavinck JN, Claas FHJ. The role of HLA molecules in the development of skin cancer. *Hum Immunol* 1994 ; 41 : 173-9.

46. Glover MT, Bodmer J, Kennedy LJ, Brown J, Navarrete C, Kwan JTC, Leigh IM. HLA antigen frequencies in renal transplant recipients and non-immunosuppressed patients with non-melanoma skin cancer. *Eur J Cancer* 1993 ; 29A : 520-4.

47. McGregor JM, Reddi G, MacDonald D, Vaughan RW, Welsh KI. HLA-A11 in renal allograft recipients with skin cancer. *J Invest Dermatol* 1992 ; 98 : 261-2.

48. Bouwes Bavinck JN, Claas FHJ, Hardie DR, Green A, Vermeer BJ, Hardie IR. Relation between skin cancer and HLA antigens in renal transplant recipients in Queensland, Australia. *J Invest Dermatol* 1997 ; 108 : 708-11.

49. Dausset J, Colombani J, Hors J. Major histocompatibility complex and cancer, with special reference to human familiar tumors (Hodgkin's disease and other malignancies). *Cancer Surv* 1982 ; 1 : 119-47.

50. von Fliedner VE, Sultan-Khan Z, Jeannet M. HLA-DRw antigens associated with acute leukemia. *Tissue Antigens* 1980 ; 16 : 399-404.

51. Bouwes Bavinck JN, Gissmann L, Claas FHJ, van der Woude FJ, Persijn GG, ter Schegget J, Vermeer BJ, Jochmus I, Müller M, Steger G, Gebert S, Pfister H. Relation between skin cancer, humoral responses to human papillomaviruses, and HLA class II molecules in renal transplant recipients. *J Immunol* 1993 ; 151 : 1579-86.

52. Euvrard S, Kanitakis J, Thivolet J, Claudy A. Retinoids for the management of dermatological complications of organ transplantation. *Biodrugs* 1997 ; 3 : 176-84.

53. Fernandez-Gonzales A, España A, Redondo P. Solid tumors after heart transplantation. *Ann Thorac Surg* 1996 ; 62 : 943-4.

54. Shuttleworth D, Marks R, Griffin PJA, Salaman JR. Treatment of cutaneous neoplasia with etretinate in renal transplant recipients. *Q J Med* 1988 ; 68 : 717-24.

55. Kelly JW, Sabto J, Gurr FW, Bruce F. Retinoids to prevent skin cancer in organ transplant recipients. *Lancet* 1991 ; 338 : 1407.

56. Bouwes Bavinck JN, Tieben LM, van der Woude FJ, Tegzess AM, Hermans J, ter Schegget J, Vermeer BJ. Prevention of skin cancer and reduction of keratotic skin lesions during acitretin therapy in renal-transplant recipients; a double-blind, placebo-controlled study. *J Clin Oncol* 1995 ; 13 : 1933-8.

57. Fa Yuan Z, Davis A, MacDonald K, Bailey RR. Use of acitretin for the skin complications in renal transplant recipients. *NZ Med J* 1995 ; 108 : 255-6.

58. Rook AH, Jaworsky C, Nguyen T, Grossman RA, Wolfe JT, Witmer WK, Kligman AM. Beneficial effect of low-dose systemic retinoid in combination with topical tretinoin for the treatment and prophylaxis of premalignant and malignant skin lesions in renal transplant recipients. *Transplantation* 1995 ; 59 : 714-9.

59. Euvrard S, Verschoore M, Touraine JL, Dureau G, Cochat P, Czernielewski J, Thivolet J. Topical retinoids for warts and keratoses in transplant recipients. *Lancet* 1992 ; 340 : 48-9.

60. Scholtens REM, van Zuuren EJ, Posma AN. Treatment of recurrent squamous cell carcinoma of the hand in immunosuppressed patients. *J Hand Surg* 1995 ; 20A : 73-6.

16

Kaposi's sarcoma

Camille FRANCÈS, Sylvie LAGRANGE
Department of Internal Medicine, Pitié-Salpêtrière Hospital, Paris, France.

In 1872, a Viennese dermatologist, Moritz Kaposi, described a multicentric, cutaneous and extra-cutaneous neoplasm with a protracted clinical course affecting predominantly the elderly. This disease is now eponymously designated Kaposi's sarcoma (KS) although it is now regarded as a polyclonal cell proliferation. Several subtypes were subsequently distinguished, including the sporadic or classic subtype initially described by Kaposi, the endemic subtype observed in black Africans, the epidemic subtype in patients infected with the human immunodeficiency virus and the iatrogenical subtype in patients treated by immunosuppressive therapy, especially organ transplant recipients. In this last group of patients, the management of KS requires a close cooperation of dermatologists with other physicians of the transplantation department.

Epidemiology

The prevalence of KS after organ transplantation varies greatly depending on the location of the institution. *Table I* summarises the main data from the recent literature [1-17]. The highest prevalence rate after renal transplantation (4.1%) has been reported in Saudi Arabia [10], the lowest one (0.45%) in the « Ile-de-France » region [1]. A comparative study of KS prevalence within the same institutions (Ile-de-France area and Toronto) shows that the prevalences are similar after renal and heart transplantation and higher after liver transplantation [1, 17].

In many countries, the geographic origin of transplant recipients with KS differs substantially from that of the general population. Indeed, posttransplant KS mainly affects patients of Mediterranean, black African or Carribean origin [1-5, 14-17], *i.e.* the same populations affected by sporadic or endemic KS. The evaluation made by the various relevant studies of

Table I. Prevalence of Kaposi's sarcoma in organ transplant recipients

Origin	Renal TR (n of TR)	Cardiac TR (n of TR)	Hepatic TR (n of TR)	Organ TR (n of TR)
France				
Ile-de-France [1]	0.45% (6,229)	0.41% (967)	1.24% (727)	0.52% (7,923)
Lyon [2-5]	0.48% (2,500)	0.25% (800)	2% (150)	0.52% (3,450)
Rennes [6]				0% (804)
Spain				
Madrid [7]	0.5% (609)			
Italy				
Milan [8]	1.5% (854)			
Rome [9]	3.3% (302)			
Saudi Arabia				
Riyadh [10]	4.1% (630)			
South Africa				
Johannesburg [11]	0.5% (989)			
Israel				
Petah Tiqva [12, 13]	2.4% (330)	11% (18)		
USA				
Cincinnati [14]				4.3% (8,191)
Pittsburgh [15]			0.12% (1,657)	
Detroit [16]		0.98% (102)		
Canada				
Toronto [17]	0.54% (1,300)	0.54% (189)	0.94% (426)	0.57% (2,099)

TR: transplant recipients; n: number of patients

transplantation-induced raise of KS risk factor is quite heterogeneous; it ranges from 25- to 400-fold in Toronto between 1979 and 1997 [17, 18] and is estimated to 224-fold in Italy [8]. In any case, the role played respectively by genetic predisposition and infectious agents such as HHV-8/KSHV, existing in all forms of KS, has not yet been entirely elucidated. No predisposing genetic factor has been so far definitely identified; the predominance of HLA-DR5 antigen, initially reported in sporadic KS, has been questioned in other KS forms, including organ-graft recipients [1, 19, 20]. According to recent epidemiologic studies [21], it seems that a high prevalence of sporadic and a fortiori endemic KS is found in the same countries, i.e. those with a high seroprevalence of HHV8. This seroprevalence is reportedly very high in some African countries (> 50% of the population), moderate in Italy and lower in other Western European countries. Although some studies provide information concerning the ethnic origin of patients, the duration of their stay in the ancestral country unfortunetaly is not mentioned.

The male predominance – well-known in sporadic, endemic and epidemic KS – also exists in post-transplant KS. In the various relevant studies, the male/female ratio ranges from 2 to 40 [1, 14, 17]. The age at KS onset depends mainly on the age at organ transplantation, about 40 years in most cases [1, 14]. Pediatric cases have been reported but no comparative study has been carried out regarding the prevalence in adult and pediatric transplant recipients of the same geographic origin [22].

The average time between organ transplantation and KS onset is 20 months, with a range of a few weeks to 18 years. This delay is reduced to 6 months after liver transplantation [5], and to about 12 months in renal transplant recipients treated with cyclosporin [1, 23]. Some data have been published concerning liver transplant recipients treated with FK 506 [24, 25]. Regarding liver transplantation the occurrence of KS seems higher in patients with preexisting viral hepatic diseases as compared with those with non viral disorders [17, 26]. This seems to correlate with the fact that the chronic prevalence of hepatitis B virus infection is higher after hepatic than renal or heart transplantation [1].

Clinical features

Mucocutaneous lesions exist in more than 90% of all cases. Similarly to other KS subtypes, cutaneous lesions have a dark blue or purplish colour. They start as macules which progress and may coalesce to form large plaques (*Figure 27, page 221*) or nodular and fungoid tumors. They are mainly localized on the lower limbs and are also frequently seen on the trunk and the upper limbs. Facial involvement is less frequent than in epidemic KS. Some lesions may be located on scars (*Figure 28, page 221*), especially the transplantation scar [27] as a result of Koebner's phenomenon. Edema of the lower limbs may be associated (*Figure 29, page 221*) and often precedes skin lesions by a few months. The diagnosis of KS is difficult at this initial edematous stage without skin lesions; in this case, serological tests for HHV8 may be useful for the diagnosis. Oral lesions involve predominantly the palate and manifest with purple macules. Gingival hyperplasia may occur and must be distinguished from the one induced by cyclosporin [28]. Genital or conjunctival involvement is less frequent. Localized involvement of the uterine cervix has been reported in one case [29].

In general, mucocutaneous lesions cause rather limited functional disability. Walking can be hampered if edema or a large subcutaneous infiltrate is present. Superinfection of ulcerated lesions should be feared since this can be serious in immunosuppressed patients; distal paraesthesia, resulting from distal nerves being included in KS lesions, rarely occurs.

Extracutaneous KS most frequently involves the lymph nodes, the gastrointestinal tract and the lungs. Enlarged lymph nodes should be examined histologically because of the possibility of an associated lymphoma. Although KS can develop throughout the entire gastrointestinal tract, it is mostly localized on stomach and duodenum. The lesions rarely cause clinical symptoms, such as nausea, heavy hemorrhage, perforation or obstruction syndrome due to tumoral compression. They are usually detected at endoscopic examination showing more or less infiltrated red lesions.

Pulmonary involvement appears at a more advanced stage of the disease; it induces diffuse interstitial infiltrates, pulmonary nodules and/or pleural effusions causing dyspnea, hypoxaemia and hypocapnia. Other localizations have been reported, especially in the hepatosplenic or cardiac areas. Bone involvement is rare. Brain involvement has not yet been reported.

Initial staging, diagnosis

Clinical examination should include ear, nose and throat, ophthalmological and genital examination. A dated scheme with photographs of all mucocutaneous lesions allows an accurate follow-up of skin lesions. Chest involvement is detected by radiography, computed tomography (CT) and measurement of arterial blood gases. If these examinations are abnormal, bronchoscopy with bronchoalveolar lavage should be performed to confirm the diagnosis of KS and exclude other diseases, especially opportunistic infections. Gastrointestinal tract involvement is detected by esogastroduodenoscopy and less frequently by colonoscopy. Deep lymph node involvement can be detected by thoracic and abdominal CT.

Regardless of the localization, the diagnosis of KS is confirmed by its characteristic histopathologic features. Early patchlike lesions show a proliferation of jagged capillaries extending out from normal vessels. As the lesions progress, a network of spindle cells and large vascular spaces develop, lined by flattened endothelial cells. Interweaving bands of spindle cells embedded in a network of reticulin associated with the vascular spaces are the prominent features of the tumor stage. Extravasated red blood cells are seen. The cellular masses are surrounded by haemosiderin-laden macrophages and a moderately dense inflammatory infiltrate.

The detection and quantification of HHV8 sequences in KS tissue samples, blood mononuclear cells and other tissues and recurrent determination of anti-HHV8 antibody levels have to be carried out for prospective studies in order to optimize the interpretation of the results over the largest possible population of organ recipients.

The detection of other viral, bacterial, fungal or parasitic infections arising as a result of iatrogenic immunosuppression, similarly to KS, is not of merely theoretical interest; indeed, these infections seem to be an aggravating factor for KS and should therefore be treated. Although they are reported in many clinical cases, no prospective study of their prevalence has been so far carried out [30].

Based on the results of the clinical work-up, KS is classified into 4 stages described by Al Khader in 1988 [31]. At stage 1, localized skin lesions involve only one limb. At stage 2, cutaneous involvement is still isolated but widespread skin lesions involve more than one limb. Stage 3 means single or multiple visceral or lymph node involvement. Stage 4 is characterized by any of the above stages associated with either life-threatening infection or other neoplasms. Lymphoma was associated in 2% of the 356 patients the series of Penn [14]. This classification is simple, widely used in the literature, and permits to evaluate KS extension. It does not take into account data essential for the therapeutic decision, such as functional disability, rate of development of KS lesions and KS-linked vital risk, which have to be evaluated on a case-by-case basis.

Treatment and prognosis

The treatment of KS in organ transplant recipients varies greatly depending on the institution, making literature analysis difficult. However, it is unequivocally agreed that immunosuppressive drugs should be tapered to the lowest possible level compatible with allograft function, which is of vital importance in case of liver or heart transplantation. The degree of immunosuppressive drug reduction will depend on the rate of development of the lesions, functional disability and vital risk linked to KS or to transplanted organ failure and should be discussed on a case-by-case basis. Associated infections must be treated whenever feasable. In one case, we observed the disappearance of extensive cutaneous KS lesions after treatment of underlying tuberculosis and without modification of immunosuppressive drugs that were already given at the lowest possible level. In many cases, reducing immunosuppressive drugs may be sufficient to induce KS regression. In the Cincinnati registry, for instance, 17% of 213 patients with mucocutaneous involvement and 16% of 143 patients with single or multiple visceral involvement experienced KS disappearance after reduction of immunosuppression [14]. These figures are likely underestimated as lesion regression was already underway in further patients at treatment initiation. An urgent need to eradicate KS is reasonable in the case of a neoplasm; however this remains questionable if no important functional disability or life-threatening risk exists, since KS is considered to be a hyperplastic process and its clonality is still controversial [32, 33]. The lesions can regress within a few weeks after immunosuppression has been tapered; however, we have often observed slower regressions that may take several months. Follow-up of mucocutaneous lesions with the help of iterative schemes gives a general view of the disease evolution during this period. In fact, cutaneous and visceral lesions do not develop in parallel, but their evolution runs a roughly parallel course. The appearance of a few cutaneous lesions does not imply that the disease is markedly progressing if other coexisting lesions regress; conversely, the disease is considered as progressive if new lesions appear and their initial area enlarges twice (if ≥ 5 lesions were present at diagnosis). Complete regression of KS lesions should not be aimed to at any price as, for instance, it may be preferable to keep a good renal function and accept that a few stable, not very unconfortable KS skin lesions persist.

Various therapies are available when KS treatment has to be considered due to lesion extension, functional or aesthetic discomfort or life-threatening risk. A small number of cutaneous or mucous-membrane lesions advocates for cryotherapy, cryosurgery, laser or surgical removal, methods providing aesthetically good results. Intralesional chemotherapy is also recommended but is painful. Radiotherapy leads to a rapid regression but increases the long-term risk for developing cutaneous carcinomas; therefore, it must be avoided since the relevant population is already at high risk for developing cutaneous carcinomas. Various single agents or combination chemo-therapies have been proposed, but none of them is clearly outstanding. The most common single chemotherapeutic agents include vinblastine at a weekly dosage of 0.1 mg/kg during 5-10 weeks and bleomycin at a dosage of 15 mg/2weeks. In the case of rapidly progressing multivisceral involvement combination chemotherapies have been used, associating e.g. adriamycin or doxorubicin, bleomycin, vinblastine or vincristine (ABV), or etoposide and cisplastin. Combination chemotherapy permits to control KS, but increases the iatrogenic immunosuppression and KS may recur after a several month- or year-long remission [17]. IFNα, which is widely used in endemic KS, is not recommended after organ transplantation, because of the risk of graft rejection [34]. It seems to be better tolerated after hepatic transplantation and has been prescribed to treat viral hepatitis recurrence on the allograft [35] and in some isolated cases of KS [36].

Although *in vitro* studies have shown that several antiherpetic molecules (foscavir, cidofovir, ganciclovir) may have an inhibitory action on HHV8 replication, an action of these antiviral agents on KS in transplant recipients has not yet been demonstrated. Their use should be limited because of toxicity, concerning especially the kidneys (foscavir) and bone marrow (ganciclovir). Whether HHV8 can be completely eradicated is doubtful as this virus may remain in the body in a latent state, similarly to other herpes viruses. A therapeutic attempt using such antiviral drugs can nevertheless be considered in critical cases, awaiting the effects of immunosuppression reduction. The same also applies to intravenous immunoglobin (IVIG), which seemingly was effective on single cases of iatrogenic KS, especially associated with polymyositis [37].

Together with a more accurate modulation of immunosuppression according to KS severity, these therapeutic modalities will hopefully permit to improve the prognosis of KS. The mortality rate due to KS varies depending on the series. In the collaborative study of the « Ile-de-France » region, 34% of 41 patients died (21% after renal, 44% after hepatic and 100% after cardiac transplantation) [1]. Similarly to the series of Penn [14], the number of deaths was higher in patients with visceral involvement than in patients with purely cutaneous KS (11% *versus* 78% in Ile-de-France, 23% *versus* 57% in the Cincinnati registry). Other series do not mention an increase of death ratio depending on the grafted organ [17] or visceral involvement [17, 25]. The cause of death is often not accurately reported; rejection, opportunistic infections or complications of visceral KS are collectively considered as KS-linked. After renal transplantation, the percentage of patients returning to dialysis ranges from 21% to 58% depending on the institution [1, 2,14].

In the literature, KS recurrence after retransplantation has been reported in all patients who previousy had a sporadic or a post-transplant KS which had disappeared for several years [38, 39]. This high recurrence risk has to be taken into account before a new transplantation is decided. It could be interesting to look for the presence of anti-HHV8 antibodies before transplantation in KS-free patients in order to evaluate the post-transplantation risk of KS development. Indeed, anti-HHV8 antibodies are detectable in the sera of most transplant recipients before initiation of the immunosuppressive treatment, suggesting that KS in these patients is primarily due to virus reactivation [40]. A possible transmission of HHV8 from the donor to the transplant recipient through the allograft has been recently reported [40]; this transmission could explain the exceptional cases when KS appeared simultaneously in two kidney recipients from the same donor [41]. Should this assumption be substantiated, then all donors should be screened for the presence of anti-HHV8 antibodies.

References

1. Farge D, and the collaborative transplantation research group of Ile-de-France. Kaposi's sarcoma in organ transplant recipients. *Eur J Med* 1993 ; 2 : 339-43.

2. Touraine JL, Raffaele P, Traeger J, Garnier JL, Lefrançois N, Pouteil-Noble C, Marrast AC, Daoud S, Euvrard S. Kaposi's sarcoma in organ transplantation (Lyon experience, 1965-1995). In : Touraine JL, et al., eds. *Cancer in transplantation, prevention and treatment*. Amsterdam : Kluwer Academic Publishers, 1996 : 73-80.

3. Curtil A, Robin J, Tronc F, Ninet J, Boissonnat P, Champsaur G. Malignant neoplasms following cardiac transplantation. *Eur J Cardiothorac Surg* 1997 ; 12 : 101-6.

4. Philit F, Mornex JF, Dureau G, Chuzel M, Euvrard S, Ecochard D, Brune J. Cutaneous Kaposi's sarcoma with pulmonary carcinomatous lymphangitis in patients with heart transplantation. *Rev Mal Respir* 1994 ; 11 : 421-3.

5. Besnard V, Euvrard S, Kanitakis J, Mion F, Boillot O, Francès C, Faure M, Claudy A. Kaposi's sarcoma after liver transplantation. *Dermatology* 1996 ; 193 : 100-4.

6. Launois B, Meunier B, Camus C, Bardaxoglou E, Lakehal M, Caulet-Maugendre S, Andrée P, Ramée MP, Chaperon J, Le Pogamp P, Messner M. Les cancers de novo après transplantation d'organe. *Bull Acad Natl Med* 1996 ; 180 : 1969-96.

7. Gomez dos Santos V, Burgos Revilla FJ, Pascual Santos J, Orofino Ascunce L, Fernandez-Juarez G, Crespo Martinez L, Clemente Ramos L, Carrera Puerta C, Marcen Letosa R, Escudero Barrilero A, Ortuno Mirete J. Neoplasm prevalence in renal transplantation. *Arch Esp Urol* 1997 ; 50 : 267-73.

8. Montagnino G, Lorca E, Tarantino A, Bencini P, Aroldi A, Cesana B, Braga M, Lonati F, Ponticelli C. Cancer incidence in 854 kidney transplant recipients from a single institution: comparison with normal population and with patients under dialytic treatment. *Clin Transplant* 1996 ; 10 : 461-9.

9. Lesnoni La Parola I, Masini C, Nanni G, Diociaiuti A, Panocchia N, Cerimele D. Kaposi's sarcoma in renal-transplant recipients: experience at the Catholic University in Rome, 1988-1996. *Dermatology* 1997 ; 194 : 229-33.

10. Qunibi WY, Barri Y, Aifurayh O, Almeshari K, Khan B, Taher S, Sheth K. Kaposi's sarcoma in renal transplant recipients: a report on 26 cases from a single institution. *Transplant Proc* 1993 ; 25 : 1402-5.

11. Margolius L, Stein M, Spencer D, Bezwoda WR. Kaposi's sarcoma in renal transplant recipients. Experience at Johannesburg Hospital, 1966-1989. *S Afr Med J* 1994 ; 84 : 16-7.

12. Shmueli D, Shapira Z, Yussim A, Nakache R, Ram Z, Shaharabani E. The incidence of Kaposi's sarcoma in renal transplant patients and its relation to immunosuppression. *Transplant Proc* 1989 ; 21 : 3209-10.

13. Zahger D, Lotan C, Admond D, Klapholz L, Kaufman B, Shimon D, Woolfson N, Gotsman MS. Very early appearance of Kaposi's sarcoma after cardiac transplantation in Sephardic jews. *Am Heart J* 1993 ; 126 : 999-1000.

14. Penn I. Sarcomas in organ allografts recipients. *Transplantation* 1995 ; 60 : 1485-91.

15. Frezza EE, Fung JJ, van Thiel DH. Non-lymphoid cancer after liver transplantation. *Hepatogastroenterology* 1997 ; 44 : 1172-81.

16. Dresdale AR, Lutz S, Drost C, Levine TB, Fenn N, Paone G, del Busto R, Silverman NA. Prospective evaluation of malignant neoplasms in cardiac transplant recipients uniformly treated with prophylactic antilymphocyte globulin. *J Thorac Cardiovasc Surg* 1993 ; 106 : 1202-7.

17. Shepherd FA, Maher E, Cardella C, Cole E, Greig P, Wade JA, Levy G. Treatment of Kaposi sarcoma after solid organ transplantation. *J Clin Oncol* 1997 ; 15 : 2371-7.

18. Harwood AR, Osoba D, Hofstader SL, Goldstein MB, Cardella CJ, Holecek MJ, Kunynetz R, Giammarco RA. Kaposi's sarcoma in recipients of renal transplants. *Am J Med* 1979 ; 67 : 759-65.

19. Tzfoni EE, Scherman L, Battat S, Brautbar H. No HLA antigen is significant in classic Kaposi's sarcoma. *J Am Acad Dermatol* 1993 ; 28 : 118-9.

20. Brunson ME, Balakrishnan K, Penn I. HLA and Kaposi's sarcoma in solid organ transplantation. *Hum Immunol* 1990 ; 29 : 56-63.

21. Gao SJ, Kingsley L, Li M, Zheng W, Parravicini C, Ziegler J, Nexton R, Rinaldo CR, Saah A, Phair J, Detels R, Chang Y, Moore PS. KSHV antibodies among Americans, Italians and Ugandans with or without Kaposi's sarcoma. *Nature Med* 1996 ; 2 : 925-8.

22. Smith L, Morris M, Wong W. Renal transplantation in children; the Auckland experience 1980-96. *N Z Med J* 1997 ; 110 : 202-4.

23. Penn I, Brunson ME. Cancers after cyclosporin therapy. *Transplant Proc* 1988 ; 20 : 885-92.

24. Rezeig MA, Fashir MB, Hainau B, Al Ashgar HI. Kaposi's sarcoma in liver transplant recipients on FK506: two case reports. *Transplantation* 1997 ; 63 : 1520-1.

25. Kadry Z, Bronsther O, Van Thiel D, Randhawa P, Fung J, Starzl T. Kaposi's sarcoma in two primary liver allograft recipients occurring under FK506 immunosuppression. *Clin Transplant* 1993 ; 7 : 188-94.

26. Bismuth H, Samuel D, Vénencie PY, Menouar G, Szekely AM. Development of Kaposi's sarcoma in liver transplants recipients: characteristics, management and outcome. *Transplant Proc* 1991 ; 23 : 1438-9.

27. Micali G, Gasparri O, Nasca MR, Sapuppo A. Kaposi's sarcoma occurring *de novo* in the surgical scar in a heart transplant recipient. *J Am Acad Dermatol* 1992 ; 27 : 273-4.

28. Quniby WY, Akhtar M, Ginn E, Smith P. Kaposi sarcoma in cyclosporin-induced gingival hyperplasia. *Am J Kidney Dis* 1988 ; 11 : 349-2.

29. Lopes P, Petit T, Audoin AF, Lenne Y. Sarcome de Kaposi du col utérin chez une transplantée cardiaque. *Presse Med* 1988 ; 17 : 1539.

30. Siegal B, Levinton-Kriss S, Schiffer A, Sayar J, Engelberg I, Vonsover A, Ramon Y, Rubinstein E. Kaposi's sarcoma in immunosuppression. Possibly the result of a dual viral infection. *Cancer* 1990 ; 65 : 492-8.

31. Al-Khader AA, Suleiman M, Al-Hasani M, Haleem A. Posttransplant Kaposi's sarcoma: staging as a guide to therapy and prognosis. *Nephron* 1988 ; 48 : 165.

32. Rabkin CS, Janz S, Lash A, Coleman AE, Musaba E, Liotta L, Biggar RJ, Zhuang Z. Monoclonal origin of multicentric Kaposi's sarcoma lesions. *N Engl J Med* 1997 ; 336 : 988-93.

33. Delabesse E, Oksenhendler O, Lebbe C, Verola O, Varet B, Turhan AG. Molecular analysis of clonality in Kaposi's sarcoma. *J Clin Pathol* 1997 ; 50 : 664-8.

34. Magnone M, Holley J, Shapiro R, Scantelbury V, McCauley J, Jordan M, Vivas C, Starzl T, Johnson J. Interferon-induced acute renal allograft rejection. *Transplantation* 1994 ; 59 : 1068-70.

35. Wright WHL, Galaver JS, Van Thiel DH. Preliminary experience with alpha-2b-interferon therapy of viral hepatitis in liver allograft recipients. *Transplantation* 1994 ; 53 : 121-4.

36. Halmos O, Inturri P, Galligioni A, Di Landro D, Rigotti P, Tedeschi U, Graziotto A, Burra P, Poletti A, Rossaro L. Two cases of Kaposi's sarcoma in renal and liver transplant recipients treated with interferon. *Clin Transplant* 1996 ; 10 : 374-8.

37. Carmeli Y, Mevorach D, Kaminski N, Raz E. Regression of Kaposi's sarcoma after intravenous immunoglobulin treatment for polymyositis. *Cancer* 1994 ; 73 : 2859-61.

38. Al-Sulaiman MH, Mousa DH, Dhar JM, Al-Khader AA. Does regressed posttransplantation Kaposi's sarcoma recur following reintroduction of immunosuppression? *Am J Nephrol* 1992 ; 12 : 384-6.

39. Doutrelepont JM, DePauw L, Gruber SA, Dunn DL, Qunibi W, Kinnaert P, Vereerstraeten P, Penn I, Abramowicz D. Renal transplantation exposes patients with previous Kaposi's sarcoma to a high risk of recurrence. *Transplantation* 1996 ; 62 : 463-6.

40. Parravicini C, Olsen SJ, Capra M, Poli F, Sirchia G, Gao SJ, Berti E, Nocera A, Rossi E, Bestetti G, Pizzuto M, Galli M, Moroni M, Moore PS, Corbellino M. Risk of Kaposi's sarcoma-associated herpes virus transmission from donor allografts among Italian posttransplant Kaposi's sarcoma patients. *Blood* 1997 ; 90 : 2826-9.

41. Bottalico D, Santabosti Barbone G, Giancaspro V, Bignardi L, Arisi L, Cambi V. Post-transplantation Kaposi's sarcoma appearing simultaneously in same cadaver donor renal transplant recipients. *Nephrol Dial Transplant* 1997 ; 12 : 1055-7.

17

Naevi and melanomas

Jane M. McGREGOR
Department of Photobiology, St Johns Institute of Dermatology, St Thomas' Hospital, London, UK,
and Center for Cutaneous Research, Royal London Hospital, London, UK.

The increase in non-melanoma skin cancer following organ transplantation is well established but there are few available data on the risk of malignant melanoma associated with iatrogenic immunosuppression. The relative rarity of melanoma in the general population means that the power of any individual transplant centre to detect a true rise in the incidence of melanoma is limited and reports to date are therefore largely anecdotal. In addition, sampling problems make statistical analysis of combined data from transplant registries unreliable. This chapter examines the evidence that organ transplantation may affect the development of benign melanocytic naevi and summarises data which indicate a possible independent effect of immunosuppression on melanoma risk.

Benign melanocytic naevi and immunosuppression

Twin studies suggest that the number and type of melanocytic naevi that develop is genetically determined to a large extent [1]. On this background however there is increasing evidence that environmental factors may also play a part. For example, the total number of benign naevi is greater in Australian children up to the age of 2 years than in age-matched children resident in the UK [2], suggesting that ultraviolet radiation (UVR) may play a role. The dysplastic naevus phenotype is also more common in Australians than in age- and skin-type matched individuals resident in the UK [3] although the distribution of atypical naevi on chronically *versus* intermittently sun-exposed sites does not indicate a direct role for UVR in this [4]. It is generally believed that differences in naevi counts with respect to sun exposure reflect the immunosuppressive effect of UVR although mutagenic and/or proliferative effects may also be involved.

Evidence that immunosuppression *per se* may play a part in determining the melanocytic naevus phenotype of an individual comes from several sources. Eruptive dysplastic naevi have been anecdotally reported in patients immunosuppressed in a variety of situations; for example those who develop HIV infection [5] and in renal allograft recipients (*Figure 30, page 221*) [6]. In one case report of identical twins, only one of whom underwent a renal transplant, excess numbers of benign melanocytic naevi appeared in the transplanted twin within several years of immunosuppression but were not seen in the healthy twin [7].

Several case control studies have also been undertaken to examine the effect of immunosuppression on numbers of benign melanocytic naevi. Significantly increased numbers of benign naevi compared with an age- and sex-matched population have been reported in children receiving chemotherapy for leukaemia and others cancers [8-11] and in children who have undergone renal transplantation [12]. Increased naevi counts on non-chronically sun exposed sites were found to be most significant, including naevi developing on the palms and soles (*Graph 6*). A strong positive correlation between naevi counts and duration of immunosuppression independent of age was observed in paediatric renal transplant recipients (*Graph 7*) [12].

Similar case control studies undertaken in adults also show significantly higher naevi counts in patients immunosuppressed by HIV infection [13] and organ transplantation than in age and sex-matched controls [13, 14]. These combined studies suggest that it is immunosuppression itself, rather than the effect of a particular chemotherapeutic regimen or disease, that is responsible for the increase in naevi observed. Anecdotally it seems that naevi may not increase equally in all individuals, but rather that some patients develop very large numbers of eruptive naevi [5, 6, 12], whilst others seem relatively unaffected. This would argue that immunosuppression, and possibly other environmental factors, predominantly affects those who have a genetic predisposition to a moley phenotype.

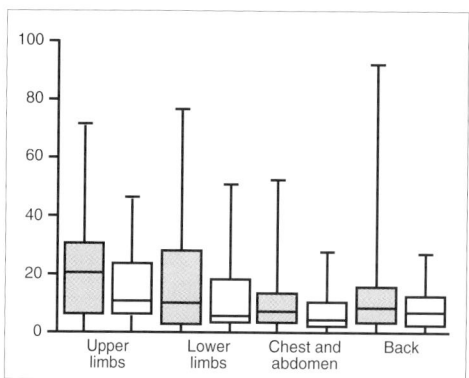

Graph 6. Regional naevi counts in children receiving renal allografts and control children. The box represents the interquartile range (*i.e.* where middle 50% of values lie) and the horizontal line within each box denotes the median value. Limits of vertical lines denote minimum and maximum values. Data from renal allograft children are shown by hatched boxes, data from control children by open boxes. Vertical axis represents number of melanocytic naevi. (From [12] with permission.)

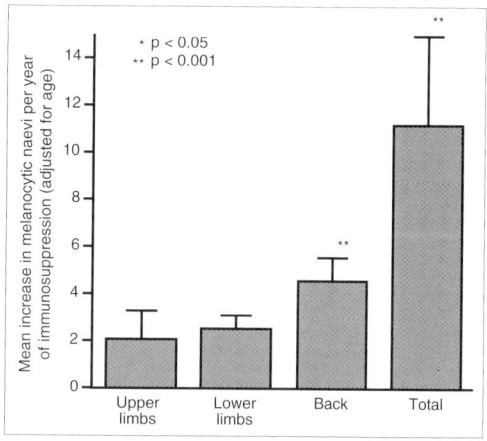

Graph 7. Increase in melanocytic naevi with duration of immunosuppression.

Malignant melanoma and immunosuppression

Melanoma occurs in organ transplant recipients in three contexts; in patients who have been treated for melanoma prior to transplantation, *de novo* tumours following transplantation and in patients in whom melanoma cells have inadvertently been transplanted along with the donor organ. Much of the data concerning these situations is necessarily anecdotal.

Melanoma treated prior to transplantation

Data accumulated by the Cincinatti Transplant Tumour Registry (CTTR) between 1968 and 1995, from an unspecified total number of transplant recipients, shows that 31 patients had malignant melanomas removed at a median time of 25 months (332-1.5 months) prior to organ transplantation [15]. The melanoma involved the skin in 30 patients and the eye in one but no information is given on Breslow thickness nor on completeness of removal. Of 31 patients, 6 (19%) died of recurrent disease within 30 months of transplantation and 25 were disease free at the time of reporting. However in 11 surviving patients (44%) the follow-up time was < 24 months and the prognosis of organ recipients previously treated for melanoma should therefore remain guarded.

Transmission of melanoma from donors

The CTTR also provides data on 20 patients who inadvertently received organs from donors with undiagnosed metastatic melanoma (most frequently misdiagnosed as primary brain tumours) [15]. Of the 20 recipients, 16 developed metastatic melanoma on average 13 months (median 10.5 months; range 2.5-42 months) after transplantation. Eleven had died at the time of reporting but 5 were said to be in remission following transplant nephrectomy and discontinuation of immunosuppression. One further patient developed local spread of melanoma beyond the allograft and remained disease-free on dialysis following nephrectomy and excision of the tumour mass. Three other patients showed no evidence of melanoma at the time of reporting.

De novo tumours in organ transplant recipients

There have been a number of studies examining the risk of malignant melanoma following organ transplantation but no single study has had sufficient power to demonstrate an unequivocal increase in this situation. Nonetheless, several transplant centres report malignant melanoma in occasional patients and some document a higher than expected incidence of melanoma in their transplant population compared to the general population (*Table 1*). Taken together, these data suggest there may be a moderate (2-10 fold) increased risk of melanoma in immunosuppressed organ transplant recipients [16-30]. It should be noted however that in many of these studies the expected number of melanomas is estimated from a population which is not directly comparable to the study population and confidence limits are therefore approximate.

The CTTR provides data on 177 patients who developed melanoma following transplantation, from many centres around the world [15]. Of these 120 were male and 57 female. The median age at diagnosis of melanoma was 46 years (9-74 years) but unusually 11 patients (6%) were aged 18 years or less. The seemingly high incidence of melanoma in children is of considerable concern although it may reflect a reporting bias to some extent. Nonetheless melanoma accounted for 14% of skin cancers in patients who received transplants in childhood compared

Table I. Malignant melanoma in renal allograft recipients: a summary of previously reported cases

Patient numbers	Observed melanoma cases	Expected melanoma cases	SMR	95% confidence limit
418 [16]	2	–	–	–
25,108 [17]	6	1.55	3.9	1.4-8.5*
3,823 [18]	5	1.0*	5.0*	–
523 [19]	3	–	–	–
580 [20]	1	–	–	–
290 [21]	2	–	–	–
200 [22]	0	–	–	–
764 [23]	0	–	–	–
223 [24]	0	–	–	–
129 [25]	0	–	–	–
598 [26]	1	–	–	–
567 [27]	2	.17	11.76	–
~ 30,000 [28]	14	–	–	–
1,158 [29]	8	4	2.0	0.9-3.9
4,241 [30]	18	N/A	~ 4.0*	

* Patients and population from which expected values were estimated are not directly comparable.

with 5% in those transplanted as adults. These preliminary data, together with possible links between immunosuppression and increased naevi in paediatric transplant recipients [12], suggest that immunosuppression commencing at an early age may be a particular risk factor for melanoma.

Of 177 patients reported to the CTTR, the median time to develop a melanoma following transplantation was 46 months (1-244 months). The majority (164 of 177) were cutaneous in origin although five (3%) arose in the eye and a further eight (5%) presented with metastatic disease from unknown primary sites. Melanoma accounted for between 4% and 10% of skin malignancies in solid organ transplant recipients but a staggering 60% of skin malignancies in bone marrow transplant patients. This figure most likely reflects the high number of children who receive bone marrow transplants, a group in whom non-melanoma skin cancer is extremely rare, but it nonetheless merits further study.

Overall 56 (32%) of all patients reported to the CTTR with *de novo* melanoma died from their disease. Thirty-two of 164 patients with cutaneous melanoma developed metastases, of whom 24 (~15%) subsequently died. No attempt can be made to compare mortality from melanoma in the transplant and immunecompetent population without accurate data on Breslow thickness; this was available in only a few cases reported to the CTTR. The seemingly high mortality rate might reflect late presentation rather than the effect of an altered immune response to the tumour. However two patients with melanomas < 1.5 mm apparently died from metastatic disease which would be unusual in an immunecompetent population.

Histological examination

Histological examination of 14 malignant melanomas in one study of renal allograft recipients with melanomas revealed an abnormal (sparse) cellular host response to the tumour [28]. Whilst it is possible that the prognosis of melanoma is worse in the immunosuppressed than the immunocompetent population, confirmation of this requires careful prospective study.

Conclusion

In conclusion there is some evidence that immunosuppression may increase numbers of benign melanocytic naevi, particularly on non-sun exposed sites. This effect may be most noticeable in children and young adults, when melanocyte activity is normally at its peak, but it is also apparent to some extent in older organ transplant recipients. Reports of large numbers of eruptive, and sometimes dysplastic, naevi in occasional patients suggests that immunosuppression may have a maximal effect in those individuals with a genetic predisposition to a moley phenotype, although this observation requires confirmation. Whether increased naevi following immunosuppression in childhood will emerge as a risk factor for the subsequent development of melanoma has yet to be established.

There is insufficient data as yet to indicate that organ transplantation alters the prognosis of patients previously treated for melanoma. However this remains a concern and requires further study. Inadvertent transmission of melanoma through organ donation, although rare, appears to carry a very poor prognosis without treatment. In the few reported cases where the affected organ was subsequently removed and immunosuppression discontinued, patients survived.

There are limited data to suggest that organ transplant recipients are at moderate (2-10 fold) increased risk of *de novo* malignant melanoma compared to the general population. Anecdotally melanoma in the immunosuppressed host appears to carry a worse prognosis than in the immunocompetent patient, although there are no reliable data to confirm this. Preliminary data from the CTTR show a higher than expected incidence of melanoma in children compared to adult transplant recipients which is of considerable concern. The incidence of melanoma in the emerging and ageing cohort of paediatric transplant recipients will need to be carefully monitored.

References

1. Easton DF, Cox GM, Macdonald AM, Ponder BA. Genetic susceptibility to naevi. A twin study. *Br J Cancer* 1991 ; 64 : 1164-7.
2. MacKie RM, Turner S, Harrison SA, MacLennan R. A comparison of the rate of development of melanocytic naevi in infants in Scotland and Australia. *Br J Dermatol* 1997 ; 137 : S50.
3. Bataille V, Grulich A, Sasieni P, Swerdlow A, Newton-Bishop J, McCarthy W, Hersey P, Cuzick J. The association between naevi and melanoma in populations with different levels of sun exposure: a joint case-control study of melanoma in the UK and Australia. *Br J Cancer* 1998 ; 77 : 505-10.
4. Stierner U, Augustsson A, Rosdahl I, Suurkula M. Regional distribution of common and dysplastic naevi in relation to melanoma site and sun exposure. A case control study. *Melanoma Res* 1992 ; 1 : 367-75.
5. Duvic M, Lowe L, Rapini RP, Rodriguez S, Levy ML. Eruptive dysplastic naevi associated with human immunodeficiency virus infection. *Arch Dermatol* 1989 ; 125 : 397-401.
6. Barker JNWN, MacDonald DM. Eruptive dysplastic naevi following renal transplantation. *Clin Exp Dermatol* 1988 ; 13 : 123-5.

7. McGregor JM, Barker JN, MacDonald DM. The development of excess numbers of melanocytic naevi in an immunosuppressed identical twin. *Clin Exp Dermatol* 1991 ; 16 : 131-2.

8. Naldi L, Adamoli L, Fraschini D, Corbetta A, Imberti L, Reseghetti A, Reciputo A, Rossi E, Cainelli T, Masera G. Number and distribution of melanocytic naevi in individuals with a history of childhood leukaemia. *Cancer* 1996 ; 77 : 1402-8.

9. Hughes BR, Cunliffe WJ, Bailey CC. Excess benign melanocytic naevi after chemotherapy for malignancy in childhood. *Br Med J* 1989 ; 299 : 88-91.

10. de Wit PE, de Vaan GA, de Boo TM, Lemmens WAT, Rampen SHJ. Prevalence of nevocytic naevi after chemotherapy for childhood cancer. *Med Pediatr Oncol* 1990 ; 18 : 336-8.

11. Baird EA, McHenry PM, MacKie RM. Effect of maintenance chemotherapy in childhood on numbers of melanocytic naevi. *Br Med J* 1992 ; 305 : 799-801.

12. Smith CH, McGregor JM, Barker JNW, Morris RW, Rigden SPA, MacDonald DM. Excess melanocytic naevi in children with renal allografts. *J Am Acad Dermatol* 1993 ; 28 : 51-5.

13. Grob JJ, Bastuji-Garin S, Vaillant L, Roujeau JC, Bernard P, Sassolas B, Guillaume JC. Excess naevi related to immunodeficiency: a study in HIV infected patients and renal transplant recipients. *J Invest Dermatol* 1996 ; 107 : 694-7.

14. Szepietowski J, Wasik F, Szepietowski T, Wlodarczyk M, Sobczak-Radwan K, Czy W. Excess benign melanocytic naevi in renal transplant recipients. *Dermatology* 1997 ; 194 : 17-9.

15. Penn I. Malignant melanoma in organ allograft recipients. *Transplantation* 1996 ; 61 : 274-8.

16. Birkeland SA. Malignant tumours in renal transplant patients. *Cancer* 1983 ; 51 : 1571-5.

17. Hoover RN. Effects of drugs: immunosuppression. In : Hiatt HH, Watson JD, eds. *Origins of human cancer*. New York : Cold Spring Harbour Laboratories 1977 : 369-79.

18. Kinlen J, Sheil AGR, Peto J, Doll R. Collaborative United Kingdom-Australia study of cancer in patients treated with immunosuppressive drugs. *Br Med J* 1979 ; 2 : 1461-6.

19. Gupta AK, Cardella CJ, Haberman HF. Cutaneous malignant neoplasms in patients with renal transplants. *Arch Dermatol* 1986 ; 122 : 1288-92.

20. Cohen EB, Komorowski RA, Clowry LJ. Cutaneous complications in renal transplant recipients. *Am J Clin Pathol* 1987 ; 88 : 32-7.

21. Hardie IR, Strong RW, Hartley LCJ, Woodruff PWH, Clunie GJA. Skin cancer in Caucasian renal allograft recipients living in a subtropical climate. *Surgery* 1980 ; 87 : 177-83.

22. Koranda FC, Dehmel EM, Kahn G, Penn I. Cutaneous complications in immunosuppressed renal homograft recipients. *J Am Med Assoc* 1974 ; 229 : 419-24.

23. Hartevelt MM, Bouwes Bavinck JN, Kootte AMM, Vermeer BJ, Vandenbroucke JP. Incidence of skin cancer after renal transplantation in the Netherlands. *Transplantation* 1990 ; 49 : 506-9.

24. Brown JH, Hutchinson T, Kelly AMT, McGeown MG. Dermatologic lesions in a transplant population. *Transplantation* 1988 ; 46 : 530-2.

25. Blohme I, Larko O. Premalignant and malignant skin lesions in renal transplant patients. *Transplantation* 1984 ; 37 : 165-7.

26. Liddington M, Richardson AJ, Higgins RM, Endre ZH, Venning VA, Murie JA, Morris PJ. Skin cancer in renal transplant recipients. *Br J Surgery* 1989 ; 76 : 1002-5.

27. McGregor JM, Morris R, Smith CH, MacDonald DM. Skin cancer morbidity amongst renal allograft recipients. A 25 year retrospective study. *Br J Dermatol* 1995 ; 133 : S45,40.

28. Greene MH, Young TI, Clark WH. Malignant melanoma in renal transplant recipients. *Lancet* 1981 ; 1 : 1196-9.

29. Bouwes Bavinck JN, Hardie DR, Green A, Cutmore S, MacNaught A, O'Sullivan B, Siskind V, Van der Woude FK, Hardie IR. The risk of skin cancer in renal transplant recipients in Queensland, Australia: a follow-up study. *Transplantation* 1996 ; 61 : 715-21.

30. Sheil AGR, Flavel S, Disney APS, Mathew TH, Hall BM. Cancer incidence in renal transplant patients treated with azathioprine and cyclosporin. *Transplant Proc* 1987 ; 19 : 2214-6.

18

Cutaneous lymphomas

Pierre SOUTEYRAND [1], Lincoln FABRICIO [2], Michel d'INCAN [1]
1. *Department of Dermatology, CHU Clermont-Ferrand, France.*
2. *Department of Dermatology, FEMPAR, Curitiba, Brazil.*

Lymphomas and organ transplantation

Epidemiology

Immunosuppressive states, whether congenital, acquired or iatrogenic, are associated with a high risk of neoplasia. The risk of developing cancer is increased 100-fold in transplant recipients as compared with age-matched individuals of the general population. Aside from cutaneous carcinomas and *in situ* carcinomas of the uterine cervix, non-Hodgkin's lymphomas are by far the most commonly observed cancers in transplant recipients. The risk of developing lymphoma in organ-graft recipients is increased from 20 to 120-fold as compared with age-matched control individuals. The incidence is higher after heart than kidney transplantation possibly because of the more aggressive immunosuppressive treatment administered to heart transplant recipients in order to prevent the more serious consequences of graft rejection [1]. The overall risk is around 2%, ranging from 1% for kidney to 5% for single lung or heart-and-lung transplantations [2]; it depends not only on the type of the organ transplanted but also on the dose of immunosuppressive drugs and the length of treatment. This would also explain why two thirds of non-Hodgkin's lymphomas occur within the first post-transplant year and why the incidence is higher for immunosuppressive regimens including cyclosporine and azathioprine. Patients who receive antithymocyte/antilymphocyte globulins or OKT3 as prophylaxis are also at greater risk of lymphoma, irrespective of the type of organ transplanted.

Characteristics of lymphomas in transplant recipients

Lymphomas in transplant recipients have several distinctive features. In the general population, lymphomas involve the lymph nodes from the outset in 52 to 76% of cases, whereas in 75% of transplant recipients the disease is extranodal; in two thirds of cases, a single organ is involved, most frequently the brain, followed by the gastrointestinal tract. As in congenital immunodeficiencies, the spectrum of lymphoid proliferations after transplantation is wide, ranging from non-specific lymphoid hyperplasia to high-grade non-Hodgkin's lymphoma [3]. Post-transplant lymphoid proliferations can be polyclonal, oligoclonal or monoclonal but there is no correlation between the histological appearance and the clonality of the tumour. Because of this heterogeneity, investigation of the tumour should include morphological, immunophenotypic and molecular studies to determine clonality by analysis of the TCR (T-cell receptor) and immunoglobulin genes and of DNA terminal sequences of EBV.

Post-transplant lymphoproliferative disorders are most commonly of B-cell origin. In 80% of the cases, they are associated with EBV and characterised by similarities in clinical and histological features and outcome [4]. About 15% of lymphoproliferative disorders are derived from T-cells [5] which, in about 20% of cases, are associated with EBV [6].

Post-transplant lymphoproliferative disorders are also different with respect to their response to treatment. A reduction in immunosuppresssion, when possible, can be successful in treating the lymphoid proliferation by restoring effective antiviral cell response. Remission was achieved in 25% of patients by simple reduction in immunosuppressive therapy [4].

Epstein-Barr virus and post-transplant lymphoproliferative disorders

Polyclonal B-cell activation, variations in the expression of latency viral proteins, possible integration and replication of EBV in lymphoid cells and loss of host-virus balance are all factors involved in the development of lymphoproliferative disorders after organ transplantation [7].

Antiviral treatment is implemented when EBV is present in the tumour. Acyclovir and ganciclovir have been widely used but the results are inconsistent [8].

The precise role of EBV in lymphomagenesis of post-transplant lymphoproliferative disorders could be determined by regular search of the virus, by studying its behaviour in tumour cells, by analysing the expression of latency and replication genes, by characterisation of the phenotypic, molecular, and in particular the oncogenic modifications caused by its presence, and also its effects on the quality of immune response. With these findings, new therapeutic strategies could be developed.

Cutaneous lymphomas and organ transplantation

Epidemiology

The real incidence of cutaneous lymphomas is unknown. Although they accounted for more than one third of lymphomas in a transplant population of 672 patients followed at Guy's Hospital (London) (4 primary cutaneous against 7 cases of systemic lymphoma), to our knowledge, only 10 cutaneous post-transplant lymphomas have been reported [9-14]. Of these, six were of B-cell and four of T-cell type. Nine cases were observed after renal [9, 10, 11, 13, 14] and one after heart transplantation [12]. Nine out of the 10 patients were men. The mean age at onset of the disease was 57 years (range: 38 to 76) and the mean time post-transplantation to the appearance of lymphoma was 5 years and 5 months (range: 0.5 to

11 years). All nine patients had received an immunosuppressive regimen including steroids; eight had taken azathioprine and six cyclosporine. Five patients were treated for graft rejection with pulse therapy.

Cutaneous B-cell lymphomas

Clinical presentation

Three of the six patients with cutaneous B-cell lymphoma had a single ulcerated nodule, respectively on the lower lip, the chest wall [14] and the anterior aspect of the left leg [10]. The other three patients had multiple nodules: in two, they were located on the forehead and were ulcerated; the last one had non-ulcerated nodules on the leg [12].

In all patients, staging was negative. On this basis, a diagnosis of primary cutaneous lymphoma was made and in the case of Whittam [14] that of multiple myeloma ruled out.

Histology, immunopathology and genotypic studies

In all cases, the infiltrate was non-epidermotropic, consisting either of blastic cells and small lymphocytes or of mature plasma cells [14] or lymphoplasmacytes [12] and a few lymphocytes and histiocytes.

The B nature of atypical cells was confirmed by immunolabelling in all but one patient [11] in whom the cells had a null phenotype. In one case [14] a polytypic proliferation was observed, but in all others the infiltrate was monotypic. The three patients with cutaneous B-cell lymphoma reported by Mc Gregor et al. [11] had atypical CD30+ lymphocytes. Rearrangement studies of immunoglobulin heavy chain genes were performed in four patients; in one patient in whom the cells had a non-T-non-B-cell phenotype, the infiltrate was monoclonal [11], and in the other three this finding was confirmed.

Treatment

Five patients [10, 11, 14] were treated successfully either by radiotherapy or by surgery. One developed a recurrent cutaneous tumour five years later, which was excised. Subsequent death was due to an unrelated cause. The clinical follow-up ranged from 1 to 5.5 years (mean: 4.1 years).

The patient of Mozzanica [12] was treated with acyclovir; azathioprine therapy was discontinued and cyclosporine dosage was reduced. A progressive reduction of the lesions was observed and after seven months the patient experienced complete remission, which was maintained during a 10-month follow-up period.

Oral cavity B-cell lymphoma

Two patients with oral presentation of posttransplantation lymphoproliferative disorders have been reported [15].

The two patients were men, respectively 62 and 41-year old when they underwent cardiac transplantation. Both had erythematous to cyanotic and hyperplastic gingiva. On gingivectomy, the fixed tissue was soft, glistening and tan-coloured, in contrast to the usual firm, white, cyclosporine-associated, benign gingival fibrous hyperplasia. Histologically, a dense, diffuse infiltrate of lymphoplasmacytoid cells with vesicular nuclei, prominent nucleoli, a moderate amount of cytoplasm, and a high mitotic activity was observed. Immunocytochemical studies confirmed that the cells were monoclonal for λ light chains in one patient and κ light chains in the other. The cells from one patient were CD45+, while both patients were negative for CD20 and all non-haematopoietic antigens tested. Both tissues were strongly positive for EBV.

Cutaneous T-cell lymphomas

Clinical presentation

Three of the four cases of cutaneous T-cell lymphomas were erythrodermic; one patient had Sézary syndrome [9] (*Figure 31, page 222*) and the other two had erythrodermic mycosis fungoides [13]. The fourth patient [11] was diagnosed as having pleomorphic T-cell lymphoma and presented with haemorrhagic plaques on the leg. In two cases, superficial lymph-node enlargement was observed [9, 13].

Histology, immunopathology and genotypic studies

In all patients the infiltrate was epidermotropic, with formation of Pautrier microabscesses typical of mycosis fungoides in two patients (*Figure 32, page 222*) [9, 13]. One patient had an infiltrate composed of a pleomorphic population of lymphoid cells with hyperchromatic nuclei [11]. Immunolabelling confirmed the T nature of the infiltrate in all cases. When performed (two patients), the search of a rearrangement of the gene encoding for the beta chain of the T-cell receptor was positive. Neither EBV- nor HTLV-1 genomic DNA were identified in the cutaneous lesions of two patients [9].

Clinical course and treatment

Each patient had a different treatment and outcome. One patient received radiotherapy and died nine months after presentation from cerebral lymphoma [11]. One of the two patients of Pascual *et al.* [13] was treated with topical steroids; he died from nodal and hepatic dissemination of the disease the day on which chemotherapy was initiated. The second patient was successfully treated with nitrogen mustard ointment followed by oral prednisone and chlorambucil; after a nine-month follow-up, remission was maintained.

After azathioprine treatment was discontinued, the patient of Euvrard *et al.* [9] was given doses of chlorambucil and etretinate and then received chemotherapy comprising cyclophosphamide, doxorubicin, vindesine and bleomycin. The outcome was unfavourable with the development of skin tumours and nodal B-cell lymphoma with a monoclonal IgAλ component.

This literature review reveals that patients with primary cutaneous lymphoma after organ transplantation present the same risk factors as patients with non-cutaneous post-transplant lymphoma, and that B-cell cutaneous lymphomas are more often associated with EBV than lymphomas of the T-cell type. Immunosuppressive therapy clearly plays a role in the development of both types of lymphomas and, as in non-cutaneous post-transplant lymphomas, especially of the B-cell type [16], tapering of the immunosuppressive treatment may lead to a reduction of cutaneous lesions [12]. By contrast, although non-cutaneous lymphomas affect equally men and women [2], nine of the ten reported cases of cutaneous lymphomas occurred in men. Another striking difference between cutaneous and non-cutaneous lymphomas is the delay between transplantation and the appearance of the disease; indeed, only one of the ten cutaneous lymphomas (contrasting with about two thirds of non-cutaneous lymphomas) appeared within the first post-transplant year [2]. This difference is all the more noteworthy that the incidence of lymphoma in the first post-transplant year was not affected by geographic location or type of (initial or maintenance) immunosuppressive therapy. Post-transplant CD30+ cutaneous lymphomas differ from those occurring in the general population since the three reported cases were of B-cell lineage whereas in non-immunosuppressed patients almost all CD30+ lymphomas are of the T-cell type [17]. Finally, post-transplant cutaneous B-cell lymphomas have usually a favourable prognosis, similarly to those developing in the general population, while cutaneous T-cell lymphomas have a much more ominous prognosis in transplant recipients as compared with non-immunosuppressed hosts.

References

1. Penn I. The changing pattern of posttransplant malignancies. *Transplant Proc* 1991 ; 23 : 1101-3.

2. Opelz G, Henderson R, for the Collaborative Transplant Study. Incidence of non-Hodgkin lymphoma in kidney and heart transplant recipients. *Lancet* 1993 ; 342 : 1514-6.

3. Griffith R, Saha B, Janney C, Ratner L, Brunt E, Gajl-Peczalska K, Hanto D. Immunoblastic lymphoma of T-cell type in a chronically immunosuppressed renal transplant recipient. *Am J Clin Pathol* 1990 ; 93 : 280-5.

4. Leblond V, Sutton L, Dorent R, Davi F, Bitker M, Gabarre J, Charlotte F, Ghoussoub JJ, Fourcade C, Fischer A, Grandjbakhch I, Binet JL, Raphael M. Lymphoproliferative disorders after organ transplantation: a report of 24 cases observed in a single center. *J Clin Oncol* 1995 ; 13 : 961-8.

5. Waller E, Ziemianska M, Bangs C, Cleary M, Kamel O. Characterization of posttransplant lymphomas that express T-cell-associated markers: immunophenotypes, molecular genetics, cytogenetics, and heterotransplantation in severe combined immunodeficient mice. *Blood* 1993 ; 82 : 247-61.

6. van Gorp J, Doornewaard H, Verdonck L, Klopping C, Vos P, van den Tweel J. *Cancer* 1994 ; 73 : 3064-72.

7. Leblond V. Virus Epstein-Barr et lymphoproliférations post-transplantation. *Ann Med Intern* 1997 ; 148 : 376-8.

8. Pirsch J, Stratta R, Sollinger H, Hafez G, D'Alessandro A, Kalayoglu M, Belzer F. Treatment of severe Epstein-Barr virus induced lymphoproliferative syndrome with ganciclovir: two cases after solid organ transplantation. *Am J Med* 1989 ; 86 : 241-4.

9. Euvrard S, Pouteil Noble C, Kanitakis J, French M, Berger F, Delecluse HJ, D'Incan M, Thivolet J, Touraine JL. Successive occurrence of T-cell and B-cell lymphomas after renal transplantation in a patient with multiple cutaneous squamous-cell carcinomas. *N Engl J Med* 1992 ; 327 : 1924-6.

10. Gonthier D, Hartman G, Holley J. Posttransplant lymphoproliferative disorder presenting as an isolated skin lesion. *Am J Kidney Dis* 1992 ; 19 : 600-3.

11. Mc Gregor J, Yu C, Lu Q, Cotter F, Levison D, MacDonald D. Posttransplant cutaneous lymphoma. *J Am Acad Dermatol* 1993 ; 29 : 549-54.

12. Mozzanica N, Cattaneo A, Fracchiolla N, Boneschi V, Berti E, Gronda E, Mangiavacchi M, Finzi AF, Neri A. Posttransplantation cutaneous B-cell lymphoma with monoclonal Epstein-Barr virus infection, responding to acyclovir and reduction in immunosuppression. *J Heart Lung Transplant* 1997 ; 16 : 964-8.

13. Pascual J, Torrelo A, Teruel JL, Bellas C, Marcen R, Ortuno J. Cutaneous T cell lymphomas after renal transplantation. *Transplantation* 1992 ; 53 : 1143-5.

14. Whittam LR, Coleman R, MacDonald DM. Plasma cell tumour in a renal transplant recipient. *Clin Exp Dermatol* 1996 ; 21 : 367-9.

15. Oda D, Persson G, Haigh W, Sabath D, Penn I, Aziz S. Oral presentation of posttransplantation lymphoproliferative disorders. An unusual manifestation. *Transplantation* 1996 ; 61 : 435-40.

16. Starzl TE, Porter KA, Iwatsuki S, Rosenthal JT, Shaw Jr BW, Atchison RW, Nalesnik MA, Griffith BP, Hakala TR, Hardesty RL, Jaffe R. Reversibility of lymphomas and lymphoproliferative lesions developing under cyclosporine-steroid therapy. *Lancet* 1984 ; 17 : 583-7.

17. Willemze R, Kerl H, Sterry W, Berti E, Cerroni L, Chimenti S, Diaz-Peréz JL, Geerts ML, Goos M, Knobler R, Rälfkiaer E, Santucci M, Smith N, Wechsler J, van Vloten WA, Meijer CJLM. EORTC classification for primary cutaneous lymphomas: a proposal from the Cutaneous lymphoma study group of the European organization for research and treatment of cancer. *Blood* 1997 ; 90 : 354-71.

19

Anogenital lesions

Michel FAURE
Department of Dermatology, Hôpital Edouard-Herriot, Lyon, France.

Human papillomavirus (HPV)-related anogenital lesions and anogenital carcinomas are observed with an increased frequency in organ transplant recipients in comparison with the general population. The first series published was only devoted to cancers, the frequency of which is increased 100-fold [1, 2]. Since then, a few other studies mentioned occasional anogenital lesions [3-14]. The best documented ones concern carcinomas of the uterine cervix [15-23]. A recent study of over 1,000 patients indicated in both men and women benign and malignant anogenital lesions after kidney, lung, liver and heart transplantation [24].

Prevalence

Although the prevalence of external anogenital lesions is much lower than that of lesions occurring on sun-exposed skin [24], anogenital lesions seem to occur with a higher frequency (2.3%) than that reported in early studies on small series [4, 6, 25, 26]; it is possible that the incidence of HPV-related benign and malignant lesions is still underestimated since patients are more likely to consult their family physicians for these problems [24]. Other studies indicated that external anogenital lesions in women occur 3 to 10 times less frequently than condylomatous, dysplastic or neoplastic lesions of the cervix [15, 17, 18]. Overall, anogenital neoplasia is about 20 times more common in renal transplant recipients than the general population [2]. Women are more often involved than men. At colposcopy, 53% of women with allografts were found to have cervical abnormalities compared with only 29% of controls [18]. Vulvar and anal cancers are increased 100-fold as compared with the general population. An increased prevalence of mainly intraepithelial neoplasms of the lower genital tract is in fact observed in organ transplant recipients [15-19].

Clinicopathological data

The diagnosis of anogenital lesions is based on both clinical and histologic examination. Some lesions with a clinical aspect of genital warts correspond histologically to bowenoid papulosis or *in situ* carcinoma, highlighting the importance of the histologic examination in each case [24].

Clinically, most lesions have an aspect of anogenital wart or condyloma acuminatum. Giant cauliflower-like tumours (giant condyloma) may also be observed (*Figure 33, page 222*). In both sexes, external genital lesions are generally multiple and extensive. Patients may present with multiple pigmented papules of the penis or the vulva suggestive of bowenoid papulosis [24] (*Figure 34, page 222*). Among anogenital carcinomas those of the uterine cervix (CIN) are the most frequently reported [15, 16, 18, 19, 22].

Both men and women may have multiple locations, with genital, anal and/or cutaneous involvement [24]. Most women have multiple locations of the anus, vagina, cervix and/or the vulva [2, 3, 17, 19, 27]; one third of women with external carcinoma also have an associated uterine cervix carcinoma.

When performed, histologic studies usually confirm the diagnosis of condyloma acuminatum in patients with genital warts or giant condylomas. The diagnosis of *in situ* carcinoma (intraepithelial neoplasia) of the cervix, vulva, penis or anus (CIN, VIN, PIN, AIN) needs in fact systematic histological examination. (Extensive) bowenoid papulosis and *in situ* carcinomas (VIN, PIN) are often misdiagnosed in the absence of histologic control [24] (*Figure 35, page 222*).

Virologic studies

Only a few studies have reported the detection of HPV DNA or antigen(s) by immunohistochemistry and/or molecular *in situ* hybridisation on tissue sections. HPV types 6 and 11 are detected within anogenital warts as in non-immunosuppressed patients. Oncogenic types 5, 16, 18 and 33 can be detected not only in dysplastic lesions, bowenoid papulosis and *in situ* carcinomas, but also in benign ones, *i.e.* anogenital warts and giant condylomas [4, 6, 10, 18, 24]. Recently, a novel HPV type, named type 74, related to the low-risk types 6, 11, 44 and 55, was found in genital specimens from immunosuppressed women but not in immunocompetent patients [28]. Furthermore, histologic signs of HPV infection or intraepithelial neoplasia and HPV DNA could be noted in respectively 24% and 47% of renal transplant patients after systematic anal biopsy, whereas only 3% of them had visible lesions [26].

In patients with both anogenital lesions and cutaneous warts, identical and in some cases oncogenic HPV types may be found in anogenital lesions and cutaneous (hand) warts [24]. It appears that organ transplant recipients harbour multiple HPV types simultaneously, with mucosal HPV types and cutaneous types detected within skin warts and mucosal lesions respectively [29, 30]. The usual tissue specificity of HPV types seems to be lost, possibly because of the immunossuppression that allows HPV types to proliferate within sites where they do not usually produce lesions [24]. Self-contamination may play a role; sexual transmission of HPV appears lower than in immunocompetent hosts, as suggested by the absence of lesions in sexual partners of the patients and by the presence of lesions in patients with no sexual activity [24, 27].

Taken together these data suggest that anogenital HPV-related lesions may represent a sign of marked immunosuppression. The presence of oncogenic HPV types within lesions that look clinically and histologically benign highlights the importance of regular follow-up of these patients.

Course and treatment

Although the course of anogenital carcinomas is variable and unpredictable, these tumours are generally more morbid and mortal as compared with the general population, because patients are younger, tumours are more undifferentiated, multifocal, and treatments induce more complications [2]. Metastases occur in 11% of the cases, and some carcinomas may undergo a fulminant course [14].

Anogenital lesions may be treated with usual methods (electrocautery, cryotherapy, laser, local podophyllotoxin, fluorouracil, surgery, depending on histology), but widespread lesions may remain refractory whatever the method used [24]. Most benign lesions and *in situ* carcinomas may be cured after the immunosuppressive treatment is tapered. This also suggests that HPV-related anogenital lesions after organ transplantation are a marker of immunosuppression, especially when they are extensive.

References

1. Penn I. Cancers of the anogenital region in renal transplant recipients: analysis of 65 cases. *Cancer* 1986 ; 58 : 611-6.
2. Sillman F, Sentovich S. Ano-genital neoplasia in renal transplant patients. *Ann Transplant* 1997 ; 2 : 59-66.
3. Blohme J, Brynger H. Malignant disease in renal transplant patients. *Transplantation* 1985 ; 39 : 23-5.
4. Rüdlinger R, Smith IW, Bunney MH, Hunter JAA. Human papillomavirus infections in a group of renal transplant recipients. *Br J Dermatol* 1986 ; 115 : 681-92.
5. Van der Leest R, Zachow K, Ostrow R, Bender M, Pass F, Faras A. Human papillomavirus heterogeneity in 36 renal transplant recipients. *Arch Dermatol* 1987 ; 123 : 354-7.
6. Cohen E, Komorowski R, Clowry L. Cutaneous complications in renal transplant recipients. *Am J Clin Pathol* 1987 ; 88 : 32-7.
7. Shuttelworth D, Roberts E, Griffin P. Renal transplantation and the skin. *Lancet* 1988 : 1 : 293-4.
8. Manias D, Ostrow R, McGlennen R, Estensen R, Faras A. Characterization of integrated human papillomavirus type 11 DNA in primary and metastatic tumors from a renal transplant recipient. *Cancer Res* 1989 ; 49 : 2514-9.
9. Couetil J, McGoldrick J, Wallwork J, English T. Malignant tumors after heart transplantation. *J Heart Transplant* 1990 ; 9 : 622-6.
10. Blessing K, McLaren KM, Morrris R, Barr B, Benton C, Alloub M, Bunney M, Smith I, Smart GE, Bird CC. Detection of human papillomavirus in skin and genital lesions of renal allograft recipients by *in situ* hybridization. *Histopathology* 1990 ; 16 : 181-5 .
11. Gentile G, Formelli G, Selva S. Atypical picture of cervico-vaginal condylomatosis in a patient submitted to hepatic transplant. *Clin Exp Obstet Gyn* 1990 ; 17 : 155-7.
12. Blohme I. Carcinoma of the vulva in renal transplant patients. *Transplant Sci* 1994 ; 4 : 6-8.
13. Gaya SBM, Rees AJ, Lechler RI, Williams G, Mason PD. Malignant disease in patients with long-term renal transplants. *Transplantation* 1995 ; 59 : 1705-9.
14. Volgger B, Marth C, Zeimet A, Muller-Holzner E, Ruth N, Dapunt O. Fulminant course of a microinvasive vulvar carcinoma in an immunosuppressed woman. *Gynecol Oncol* 1997 ; 65 : 177-9.
15. Schneider V, Kay S, Lee HM. Immunosuppression as a high-risk factor in the development of condyloma acuminatum and squamous neoplasia of the cervix. *Acta Cytol* 1982 ; 27 : 220-4.
16. Sillman F, Stanek A, Sedlis A, Rosenthal J, Lanks KW, Buchhagen D, Nicastri A, Boyce J. The relationship between human papillomavirus and lower genital intraepithelial neoplasia in immunosuppressed women. *Am J Obstet Gynecol* 1984 ; 150 : 300-8.

17. Halpert R, Fruchter RG, Sedlis A, Butt K, Boyce J, Sillman FH. Human papillomavirus and lower genital neoplasia in renal transplant patients. *Obstet Gynecol* 1986 ; 68 : 251-8.
18. Alloub MI, Barr BB, McLaren KM, Smith IW, Bunney MH, Smart GE. Human papillomavirus infection and cervical intraepithelial neoplasia in women with renal allografts. *Br Med J* 1989 ; 298 : 153-6.
19. Touraine JL, Lavagna-Maurice C, Dargent D. Infections à HPV, dysplasies et néoplasies intra-épithéliales du col utérin chez les femmes immunodéprimées. *Gynécologie* 1990 ; 41 : 323-6.
20. Fairley CK, Chen S, Tabrizi SN, McNeil J, Becker G, Walker R, Atkins RC, Thomson N, Allan P, Woodburn C, Garland SM. Prevalence of HPV DNA in cervical specimens in women with renal transplants: a comparison with dialysis-dependant patients and patients with renal impairment. *Nephrol Dial Transplant* 1994 ; 9 : 416-20.
21. Birkeland SA, Storm HH, Lamm LU, Barlow L, Blohmé I, Forsberg B, Eklund B, Fjeldborg O, Friedberg M, Frödin L, Glattre E, Halvorsen S, Holm NV, Jakobsen A, Jørgensen HE, Ladefoged J, Lindholm T, Lundgren G, Pukkala E. Cancer risk after renal transplantation in the nordic countries, 1984-1986. *Int J Cancer* 1995 ; 60 : 183-9.
22. Ter Haar-Van Eck SA, Rischen-Vos J, Chadha-Ajwani S, Huikeshoven FJM. The incidence of cervical intraepithelial neoplasia among women with renal transplant in relation to cyclosporin. *Br J Obstet Gynaecol* 1995 ; 102 : 58-61.
23. Morrison EAB, Dole P, Sun XW, Stern L, Wright TC. Low prevalence of human papillomavirus infection of the cervix in renal transplant recipients. *Nephrol Dial Transplant* 1996 ; 11 : 1603-6.
24. Euvrard S, Kanitakis J, Chardonnet Y, Pouteil Noble C, Touraine JL, Faure M, Thivolet J, Claudy A. External anogenital lesions in organ transplant recipients. *Arch Dermatol* 1997 ; 133 : 175-8.
25. Sheil AGR, Flavel S, Disney APS, Mathew TH, Hall BM. Cancer incidence in renal transplant patients treated with azathioprine or cyclosporin. *Transplant Proc* 1987 ; 19 : 2214-6.
26. Ogunbiyi OA, Scholefield H, Raftery AT, Smith JHF, Duffy S, Sharp F, Rogers K. Prevalence of anal human papillomavirus infection and intraepithelial neoplasia in renal allograft recipients. *Br J Surg* 1994 ; 81 : 365-7.
27. Arends MJ, Benton EC, McLaren KM, Stark LA, Hunter JAA, Bird CC. Renal allograft recipients with high susceptibility to cutaneous malignancy have an increased prevalence of human papillomavirus DNA in skin tumours and a greater risk of anogenital malignancy. *Br J Cancer* 1997 ; 75 : 722-8.
28. Longuet M, Cassonnet P, Orth G. A novel genital human papilomavirus (HPV), HPV type 74, found in immunosuppressed patients. *J Clin Microbiol* 1996 ; 34 : 1859-62.
29. Soler C, Chardonnet Y, Allibert P, Euvrard S, Schmitt D, Mandrand B. Detection of mucosal human papillomavirus types 6/11 in cutaneous lesions from transplant recipients. *J Invest Dermatol* 1993 ; 101 : 286-91.
30. Soler C, Chardonnet Y, Allibert P, Euvrard S, Mandrand B, Thivolet J. Detection of multiple types of human papillomavirus in a giant condyloma from a grafted patient. *Virus Res* 1992 ; 23 : 193-208.

20

Rare cutaneous tumours

Brigitte DRÉNO
Department of Dermatology, Nantes, France.

The incidence of premalignant and malignant skin lesions in transplant patients is higher than in the general population. Among them, basal cell and squamous cell carcinomas are the most frequent forms of cutaneous tumours. The frequency of melanoma is also reportedly higher than in the general population, however lower than that of skin carcinomas.

Other rarer skin lesions have also been reported in the literature. They include dysplastic epithelial proliferations without malignant potential (*e.g.* sebaceous hyperplasia) or with malignant potential (*e.g.* porokeratosis) and malignant skin tumours (*e.g.* Merkel cell carcinoma).

Merkel cell carcinoma

Merkel cell carcinoma, first described in 1972 by Toker, is a rare malignant tumour of the skin. It is believed to originate from Merkel cells, considered as a component of the amine precursor uptake and decarboxylation (APUD) system, and is related to neuroendocrine-derived neoplasia of the skin. Subsequent ultrastructural studies revealed neurosecretory-type granules similar to those found in Merkel cells, and neuron-specific enolase has been identified within tumour cells by immunohistochemistry. However the epithelial origin of Merkel cell carcinoma is also suggested by the identification of cytokeratin filaments within tumour cells; moreover, pseudoepitheliomatous hyperplasia or true *in situ* carcinoma in the epidermis overlying the tumour have been described. Foci of squamous differentiation or bowenoid changes may exist even within the tumour itself.

Merkel cell carcinoma in immunocompetent patients has a reported mortality rate of 25% or more. It shows a high incidence of local recurrence (40%) within a few months to several years after initial diagnosis. Local or distant lymph node metastases are observed in 18-45% of patients. The most frequently involved metastatic sites are lung, liver and bone. Mean survival is 60% at 3 years.

Eight cases of Merkel carcinoma have been described in transplant recipients:
– Formica [1] reported the case of a patient developing a chest lesion after 3 years of transplantation, with distant lymph node metastases and in association with a malignancy of the prostate;
– Stempfle [2] described the rapid growth of a neuroendocrine carcinoma promoted by OKT3 monoclonal antibody in a patient with a refractory cardiac allograft rejection;
– Douds [3] reported a fatal issue of a Merkel cell carcinoma two years after renal transplantation;
– Vazquez-Mazariego [4] found an abnormal caryotype in a metastatic lymph node of Merkel cell carcinoma that appeared in a patient one year after heart transplantation. The abnormality included two markers derived from the long arm of chromosome 1;
– Gooptu [5] reported two cases of rapidly fatal Merkel cell carcinoma, in two transplant patients treated by both azathioprine and cyclosporin;
– Pham [6] among 608 cardiac transplant recipients identified one case of Merkel cell carcinoma;
– Jonas [7] described one case of Merkel cell tumour 21 months after liver transplantation. The patient died in spite of combined chemotherapy and radiotherapy 19 months after diagnosis of the tumour.

Merkel cell carcinoma typically presents as a firm erythematous nodule (*Figures 36 and 37, page 223*) occurring on the extremities in over one-third of cases. It has an aggressive evolution with a rapid growth of lesions and a fatal issue in transplant patients, probably related to the immunosuppression. Various mechanisms have been suggested to explain the effect of immunosuppression. Immunosuppressive drugs may decrease immune surveillance. Azathioprine, being a derivative of the purine analogue 6-mercaptopurine, may act directly by inhibiting purine synthesis, or may act *via* its metabolite 6-thioguanine which is incorporated into DNA as a guanine analogue, thereby disrupting DNA synthesis.

Treatment of primary tumours [8] consists in surgical removal with at least 2 cm-free margins. Improved locoregional control has been reported by several authors using postoperative irradiation to the primary site as well as to the regional draining lymph nodes, but this has to be confirmed by further studies. At a metastatic stage, different chemotherapeutic agents may be used; the commonest include cyclophosphamide (600mg/m^2), methotrexate (40 mg/m^2), 5 fluorouracil (600 mg/m^2) and cisplatin or etoposide. However, at this disseminated stage the response is generally low. Furthermore, decrease or discontinuation of the immuno-suppressive treatment is necessary if control of the tumour is to be expected.

Mesenchymal cutaneous tumours

Benign vascular tumours

An eruptive vascular proliferation resembling acquired tufted angioma has been described in a liver transplant patient [9]. The cutaneous lesions were erythematous papules of the right axilla and arm which appeared rapidly after transplantation. Histology showed capillary lobules studding the dermis. Spontaneous regression was noted several months later. The diagnosis of Kaposi's sarcoma and bacillary angiomatosis were excluded. This lesion could be related to eruptive pyogenic granuloma (*Figure 38, page 223*), one case of which has been reported in a kidney transplant patient [10]. This lesion appeared following injury on the right thumb

70 days after transplantation. The dermis contained a lobular vascular proliferation, without cell atypia or necrosis. The lesion recurred rapidly with multiple satellite lesions after surgical excision and radiotherapy was administered inducing a regression in two months. The immunosuppressive treatment could account for the extensive and rapid growth of the tumour.

Angiosarcoma

This is a rare malignant tumour accounting for less than 1% of all sarcomas in the general population. Seven cases of angiosarcoma have been reported in transplant patients but only one concerned the skin. Kibe reported a case of angiosarcoma developed in a male 12 years after renal transplantation [11]. This lesion was located on the scalp and characterised by multiple violaceous nodules surrounded by poorly-demarcated red to purple discoloration of the skin. The immunosuppressive treatment consisted of azathioprine and prednisolone. The treatment of this tumour is similar to the one performed in immunocompetent patients, *i.e.* wide surgical excision with 3 cm margins. Moreover this patient was treated postoperatively with systemic recombinant interleukin-2, but he refused to continue this treatment because the drug induced an acute rejection of the transplanted kidney. Post-operative radiotherapy may be considered although its real benefit has never been demonstrated. It was introduced for this patient but he developed lung metastasis and died. Histologically, angiosarcoma should be differentiated from Kaposi's sarcoma. Angiosarcoma is associated with a rapidly progressive course and poor prognosis. Among the other six cases of angiosarcoma reported in the literature, there were five men aged 28 to 50 years, and the average interval between renal transplantation and the onset of angiosarcoma was 6.5 years. Three of the six tumours arose at the site of the arteriovenous fistulae. The survival was 5 to 12 months [12-16].

Atypical fibroxanthoma

This is a low-grade malignant tumour which runs usually an indolent course after surgical excision. Metastases are rare. It presents as a solitary ulcerated nodular lesion on sun-exposed area in old people. The role of UV radiation, suspected on clinical grounds, has been confirmed by the frequent finding of p53 mutations at dipyrimidine sites.

Two cases of atypical fibroxanthoma [17, 18] have been reported in transplant patients. One case was associated with eruptive actinic keratoses following heart transplantation [17]. This lesion recurred after excision with a destruction of large vessels. The location of this tumour on sun-exposed skin argues for a combined role of both immunosuppression and UV light in the evolution of this lesions. The invasive evolution might be related to the immunosuppressive treatment. The second case of atypical fibroxanthoma [18] was observed in a renal transplant patient that necessitated multiple excisions and reduction of the immunosuppressive treatment.

Malignant fibrous histiocytoma has been noted in a long-term renal transplant [19] concomitantly with skin carcinoma and non Hodgkin's lymphoma, highlighting the inducing role of immunosuppression in the development of this tumour. Another case of malignant histiocytoma has also been mentioned in the literature but no details concerning the course of the lesion were given [20].

Dermatofibrosarcoma protuberans

Lai [21] reported a case of dermatofibrosarcoma that developed four years after renal transplantation; the patient remained disease-free after two years of follow-up. One case of fibrosarcoma of the left temple after radiotherapy for basal cell carcinoma of the skin is mentioned in a review of 8,724 *de novo* malignancies that occurred in 8,191 organ allograft recipients. 7.4% of these malignancies were sarcomas [22]. This soft tissue tumour is characterised by local recurrence and rarely metastatic spread. A wide and depth excision (margins 3-5 cm) is necessary to prevent the recurrences.

Sweat gland carcinoma

Syringomatous carcinoma is an adnexal tumour derived from eccrine sweat glands the diagnosis of which is often difficult both clinically and microscopically. Its growth is slow but extremely invasive with very frequent local recurrences due to extensive perineural invasion. Thus mutilating procedures are often necessary and the best surgical technique inducing the less of recurrence consists of a wide and complete microscopically controlled surgical excision. A case of syringomatous carcinoma has been described after kidney transplantation in a patient receiving cyclosporin [23]. He presented a firm mass in the eyebrow region and in the nasal area of the orbit. Exenteration was recommended. Sweat gland carcinoma of the trunk was found in 98 renal-transplant patients receiving 10-23 years of continuous immunosuppressive therapy [20].

In conclusion, rare malignant cutaneous tumours in transplant patients often raise diagnostic and therapeutic problems. Dermatologists have an important role in the follow-up of these patients. These tumours mainly raise the question of local recurrences and therefore wide surgical excision should be rapidly performed. The benefit of radiotherapy has to be determined. Finally, at a metastatic stage, chemotherapy induces a low rate of remission. A decrease and when possible discontinuation of immunosuppressive drugs should be attempted.

References

1. Formica M, Basolo B, Funaro L, Mazzucco G, Segoloni GP, Piccoli G. Merkel cell carcinoma in renal transplant recipient. *Nephron* 1994 ; 68 : 399.

2. Stempfle HU, Mudra H, Angermann CE, Weiss M, Reichart B, Theisen K. Rapid growth of cutaneous neuroendocrine (Merkel cell) carcinoma during treatment of refractory cardiac allograft rejection with OKT3, monoclonal antibody. *J Heart Lung Transplant* 1993 ; 12 : 501-3.

3. Douds AC, Mellotte GJ, Morgan SH. Fatal Merkel-cell tumour (cutaneous neuroendocrine carcinoma) complication renal transplantation. *Nephrol Dial Transplant* 1995 ; 10 : 2346-8.

4. Vazqua-Mazariego Y, Vallcorba I, Ferro MT, Lopez-Yarto A, Garcia-Sagredo JM, Cabello P, Resino M, Munoz R, Mayayo M, San Roman C. Cytogenetic study of neuroendocrine carcinoma of Merkel cells. *Cancer Genet Cytogenet* 1996 ; 92 : 79-81.

5. Gooptu G, Waalans A, Ross J, Price M, Wojnarowska F, Morris PJ, Wall S, Bunker CB. Merkel cell carcinoma arising after therapeutic immunosuppression. *Br J Dermatol* 1997 ; 137 : 637-41.

6. Pham SM, Karmas RL, Landreneau RJ, Kawai A, Gonzalez-Cancel I, Hardesty RL, Hattler BG, Griffith BP. Solid tumors after heart transplantation: lethality of lung cancer. *Ann Thorac Surg* 1995 ; 60 : 1623-6.

7. Jonas S, Rayez N, Neumann U, Neuhaus R, Bechstein WO, Guckelberger O, Tullius SG, Serke S, Neuhaus P. *De novo* malignancies after liver transplantation using Tacrolimus-based protocols or cylosporine-based quadruple immunosuppression with an interleukin-2 receptor antibody or antithymocyte globulin. *Cancer* 1997 ; 80 : 1141-50.

8. Fenig E, Brenner B, Katz A, Rakovsky E, Hana MB, Sulkas A. The role of radiation therapy and chemotherapy in the treatment of Merkel cell carcinoma. *Cancer* 1997 ; 80 : 881-5.

9. Chu P, Le Boit PE. An eruptive vascular proliferation resembling acquired tufted angioma in the recipient of a liver transplant. *J Am Acad Dermatol* 1992 ; 26 : 322-5.

10. Le Meur Y, Bédane C, Clavere P, Peyronnet P, Leroux-Robert C. A proliferative vascular tumour of the skin in a kidney-transplant recipient (recurrent pyogenic granuloma with satellitosis). *Nephrol Dial Transplant* 1997 ; 12 : 1271-2.

11. Kibe Y, Kishimoto S, Katoh N, Yasuno H, Yasumura T, Oka T. Angiosarcoma of the scalp associated with renal transplantation. *Br J Dermatol* 1997 ; 136 : 752-6.

12. Askari A, NovickA, Braun W, Steinmuller D. Late ureteral obstruction and hematuria and treatment. *Cancer* 1987 ; 59 : 1046-57.

13. Alpers CE, Biava CG, Salvatierra O. Angiosarcoma following renal transplantation. *Transplant Proc* 1982 ; 14 : 717-9.

14. Byers RJ, McMahon RFT, Freemont AJ. Epithelioid angiosarcoma arising in an arteriovenous fistula. *Histopathology* 1992 ; 21 : 87-9.

15. Keane MM, Carney DN. Angiosarcoma arising from a defunctionalized arteriovenous fistula. *J Urol* 1993 ; 149 : 364-5.

16. Conlon PJ, Daly T, Doyele G. Angiosarcoma at the site of a ligated arteriovenous fistula in a renal transplant recipient. *Nephrol Dial Transplant* 1993 ; 8 : 259-62.

17. Paquet P, Piérard GE. Invasive atypical fibroxanthoma and eruptive actinic keratoses in a heart transplant patient. *Dermatology* 1996 ; 192 : 411-3.

18. Kanitakis J, Euvrard S, Montazeri A, Garnier JL, Faure M, Claudy A. Atypical fibroxanthoma in a renal graft recipient. *J Am Acad Dermatol* 1996 ; 35 : 262-4.

19. Barroso-Vicens E, Ramirez G, Rabb H. Multiple primary malignancies in a renal transplant patient. *Transplantation* 1996 ; 61 : 1655-6.

20. Blöhme I, Larkö O. Skin lesions in renal transplant patients after 10-23 years of immunosuppressive therapy. *Acta Derm Venereol* 1990 ; 70 : 491-4.

21. Lai KN, Lai FM, King WW, Li PK, Siu D, Leung CB, Lui SF. Dermatofibrosarcoma protuberance in a renal transplant patient. *Aust N Z J Surg* 1995 ; 65 : 900-2.

22. Penn I. Sarcomas in organ allograft recipients. *Transplantation* 1995 ; 60 : 1485-91.

23. Happenreijs VPT, Reuser TTQ, Maay CM, De Keizer RJW, Maurits MPh. Syringomatous carcinoma of the eyelid and orbit: a clinical and histopathological challenge. *Br J Ophtalmol* 1997 ; 81 : 668-72.

21

Photoprotection

Marie-Thérèse LECCIA, Jean-Claude BÉANI, Pierre AMBLARD
Department of Dermatology, Albert-Michallon Hospital, Grenoble, France.

Why is photoprotection necessary for transplant recipients?

Three factors appear to participate in the increased incidence of skin cancers of organ transplant recipients: the immunosuppressive therapy, infection of the skin with human papillomaviruses (HPV) and solar radiation. Sunlight exposure is certainly the most important risk factor for the development of skin cancers in transplant recipients and this factor can be avoided.

Most precancerous lesions such as actinic keratoses and malignant skin tumors develop on sun-exposed areas of the skin (face and ears, forearms and dorsum of hands). Previous studies have shown that squamous cell carcinomas (SCC) are more frequent than basal cell carcinomas (BCC). In fact, the ratio SCC/BCC depends on sun exposure, varying from 0.7 at Glasgow to 5.9 at Brisbane [1]. Similarly, within the same country, the incidence of skin carcinomas in transplant recipients increases as the latitude decreases. On the other hand, comparing a very sunny country such as Australia to a country such as the Netherlands with more limited sunlight, the cumulative rate to develop skin cancers after 5 years of graft survival is 23% in Australia *versus* 2% in the Netherlands. After nine years, the risk is 44% in Australia and 9% in the Netherlands. Interestingly, however, the risk reaches 40% in this last country after 20 years of graft survival [2].

Chronic cumulative sun exposure before organ transplantation seems to be determinant. Boyle *et al.* compared transplant recipients with high sun exposure (more than 3 months in a tropical or subtropical climate, or more than 5 years for a outdoor worker) [3]. They found a significant risk for development of viral lesions, actinic keratoses and non-melanoma skin cancers in transplant recipients with a high past sun exposure. In another retrospective follow-up study, Bouwes-Bavinck *et al.* found that the exposure to sunlight before the age of 30 contributes more to the risk of skin cancer in renal transplant recipients than exposure after the age of 30 [4]. However, in this study, cumulative life-time exposure to sunlight did not appear to be associated with an increased number of keratotic skin lesions. Nevertheless, these lesions appear closely associated with the development of skin cancers and their preferential location on sun-exposed areas suggests a possible role of recent exposure to sunlight.

Additional risk factors for the development of non-melanoma skin cancers in transplant recipients are represented by the immunosuppressive therapy and HPV infection of the skin. In transplant recipients, HPV-specific nucleotide sequences are often found in warts and occasionally in skin carcinomas suggesting a pathogenic role of HPV in the development of skin cancer [5]. In addition, viral antigens can be modulated by ultraviolet radiation. Integration of the HPV genome, particularly the subgenomic fragments E6 and E7, seems to be an important event in malignant transformation. The E6 and E7 oncoproteins can bind p53 and the retinoblastoma gene product Rb, *i.e.* proteins involved in the control of the cell cycle known to be modulated by ultraviolet radiation [6]. Ultraviolet radiation-induced changes in epidermal DNA and immune response may thus be perpetuated by the HPV-stimulated cellular proliferation.

The synergistic action of multiple carcinogenic risk factors such as immunosuppression, HPV infection and sunlight seems to be essential for the development of skin cancers in organ transplant recipients. Immunosuppressive drugs are required to maintain the transplant functional and today there is no efficient antiviral treatment to eliminate HPV. Thus, the only strategy to reduce the risk of skin cancers substantially for these patients goes through a decreased sunlight exposure associated with a correct photoprotection.

How to protect transplant recipients against sunlight?

Prevention of skin cancer has to take into account that the development of cutaneous solar damage depends both on the amount of sun exposure and on individual sensitivity to sunlight.

Natural pigmentation represents the main factor of interindividual variations in the ability to develop sun-induced damage and therefore individual sun sensitivity is usually appreciated by skin phototype [7]. Clearly, fair phototypes have a higher risk of skin cancers. Other phenotypic attributes, such as inability to tan and easy burning after sun exposure, also put the individual at high risk for both melanoma and non-melanoma skin cancer. All these parameters have to be taken into consideration for an efficient photoprotection of transplant recipients, even if other factors, namely immunodepression or viral infection, induce a specific susceptibility.

As an evidence, to avoid skin carcinoma the higher the individual sun sensitivity, the higher the measures have to be to limit the quantity of sunlight which may reach crucial cutaneous targets.

Strategies to protect the skin against sunlight

The prevention of cutaneous precancerous conditions and skin cancers of transplant recipients includes correct sun protection and a thorough and regular dermatological examination.

There are three strategies to reduce sun exposure: avoiding the sun, wearing protective clothing and using sunscreens. The first two strategies require substantial lifestyle changes and reduce not only the risks, but also some of the pleasures and benefits associated with sun exposure. Sunscreens interfere less with outdoor activity but are costly and their effectiveness as cancer-preventing agents in adults is not well established. Specific data on these protective means are discussed below.

UV-protective clothing

Appropriate clothing can provide an optical filter against the penetration of harmful radiations. Broad-brimmed hats protect the ears, nose and cheeks in addition of the scalp. The sun protective effect of clothing is highly variable depending on the texture, color and thickness [8]. Dark, especially black, clothes are excellent but they absorb infrared radiations and thus may be quite uncomfortable. Wet clothing, especially after perspiring or swimming, may become more transparent and ineffective against impinging UV radiations. Robson and Diffey showed that the protection offered by fabric against UV light is influenced by a number of factors including the color, the nature of the textile, structure of the fabric and above all the type of weave [9]. There was an enormous range in sun protective factor (SPF) from 2 for a polyester blouse to more than 1,000 for cotton twill jeans; for maximum protection the authors recommended to avoid wool and some human-made fibers such as viscose or acrylic, to avoid open weaves such as crepe and to select tightly woven fabrics such as cotton twill or silk or high-lustre polyester materials. Some recent studies focused on the protection of some fabrics against skin cancer. Bech-Thomsen concluded that there is a direct relationship between UV transmission of clothes and the appearance of skin tumors in a patient with *Xeroderma pigmentosum* [10]. Menter *et al.* showed that a typical summer tee-shirt provides only « moderate » protection from sunburn SPF (between 5 and 9) and does not protect against tumor induction in mice. On the contrary, a new special « highly UV-protective » fabric that offers broad-spectrum high UV protection (SPF > 30) completely protected mice against carcinoma under the same experimental conditions [11]. Therefore, typical summer clothing fabrics offer an inadequate protection against skin cancer. In the same way, Bowen's disease, squamous and basal cell carcinoma and malignant melanoma occur more frequently on the lower legs of women compared with men, perhaps because of increased solar UV exposure as a consequence of dress. Sinclair and Diffey have measured the spectral transmission of UV radiation through a range of thickness and colors of plain-knit ladies stockings and calculated the SPF [12]. They found:
– that SPFs increased from about 1.5 to 3 for black stockings ranging from 10 to 40 deniers,
– that there were statistically significant differences in SPFs with color (higher for darker color),
– that UVA and UVB were absorbed equally.

They concluded that the most popular type of stocking (15 deniers) does not provide good protection of the legs; this protection requires at least a 40 denier stocking or better wearing trousers.

Topical sunscreening agents

Sun-protective topical preparations are chemical agents in the form of solutions (clear or milky lotions), gels, creams, or ointments that absorb and screen UV radiation [13, 14]. Protection is afforded through absorption, reflection and scattering of solar radiation impinging on the skin. Topical sunscreens can be subdivided into three categories: chemical sunscreens, physical sunscreens and combinations of sunscreens containing two or more UV-absorbing chemicals and UV-scattering agents.

Chemical sunscreens act as UV-absorbing filters that partially or totally block the penetration of UV radiations to the viable cells of epidermis [15]. They are categorized into narrow-band filters that only prevent the penetration of UVB into the skin and broad-band filters with an absorbing spectrum extending up to UVA wavelengths. The majority of available UV filters belong to the first class: para-aminobenzoic acid (PABA) and its derivatives called PABA esters (Padimate A or Escalol 506 ; Padimate O or Escalol 507), cinnamates (octylmethoxycinnamate, cinnoxate, p-methoxy-2-ethylhexylcinnamate or Parsol MCX), salicylates (homomenthyl salicylate), 2-phenylbenzimidazole, 5-sulfonic acid and salts, methyl-benzylidene and benzylidene camphre. The first real UVA filter available in Europe in the early eighties was 4-tert-butyl-4'-methoxy-dibenzoylmethane or Parsol 1789. Benzophenones are broad-spectrum filters with an absorbance both in the UVB and UVA spectrum; unfortunately, these molecules often induce contact or photoallergic reactions and have been excluded of formulations by many manufacturers. Recently, a new filter (Mexoryl SX®) has been available in Europe, which absorbs longer UVB and shorter UVA wavelengths (UVA_2); one of its major qualities is its photostability (photodegradation may change the absorption profile and thereby reduce efficiency). Physical sunscreens, also referred to as physical blockers, contain mineral particulates (zinc oxide, titanium dioxide, mica titanium, magnesium silicate, ferrous and ferric oxide) that reflect and scatter not only UV radiation but also visible and infrared radiations. Recently, mineral particles have been micronized and cosmetic inconvenients of physical sunscreens are now partly overcome.

Therefore, in order to provide broad-spectrum protection in the UVB and UVA range, and high SPF values, Parsol 1789 and/or Mexoryl SX® are usually combined with UVB absorbers (for instance Parsol MCX or methyl benzylidene camphre) or, more often, with physical agents. The vehicle in which the UV-absorbing chemical is crucial for ensuring that a sunscreen remains effective under general use conditions such as prolonged sunbathing, sweating caused by sporting activities and swimming. This property, known as substantivity, has to be evaluated and to be labelled on packaging [16]. New formulations with polyacrylamide base are highly substantive.

Taking all theses factors into account, the ideal characteristics of a sunscreen should be as follows:
– cosmetically pleasant,
– water resistant,
– photostable during sun exposure time,
– not inducing undesirable effects,
– broad-spectrum to prevent all deleterious sun effects with the same effectiveness.

Unfortunately, if the first three conditions can be reached nowadays, the last two remain problematic limiting the place of sunscreens in the prevention of chronic sun damages. Chemical sunscreens have been reported to induce contact or photocontact allergic reactions [17]. The greatest inductors of these reactions were benzophenones. Sunscreen preparation excipients, particularly preservatives and fragrances, can also cause contact allergic and irritant contact dermatitis. The daily use significantly increases the frequency of these adverse effects, particularly irritation [18]. The risk of vitamin D3 depletion with chronic use of sunscreens is not clearly demonstrated but should be considered in the case of elderly patients [19]. Finally, the daily application of sunscreens can be expensive.

The « sun protection factor » (SPF) represents the protective value or potency of a sunscreen. It is defined as the ratio of the exposure dose of the erythemogenic UV radiation required to produce the minimal erythema reaction through the applied sunscreen product to the UV dose required to produce the same reaction without topical application of the sunscreen [20]. Since UVA radiation has been shown to produce many of the potentially deleterious effects in human skin [21], two SPF are now labelled on sunscreen formulation : SPF against UVB and SPF against UVA. The protection against UVA is always very much lower than UVB protection and this imbalance increases in very high SPF sunscreen.

Several lines of evidence exist suggesting that sunscreens can completely prevent erythema whereas it has not been shown that they prevent other deleterious effects of sunlight. Photoimmunosuppression is a good example of this situation. It has been clearly demonstrated that UV exposure induces immunosuppression which can play an important role in the development of UVB-induced skin tumors in mice [22]. Although there is no direct evidence that UVB-induced immunosuppression plays a role in the growth of sunlight-associated skin malignancies in humans, the role of the immune system in regulating the appearance of skin cancers is highlighted by findings that immunosuppressed patients have highly increased rates of skin cancer. Organ transplant recipients are directly concerned. Many studies have shown a lack of correlation between protection against inflammation and immunosuppression and sunscreens appear ineffective or only partially effective in preventing UV-induced immunosuppression [22-25]. The reasons for this remain unclear but, recently, Walker showed that the failure of the sunscreen to protect completely against UV-induced immunosuppression was due to the ability of subedemal doses of UVB to induce substantial immunosuppression [26]. Therefore the suppression of the erythemal alarm by high SPF sunscreens could be perverse. On the other hand, Fourtanier showed in mice that a broad-spectrum sunscreen was much more effective than a UVB filter but also that SPF did not correctly predict protection against photocarcinogenesis [27]. Similarly, several epidemiological studies have examined the relationship of sunscreen use and melanoma or non-melanoma skin cancer and suggested that sunscreens may not be effective in preventing skin cancer [28-32]. However, two recent studies have demonstrated that high SPF sunscreens can protect against the development of actinic keratoses [33, 34].

Further studies are necessary to evaluate the efficacy of recent formulations of sunscreens including a better UVA protection in the prevention of carcinoma and melanoma [35]. External photoprotection is still a moving subject and the controversy surrounding sunscreens is not yet resolved. In the present state of our knowledge, dermatologists should remember that:
– sunscreens with high UVB SPF suppress the natural warnings of overexposure to the sun and may thus facilitate excessive exposure to the same wavelengths that they do not block sufficiently (*id.* UVA); they could create a false sense of security;
– limiting time spent in the sun and clothing photoprotection remain the two most reliable ways to prevent the harmful effects of sun, particularly induction of skin cancer.

Novel approaches to photoprotection?

New photoprotective molecules could represent a novel approach to photoprotection but require investigations on humans. Greenberg *et al.* studied the effect of a 5-year supplementation with β-carotene (50 mg/day) on the incidence of skin carcinoma but did not find any decrease in the supplemented-group [36]. A recent randomized double-blind study investigated the effects of an internal photoprotection with selenium during 4.5 years (200 mg/day) for the prevention of skin cancers [37]. Selenium treatment did not protect against the development of skin carcinoma but it did decrease the incidence of carcinoma of other organs. Experimental studies in mice have shown the decreased incidence of UV-induced skin carcinoma after treatment with various antioxidant compounds such as selenium, thiols or green tea polyphenols [38,39]. Moreover, polyphenols prevent UV-induced immunosuppression [40]. The question whether oral intake of antioxidants could prevent skin cancers in transplant recipients is of particular interest and current studies should bring new data in the years to come.

Photoprotection in practice...

Organ transplant recipients have pathologies and heavy treatments that make sun protective measures an additional restricting factor. However, dermatologists have to play a crucial role not only in the diagnosis and treatment of skin problems but also in educating these patients about skin care and the need of an efficient photoprotection. An appropriate photoprotection can be achieved by individualizing our recommendations according to the patient's risks of skin cancers based on that individual's phototype, past sun exposures and current habits. Dermatologists have to explain to each patient that not only exposures received during a summer spent at the seaside but also recreational and occupational exposures during sunny days are equally harmful. Natural protection must be privileged as the best photoprotection. This includes avoiding the sun, at least around the middle of the day, using appropriate clothing and hats, and seeking shade during outdoor activities such as gardening. Sunscreens should be viewed as an adjunct to natural protection and not as a substitute for it and chosen according to the patient's phototype and activities.

Finally, every candidate for organ transplantation should be examined and informed of the necessity of a regular dermatological surveillance. Individuals at high risk for skin cancers, including those with a history of skin cancer, multiple actinic keratoses, and those who work or spend a long time outdoors, especially if they have a fair phototype, need repeated consultations after transplantation. Any suspicious lesion should be examined histologically. Such an educational and medical follow-up can certainly be carried out only with the co-operation of the transplantation team.

References

1. Gupta A, Cardella I, Haberman H. Cutaneous malignant neoplasms in patients with renal transplants. *Arch Dermatol* 1986 ; 122 : 1288-93.

2. Hartevelt MM, Bouwes Bavinck JN, Kootte AM, Vermeer BJ, Vandenbroucke JP. Incidence of skin cancer after renal transplantation in the Netherlands. *Transplantation* 1990 ; 49 : 506-9.

3. Boyle J, Mackie RM, Briggs JD, Junor BJR, Aitchison TC. Cancer, warts, and sunshine in renal transplant patients. A case-control study. *Lancet* 1984 ; 1 : 702-4.

4. Bouwes-Bavinck JN, De Boer A, Vermeer BJ, Hartevelt MM, Van der Woude FJ, Claas FHJ, Wolterbeek R, Vandenbroucke JP. Sunlight, keratotic skin lesions and skin cancer in renal transplant recipients. *Br J Dermatol* 1993 ; 124 : 242-45.

5. Höpfl R, Bens G, Wieland U, Petter A, Zelger B, Fritsch P, Pfister H. Human papillomavirus DNA in non-melanoma skin cancers of a renal transplant recipient: detection of a new sequence related to epidermodysplasia verruciformis associated types. *J Invest Dermatol* 1997 ; 108 : 53-6.

6. zur Hausen H. Papillomavirus infections: a major cause of human cancers. *Biochem Biophys Acta* 1996 ; 1288 : F55-78.

7. Pathak MA. Intrinsic photoprotection in human skin. In : Lowe NJ, Shaath NA, eds. *Sunscreens: development, evaluation, and regulatory aspects*. New-York : Marcel Dekker, 1990 : 73-83.

8. Jevtic AP. The sun protective effect of clothing, including beachwear. *Aust J Dermatol* 1990 ; 21 : 5-7.

9. Robson J, Diffey B. Textiles and sun protection. *Photodermatol Photoimmunol Photomed* 1990 ; 7 : 32-4.

10. Bech-Thomsen N, Wulf HC, Ullman S. Xeroderma pigmentosum lesions related to ultraviolet transmittance by clothes. *J Am Acad Dermatol* 1991 ; 24 : 365-8.

11. Menter JM, Hollins TD, Sayre RM, Etemadi AA, Willis I, Hughes NG. Protection against UV photocarcinogenesis by fabric material. *J Am Acad Dermatol* 1994 ; 31 : 711-6.

12. Sinclair SA, Diffey BL. Sun protection provided by ladies stocking. *Br J Dermatol* 1997 ; 136 : 239-41.

13. Barker MO. Sunscreens update. *Am J Contact Dermatol* 1997 ; 8 : 247-9.

14. Pathak MA. Topical and systemic photoprotection of human skin against solar radiation. In : Lim HW, Soter NA, eds. *Clinical photomedicine*. New York : Marcel Dekker Inc, 1993 : 287-306.

15. Shaath NA. The chemistry of sunscreens. In : Lowe NJ, Shaath NA, eds. *Sunscreens: development, evaluation, and regulatory aspects*. New York : Marcel Dekker, 1990 : 211-33.

16. Kaidbey K. Substantivity and water resistance of sunscreens. In : Lowe NJ, Shaath NA, eds. *Sunscreens: development, evaluation, and regulatory aspects*. New York : Marcel Dekker, 1990 : 405-9.

17. Dromgoole SH, Maibach IH. Sunscreening agent intolerance: contact and photocontact sensitization and contact urticaria. *J Am Acad Dermatol* 1990 ; 22 : 1068-72.

18. Foley P, Nixon R, Marks R, Frowen K, Thompson S. The frequency of reactions to sunscreens: results of a longitudinal population based study on the regular use of sunscreens in Australia. *Br J Dermatol* 1993 ; 126 : 512-8.

19. Matsuoka LU, Ide L, Wortsman J, McLaughlin J, Holick MF. Sunscreens suppress cutaneous vitamin D3 synthesis. *J Clin Endocrinol Metab* 1987 ; 64 : 1165-8.

20. Lowe NJ. Sun protective factors: comparative techniques and selection of UV sources. In : Lowe NJ, Shaath NA, eds. *Sunscreens: development, evaluation, and regulatory aspects*. New York : Marcel Dekker, 1990 : 379-93.

21. Danby FW. Cumulative effects of UVA in human skin. *J Am Acad Dermatol* 1995 ; 33 : 691.

22. Kripke ML. Immunologic mechanisms in UV radiation carcinogenesis. *Adv Cancer Res* 1987 ; 34 : 34-69.

23. Bestak R, Barnetson RSC, Nearn MR, Halliday GM. Sunscreen protection of contact hypersensitivity responses form chronic solar-simulated ultraviolet irradiation correlates with the absorption spectrum of the sunscreen. *J Invest Dermatol* 1995 ; 105 : 345-51.

24. Reeve VE, Bosnic M, Boham-Wilcox C, Ley RD. Differential protection by two sunscreens from UV radiation-induced immunosuppression. *J Invest Dermatol* 1991 ; 97 : 624-8.

25. Wolf P, Donawho CL, Kripke ML. Effect of sunscreen on UV radiation-induced enhancement of melanoma growth in mice. *J Natl Cancer Inst* 1994 ; 86 : 99-105.

26. Walker SL, Young AR. Sunscreens offer the same UVB protection factors for inflammation and immunosuppression in the mouse. *J Invest Dermatol* 1997 ; 108 : 133-8.

27. Fourtanier A. Meroxyl SX protects against solar-simulated UVR-induced photocarcinogenesis in mice. *Photochem Photobiol* 1996 ; 64 : 688-93.

28. Autier P, Doré JF, Lejeune F, Koelmel K, Geffeler O, Hille P, Cesarini JP, Liénard D, Liabeuf A, Joarlette M, Chemaly P, Hakin K, Koekn A, Kleeberg U. Recreational exposure to sunlight and lack of information as risk factors for cutaneous malignant melanoma. Results of an EORTC case-control study in Belgium, France and Germany. *Melanoma Res* 1994 ; 4 : 79-85.

29. Beitner H, Norell S, Ringborg U, Wennesten G, Mattson B. Malignant melanoma: aetiological importance of individual pigmentation and sun exposure. *Br J Dermatol* 1990 ; 122 : 43-51.

30. Graham S, Marshall J, Haughey B, Stoll H, Zielezny M. An enquiry into the epidemiology of melanoma. *Am J Epidemiol* 1985 ; 122 : 606-19.

31. Hunter D, Colditz G, Stampfer M. Risk factors for basal cell carcinoma in a prospective cohort of women. *Ann Epidemiol* 1990 ; 1 : 13-23.

32. Westerdahl J, Olson H, Masback A, Ingvar C, Johnson N. Is the use of sunscreens a risk factor for malignant melanoma? *Melanoma Res* 1995 ; 5 : 59-65

33. Naylor M, Boyd A, Smith D, Cameron G, Hubbard D, Neldmer K. High sun protection factor sunscreens in the suppression of actinic neoplasia. *Arch Dermatol* 1995 ; 131 : 170-5.

34. Thompson S, Jolley D, Marks R. Reduction of solar keratoses by regular sunscreen use. *N Engl J Med* 1993 ; 329 : 1147-51.

35. Béani JC. Photoprotecteurs externes et cancers cutanés. *Ann Dermatol Venereol* 1996 ; 123 : 666-74.

36. Greenberg ER, Baron JA, Stukkel TA. A clinical trial of beta-carotene to prevent basal cell and squamous cell cancers of the skin. *N Engl J Med* 1990 ; 323 : 789-95.

37. Clark LC, Combs GF, Turnbull BW, Slate EH, Chalker DK, Chow J, Davis LS, Glover RA, Graham GF, Gross BG, Krongrad A, Lesher JL, Park HK, Sanders BB, Smith CL, Taylor JR. Effects of selenium supplementation for cancer prevention in patients with carcinoma of the skin. *JAMA* 1996 ; 276 : 1957-63.

38. Steenvoorden DPT, Beijersbergen van Henegouwen GMJ. The use of endogenous antioxidants to improve photoprotection. *J Photochem Photobiol* 1997 ; 41 : 1-10.

39. Wang ZY, Huang MT, Lou YR, Xie JG, Reuhl KR, Newmark HL, Ho CT, Yang CS, Conney AH. Inhibitory effects of black tea, green tea, decaffeinated black tea, and decaffeinated green tea on ultraviolet B light-induced skin carcinogenesis in 7,12-dimethylbenz(a)anthracene-initiated SKH-1 mice. *Cancer Res* 1994 ; 54 : 3428-35.

40. Katiyar SK, Elmets CA, Agarwal R, Mukhtar H. Protection against ultraviolet-B radiation-induced local and systemic suppression of contact hypersensitivity and edema responses in CEH/HeN mice by green tea polyphenols. *Photochem Photobiol* 1995 ; 62 : 855-61.

22

Systemic retinoids for the treatment of skin cancer

Christoph C. GEILEN, Brigitte ALMOND-ROESLER, Constantin E. ORFANOS
Department of Dermatology, University Medical Center Benjamin Franklin,
The Free University of Berlin, Berlin, Germany.

Skin cancers are the most common malignancies in humans and a worldwide increased incidence of all forms has been recognized. In recent years especially organ transplant recipients have an increased risk to develop skin cancer due to prolonged immunosuppressive treatment. For Caucasian renal allograft recipients living in Australia a 20.6 fold increased risk of skin cancer has been estimated [1]. Although distant metastasis from light-induced squamous cell carcinoma is uncommon, it occurs in 3% to 5% of all patients [2] and transplant recipients have a tenfold higher mortality from skin cancer, thus suggesting increased metastatic potential [3, 4]. With this background the development of cancer prevention and anticancer strategies appear necessary, especially for this group of patients. Retinoids, the natural and synthetic analogues of vitamin A, accumulate primarily in the skin and have been therefore used to manage various skin disorders including skin cancer [5].

Mechanisms of action

The mechanisms underlying the beneficial effect of systemic retinoids in skin neoplasia and/or in prevention of skin cancer are still largely unknown, but promotion of terminal epithelial cell differentiation and induction of apoptosis may lead to tumor regression. Retinoids are known to modulate epidermal growth and to control epidermal cell differentiation. Furthermore, retinoids are known to increase the formation of extracellular matrix and to suppress production of sebum (*Graph 8*).

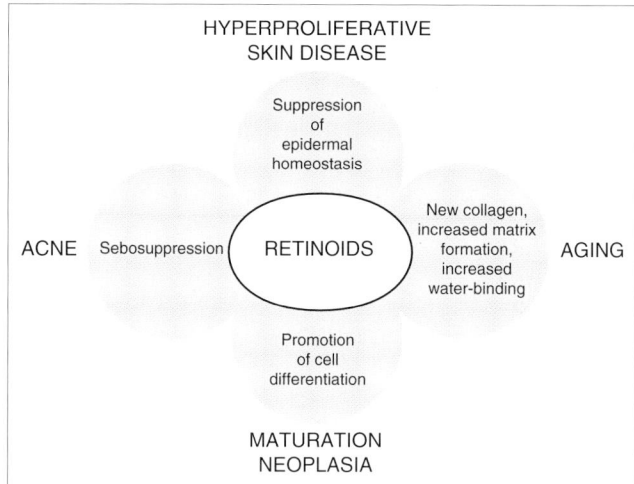

Graph 8. Action spectrum of synthetic retinoids.

Retinoid receptors are members of the steroid hormone superfamily and act as ligand-dependent transcription factors. Two classes of nuclear retinoid receptors (RARs and RXRs) were suggested to mediate retinoid action at the molecular level. Retinoid receptors regulate the transcription of genes containing DNA sequences in their promoter regions, known as retinoid-responsive elements (RAREs and RXREs); they are able to bound receptor heterodimers (e.g. RXR/RAR) as well as homodimers (e.g. RXR/RXR). In general, different types of retinoids may be characterized by their receptor binding properties (*Table I*).

Table I. Three retinoid types and their receptor binding as possible candidates for anticancer action

Type I	RARα,β,γ panagonist: all-trans-retinoic acid	Strong action on keratinizing epithelia and blood cell maturation; no sebosuppression
Type II	RAR β,γ agonists: tazarotene, adapalene	(Selective) action on keratinizing epithelia; no sebosuppression
Type III	RXR agonist: isotretinoin	Action on keratinizing epithelia; strong sebosuppression

Based on our current knowledge, three distinct mechanisms exist through which retinoid receptors modulate gene expression and thereby cellular processes such as growth and differentiation:
– transactivation by direct binding to retinoic acid response elements (RARE) in the promotor region of the target gene,
– competition with other nuclear receptors, e.g. vitamin D receptor, for heterodimerization with the retinoid X receptor (RXR),
– transrepression of activator protein 1 (AP-1) and perhaps other, yet unknown transcription factors, by protein-protein interactions [5, 6].

AP-1 is a complex of the two proto-oncogenes c-*fos* and c-*jun* and plays a crucial role in cell cycle progression [7, 8]. Therefore, anti-AP-1 synthetic retinoids may represent a promising novel therapeutic concept for hyperproliferative skin diseases including skin cancer.

With respect to these distinct molecular effects of different retinoid receptors, it was suggested that receptor-selective retinoids could contribute to a better discrimination of their biological activity. *Table II* gives an overview of the receptor selectivity of various retinoids. However, the question is whether receptor-selective retinoids are better targeting distinct cellular dysfunctions and enlarge their therapeutic window by minimizing their adverse effects.

Table II. Receptor selectivity of old and new retinoids

RARα	CD 336, Ro 41-5253
RARβ	CD 2314
RARγ	CD 437, CD 666
RARα,β,γ	All-*trans*-retinoic acid
RARβ,γ	Tazarotene, TTNT
RARβ,γ/RXRs	Adapalene
RXRa	Ro 26-4453
RXRs (high affinity)	9-*cis*-retinoic acid
RXRs (low affinity)	13-*cis*-retinoic acid (isotretinoin)
RXRα,β,γ	LGD 1069

As indicated above, UV radiation ranks high as a possible factor to increase the risk of skin cancer, especially in kidney transplant recipients. In this context, the dysfunction of the tumor suppressor protein p53 has been suggested as a mechanism underlying epithelial neoplasia. It is known, that UV radiation may lead to a mutation of the *p53* gene which can cause an abnormal function of this tumor protective protein [9, 10]. In p53-deficient mice, the induction of squamous cell carcinomas was seen after UV irradiation [11]. In a very recent study, the expression of the p53 protein in premalignant and malignant cutaneous lesions in kidney transplant recipients has been investigated and the effect of low-dose oral etretinate was determined. An immunoreactivity of p53 was observed in approximately 60% of basal cell carcinomas and squamous cell carcinomas, but there were no differences as compared to the expression of p53 protein in viral warts or Bowen's disease. It is interesting to note that the expression of the p53 tumor suppressor gene protein was not influenced by etretinate therapy [12]. The high prevalence of p53 protein detected in hyper-proliferative skin disorders of transplant recipients supports the opinion that p53 may play a contributing role in the development of skin cancer. However, the mechanism(s) underlying these high p53 protein levels has not been investigated in detail. Furthermore, the missing effect of etretinate treatment on p53 protein expression suggests that p53 expression is not one of the main targets of retinoid action.

Recently, the significance of the sphingomyelin cycle has been demonstrated in our laboratories as an important growth and differentiation control mechanism in human epidermis [13, 14]. This mechanism leads to elevation of intracellular ceramide levels and thereby to inhibition of cell growth, induction of differentiation and apoptosis. For retinoids, elevation of intracellular ceramide levels was also shown. This was paralleled by inhibition of cell proliferation [15]. Whereas retinoids may increase the *de novo* biosynthesis of ceramide, $1\alpha,25$-dihydroxyvitamin D_3 and its analogue calcipotriol have been shown to elevate the ceramide pool *via* degradation of the membrane lipid sphingomyelin [13, 16]. Therefore, a synergistic effect of vitamin A and D analogues should be considered under these conditions.

This synergistic effect was also shown for the plasma membrane NADH oxidase [17]; regulation of this enzyme seems to be closely associated with cellular growth [18] and it may be an interesting target for anticancer therapy. Very recently, it was found that different natural and synthetic retinoids may inhibit the activity of NADH oxidase, paralleled by growth inhibition [19].

Clinical applications

The described antiproliferative and differentiating effects of retinoids are a major rationale for the use of various retinoids for prevention and treatment of skin cancer. Over 1,500 different retinoid compounds have been synthesized by modifying different parts of the molecule in order to obtain retinoids with higher efficacy and fewer adverse effects. Synthetic retinoids have been applied not only for therapy of skin malignancies, but also in several randomized trials for tumor chemoprevention. It is important to stress that drug tolerability is a major issue for such trials. The adverse effect profile of oral retinoids is closely associated with hypervitaminosis A. It includes reversible dose-dependent mucocutaneous side effects such as skin and mucosal dryness, skin fragility, retinoid dermatitis, pruritus and hair loss. Furthermore, elevation of serum triglycerides, hyperostosis and extraskeletal calcification may occur. Retinoids are teratogenic if given orally during embryogenesis [5]. Therefore, combinations between low-dose systemic retinoid therapy with topical retinoids or with systemic interferons have been tested in various chemoprevention trials. Based on current information both topical or systemic administration of synthetic retinoids have a significant effect in reversing premalignant skin lesions and maintaining normal differentiation [20-23]. For long-term systemic isotretinoin [24] and systemic etretinate [25] successful prevention of basal cell carcinomas and squamous cell carcinomas in patients with xeroderma pigmentosum has been described. Isotretinoin was shown to reduce the occurrence of basal cell carcinomas by 80% and of squamous cell carcinomas by 60% over a period of two years. A similar clinical response was seen for etretinate. Furthermore, in the nevoid basal cell carcinoma syndrome both retinoids have been shown to prevent cutaneous tumors [26, 27]. In a large prospective study in patients with previously treated basal cell carcinomas, the use of long-term low dose isotretinoin was no more effective than placebo in reducing the occurrence of new basal cell carcinomas, over a 36 month period [28].

As mentioned above, organ transplant recipients under immunosuppressive therapy have an increased risk to develop skin cancer. Therefore, systemic retinoid administration of etretinate in doses of 25-50 mg/d appears an important improvement for managing this group of patients. Aside from several isolated case reports [29, 30] some observations on larger patient series are available (*Table III*). Kelly *et al.* treated four male renal transplant recipients with etretinate (50 mg/d) for 8-13 months [3]. As compared to the development of squamous cell carcinomas 12 months before and 12 months after this therapy, etretinate suppressed squamous cell carcinoma formation. No patient in this study showed renal dysfunction or increase of serum triglycerides and also cholesterol. It is interesting to note that 2 out of 4 patients developed an increased number of squamous cell carcinomas after oral etretinate treatment was stopped. This is in agreement with data obtained in patients with xeroderma pigmentosum treated with isotretinoin [24]. In this study, 2 out of 5 patients showed a similar early acceleration in tumor formation after cessation of oral retinoid therapy. Of course, from these incomplete data it is not possible to conclude whether or not there is an increase of skin cancer formation when oral retinoid therapy is discontinued over a longer period of time.

Shuttleworth *et al.* used etretinate in 6 renal transplant recipients with recurrent skin malignancies [31]. They found that 5 responded, although 2 patients developed further tumors within 6 months after discontinuing drug medication. None of these patients showed any evidence of graft dysfunction.

Table III. Systemic retinoids in chemoprevention of renal transplant recipients

Retinoid	Daily dose	Treatment period (months)	Number of patients	Response rate (reduction of lesions)	Reference
Etretinate	1 mg/kg	6	6	5/6	[31]
Etretinate	50 mg	8-13	4	74%	[3]
Etretinate	0.2-0.4 mg/kg	3-13	6	reduction of frequency of surgery	[33]
Etretinate and topical tretinoin	10 mg	3-9	7/11 etretinate+tretinoin 4/11 tretinoin alone	3 mo.: 9/11 (82%) decrease of 25% 6 mo.: 6/8 (75%) decrease of 50%	[32]
Acitretin	30 mg	6	19/38 acitretin, 19/38 placebo	13% relative decrease of lesions, 28% increase in placebo group	[34]
Acitretin	10-50 mg	< 6, 6-12 or >12	15	decrease of lesions in all patients	[35]

Furthermore, a combination of topical tretinoin and low-dose oral etretinate (10 mg/d) has been proposed for chemoprevention with reduced side effects [32]. However, only limited data were available on chemoprevention of basal and squamous cell carcinoma in organ transplant recipients using systemic retinoids [33-35]. It was shown in a series of patients that long-term treatment with etretinate led to a marked reduction in the frequency of surgery for epithelial tumors in renal transplant recipients [33]. A daily dose of 30 mg acitretin was significantly effective to prevent squamous cell carcinoma and to reduce the occurrence of keratotic skin lesions in a study of 38 renal transplant patients [34]. An improvement in actinic keratoses, in skin texture, and reduction of skin malignancies was shown with long-term treatment of 10 to 50 mg/day acitretin [35].

Systemic retinoids were also used for the therapy of precanceroses. Oral leukoplakia was shown to be sensitive to etretinate as well as to isotretinoin. Thereby, regressions between 61% (isotretinoin) and 92% (etretinate) have been reported [36, 37]. For treatment of oral leukoplakia also fenretinide (200 mg daily with a 3-day drug holiday each month) was investigated. Preliminary results in a controlled study with 153 patients showed that the risk of recurrence and of new localizations was lower in the fenretinide group as compared to the control group [38].

Squamous cell carcinomas did not respond to systemic retinoid monotherapy. This is in contrast to the benefits of chemoprevention. However, effective combinations of isotretinoin with interferon alpha-2a were reported in advanced squamous cell carcinomas. Twenty-three percent of the patients showed complete, and 41% partial remission [39, 40]. Another trial using 13-cis-retinoic acid (1mg/kg/d) and interferon alpha-2a (3 or 6 x 10^6 IU) showed beneficial response in 68% of the patients [41].

For other skin neoplasias, systemic retinoid therapy has been also investigated. In malignant melanoma, monotherapy with isotretinoin, etretinate, tretinoin or fenretinide as well as combination of isotretinoin with interferon alpha-2a were shown to be ineffective [42, 43]. In contrast, in cutaneous T-cell lymphoma successful therapy has been reported with etretinate, isotretinoin and also with the arotinoid Ro 13-6298 [44-49]. A new promising approach for systemic treatment of cutaneous T-cell lymphoma is a combination treatment with etretinate and interferon alpha [50-53]. Depending on the interferon alpha type used remission rates between 77% and 53% were reported. Combination of systemic isotretinoin and interferon alpha-2b also showed good therapeutic results with a remission rate of 57% [54].

Recently, the beneficial effect of systemic tretinoin in patients with HIV-related Kaposi's sarcoma was reported in first pilot study [55]. From *in vitro* studies [56], it was suggested that systemic retinoids may decrease endothelial proliferation also *in vivo*. As shown in cutaneous T cell lymphomas, it seems that retinoids and interferons may act synergistically. The mechanisms underlying this synergistic effect were thought to be an induction of the expression of RARs and *vice versa* the expression of interferon-receptors by retinoids. Therefore, combination therapy of HIV-related Kaposi's sarcoma with interferon alpha and systemic tretinoin may be a promising concept.

In summary, the clinical data available for prevention and therapy of basal cell carcinomas and squamous cell carcinomas in organ transplant recipients indicate that systemic retinoids have a beneficial effect in suppressing skin cancer formation. The development of new retinoids and new combination regimens, *e.g.* with vitamin D analogues, will improve the management of organ transplant recipients and reduce skin cancer formation in these patients. Further basic and clinical research is necessary to elucidate the mechanisms underlying the promotion of skin cancer and the action of chemopreventive concepts. Especially, placebo-controlled clinical studies on the effect of systemic retinoids for chemoprevention of skin cancer in organ transplant recipients will be necessary.

References

1. Hardie IR, Strong RW, Hartley LCJ, Woodruff PWH, Clunie GJA. Skin cancer in Caucasian renal allograft recipients living in a subtropical climate. *Surgery* 1980 ; 87 : 177-83.
2. Ko CB, Walton S, Keczkes K, Bury HP, Nichloson C. The emerging epidemic of skin cancer. *Br J Dermatol* 1994 ; 130 : 269-72.
3. Kelly JW, Sabto J, Gurr FW, Bruce F. Retinoids to prevent skin cancer in organ transplant recipients. *Lancet* 1991 ; 338 : 1407.
4. Euvrard S, Kanitakis J, Pouteil-Noble C, Disant F, Dureau G, Finaz de Villaine J, Claudy A, Thivolet J. Aggressive squamous cell carcinoma in organ transplant recipients. *Transplant Proc* 1995 ; 27 : 1767-8.
5. Orfanos CE, Zouboulis ChC, Almond-Roesler B, Geilen CC. Current use and future potential role of retinoids in dermatology. *Drugs* 1997 ; 53 : 358-88.
6. Fisher GJ, Voorhees JJ. Molecular mechanisms of retinoid actions in skin. *FASEB J* 1996 ; 10 : 1002-13.
7. Pfahl M. Nuclear receptor/AP-1 interaction. *Endocr Rev* 1993 ; 14 : 651-8.
8. Fanjul A, Dawson MI, Hobbs PD, Jong L, Cameron JF, Harlev E, Graupner G, Lu XP, Pfahl M. A new class of retinoids with selective inhibition of AP-1 inhibits proliferation. *Nature* 1994 ; 372 : 107-11.
9. Brash DE, Rudolph JA, Simon JA, Lin A, McKenna GJ, Baden HP, Halperin AJ, Ponten J. A role for sunlight in skin cancer: UV-induced p53 mutations in squamous cell carcinoma. *Proc Natl Acad Sci USA* 1991 ; 88 : 10124-8.
10. Henseleit U, Zhang J, Wanner R, Haase I, Kolde G, Rosenbach T. Role of p53 in UVB-induced apoptosis in human HaCaT keratinocytes. *J Invest Dermatol* 1997 ; 109 : 722-7.
11. Li G, Tron V, Ho V. Induction of squamous cell carcinoma in p53-deficient mice after ultraviolet irradiation. *J Invest Dermatol* 1998 ; 110 : 72-5.
12. Gibson GE, O'Grady A, Kay EW, Leader M, Murphy GM. p53 tumor suppressor gene protein expression in premalignant and malignant skin lesions of kidney transplant recipients. *J Am Acad Dermatol* 1997 ; 36 : 924-31.

13. Geilen CC, Bektas M, Wieder Th, Orfanos CE. The vitamin D3 analogue, calcipotriol, induces sphingomyelin hydrolysis in human keratinocytes. *FEBS Lett* 1997 ; 378 : 88-92.

14. Geilen CC, Wieder T, Orfanos CE. Ceramide signalling: regulatory role in cell proliferation, differentiation and apoptosis in human epidermis. *Arch Dermatol Res* 1997 ; 289 : 559-66.

15. Kalen A, Borchardt RA, Bell RM. Elevated ceramide levels in GH4C1 cells treated with retinoic acid. *Biochem Biophys Acta* 1992 ; 1125 : 90-6.

16. Geilen CC, Bektas M, Wieder T, Kodelja V, Goerdt S, Orfanos CE. 1α,25 dihydroxy-vitamin D3 induces sphingomyelin hydrolysis in HaCaT cells *via* tumor necrosis factor α. *J Biol Chem* 1997 ; 272 : 8997-9001.

17. Morré DJ, Morré DM, Paulik M, Batova A, Broome AM, Pirisi L, Creek E. Retinoic acid and calcitriol inhibition of growth and NADH oxidase of normal immortalized human keratinocytes. *Biochem Biophys Acta* 1992 ; 1134 : 217-22.

18. Morré DJ, Brightman AO. NADH oxidase of plasma membranes. *J Bioenerg Biomemb* 1991 ; 23 : 469-89.

19. Dai S, Morré DJ, Geilen CC, Almond-Roesler B, Orfanos CE, Morré DM. Inhibition of plasma membrane NADH oxidase activity and growth of HeLa cells by natural and synthetic retinoids. *Mol Cell Biochem* 1997 ; 166 : 101-9.

20. Lippman SM, Brenner SE, Hong WK. Cancer chemoprevention. *J Clin Oncol* 1994 ; 12 : 851-73.

21. Gollnick H, Orfanos CE. Theoretical aspects of the use of retinoids as anticancer agents. In : Marks R, ed. *Retinoids in cutaneous malignancy*. Oxford : Blackwell, 1991 : 41-65.

22. Bollag W, Holdener EE. Retinoids in cancer prevention and therapy. *Ann Oncol* 1992 ; 3 : 513-26.

23. Lippman SM, Heyman RA, Kurie JM, Benner SE, Hong WK. Retinoids and chemoprevention: clinical and basic studies. *J Cell Biochem* 1995 ; 22 : 1-10.

24. Kraemer KH, Di Giovanna JJ, Moshella AN, Tarone RE, Peck GL. Prevention of skin cancer in xeroderma pigmentosum with the use of oral isotretinoin. *N Engl J Med* 1988 ; 318 : 1633-7.

25. Berth-Jones J, Cole J, Lehmann AR, Arlett CF, Graham-Brown RA. Xeroderma pigmentosum variant: 5 years of tumour suppression by etretinate. *J R Soc Med* 1993 ; 86 : 355-6.

26. Hodak E, Ginzburg A, David M, Sandbank M. Etretinate treatment of the nevoid basal cell carcinoma syndrome. *Int J Dermatol* 1987 ; 26 : 606-9.

27. Goldberg L, Hsu S, Alcalay J. Effectiveness of isotretinoin in preventing the appearance of basal cell carcinomas in basal cell nevus syndrome. *J Am Acad Dermatol* 1989 ; 21 : 144-5.

28. Tangrea JA, Edwards BK, Taylor PR, Hartman AM, Peck GL, Salasche SJ, Menon PA, Benson PM, Mellette JR, Guill MA, Robinson JK, Guin JD, Stoll HL, Grabski WJ, Winton GB. Long-term therapy with low dose isotretinoin for prevention of basal cell carcinoma: a multicenter clinical trial. *J Natl Cancer Inst* 1992 ; 84 : 328-32.

29. Mc Lelland J, Chu AC. Skin tumors in renal allograft recipient. *J R Soc Med* 1989 ; 82 : 110-1.

30. Vanderghinste N, De Bersaques J, Geerts ML, Kint A. Acitretin as cancer chemo-prophylaxis in renal transplant recipient. *Dermatol* 1992 ; 185 : 307-8.

31. Shuttleworth D, Marks R, Griffin PJA, Salaman JR. Treatment of cutaneous neoplasia with etretinate in renal transplant recipients. *Q J Med* 1988 ; 68 : 717-25.

32. Rook AH, Jaworsky C, Nguyen T, Grossmann RA, Wolfe JT, Witmer WK, Kligman AM. Beneficial effect of low-dose systemic retinoid in combination with topical tretinoin for the treatment and prophylaxis of premalignant and malignant skin lesions in renal transplant recipients. *Transplantation* 1995 ; 59 : 714-9.

33. Glover MT, Niranjan N, Kwan JT, Leigh IM. Non-melanoma skin cancer in renal transplant recipients: the extent of the problem and strategy for management. *Br J Plast Surg* 1994 ; 47 : 86-9.

34. Bouwes-Bavinck JN, Tieben LM, Van der Woude FJ, Tegzess AM, Hermans J, ter Schegget J, Vermeer BJ. Prevention of skin cancer and reduction of keratotic skin lesions during acitretin therapy in renal transplant recipients: a double-blind, placebo-controlled study. *J Clin Oncol* 1995 ; 13 : 1933-8.

35. Yuan Z, Davis A, Macdonald K, Bailey RR. Use of acitretin for the skin complications in renal transplant recipients. *N Z Med J* 1995 ; 108 : 255-6.

36. Hong WK, Endicott J, Itri LM, Doos W, Batsakis JG, Bell R, Fofonoff S, Byers R, Atkinson EN, Vaughan C. 13-cis-retinoic acid in the treatment of oral leukoplakia. N Engl J Med 1986 ; 315 : 1501-5.
37. Toma S, Mangiante PE, Margarino G, Nicolo G, Palumbo R. Progressive 13-cis-retinoic acid dosage in the treatment of oral leukoplakia. Oral Oncol Eur J Cancer 1992 ; 28B : 121-3.
38. Costa A, Formelli F, Chiesa F, Decensi A, De Palo G, Veronesi U. Prospects of chemoprevention of human cancers with the synthetic retinoid fenretinide. Cancer Res 1994 ; 54 : 2032-7.
39. Lippman SM, Parkinson DR, Itri LM, Weber RS, Schantz SP, Ota DM, Schustermann MA, Krakoff IH, Guttermann JU, Hong WK. 13-cis-retinoic acid and interferon alpha-2a: effective combination therapy for advanced squamous cell carcinoma of the skin. J Natl Cancer Inst 1992 ; 84 : 241-5.
40. Toma S, Palumbo R, Vincenti M, Aitini E, Paganini G, Pronzato P, Grimaldi A, Rosso R. Efficiency of recombinant alpha-interferon 2a and 13-cis-retinoic acid in the treatment of squamous cell carcinoma. Ann Oncol 1994 ; 5 : 463-5.
41. Eisenhauer EA, Lippman SM, Kavanagh JJ, Parades-Espinoza M, Arnold A, Hong WK, Massimini G, Schleuniger U, Bollag W, Holdener EE, Krakoff I. Combination 13-cis-retinoic acid and interferon alpha 2a in the therapy of solid tumours. Leukemia 1994 ; 8 : 1622-5.
42. Modiano M, Dalton W, Lippman SM, Joffe L, Booth AR, Meyskens FL Jr. Phase II study of fenretinide N-(4-hydroxyphenyl)retinamide in advanced breast cancer and melanoma. Invest New Drugs 1990 ; 8 : 317-9.
43. Dhingra K, Papadopoulos N, Lippman SM, Lotan R, Legha SS. Phase II study of alpha-interferon and 13-cis-retinoic acid in metastatic melanoma. Invest New Drugs 1993 ; 11 : 39-43.
44. Kessler JF, Jones SE, Levine N, Lynch PJ, Booth AR, Meyskens FL Jr. Isotretinoin and cutaneous helper T-cell lymphoma (mycosis fungoides). Arch Dermatol 1987 ; 123 : 201-20.
45. Molin L, Thomsen K, Volden G, Aronsson A, Hammar H, Hellbe L, Wantzin GL, Roupe G. Oral retinoids in mycosis fungoides and Sézary syndrome: a comparison of isotretinoin and etretinate. Acta Derm Venereol 1987 ; 67 : 232-6.
46. Molin L, Thomsen K, Volden G, Jensen P, Knudsen E, Nyfors A, Schmidt H. Retinoids and systemic chemotherapy in cases of advanced mycosis fungoides. Acta Derm Venereol 1987 ; 67 : 179-82.
47. Neely SM, Mehlmauer M, Feinstein DI. The effect of isotretinoin in six patients with cutaneous T-cell lymphoma. Arch Intern Med 1987 ; 147 : 529-31.
48. Zachariae H, Thestrup-Pedersen K. Interferon alpha and etretinate combination treatment of cutaneous T-cell lymphoma. J Invest Dermatol 1990 ; 95 : 206-8.
49. Tousignant J, Raymond GP, Light MJ. Treatment of cutaneous T-cell lymphoma with the arotinoid Ro 13-6298. J Am Acad Dermatol 1987 ; 16 : 167-71.
50. Altomare GF, Capella GL, Pigatto PD, Finzi AF. Intramuscular low dose alpha-2b interferon and etretinate for treatment of mycosis fungoides. Int J Dermatol 1993 ; 32 : 138-41.
51. Dréno B, Célérier P, Litoux P. Roferon, a in combination with Tigason, in cutaneous T-cell lymphomas. Acta Haematol 1993 ; 89 : 28-32.
52. Dréno B, Claudy A, Meynadier J, Verret JL, Souteyrand P, Ortonne JP, Kalis B, Godefroy WY, Beerblock K, Thill L. The treatment of 45 patients with cutaneous T-cell lymphoma with low doses of interferon-alpha-2a and etretinate. Br J Dermatol 1991 ; 125 : 456-9.
53. Braathen LR, McFadden N. Successful treatment of mycosis fungoides with the combination of etretinate and human recombinant interferon alpha-2a. J Dermatol Treat 1989 ; 1 : 29-32.
54. Knobler RM, Trautinger F, Radaszkiewicz T, Kokoschka EM, Micksche M. Treatment of cutaneous T-cell lymphoma with combination of low-dose interferon alpha-2b and retinoids. J Am Acad Dermatol 1991 ; 24 : 247-52.
55. Bonhomme L, Fredj G, Ecstein E, Maurisson G, Farabos C, Misset JL, Jasmin C. Treatment of AIDS-associated Kaposi's sarcoma with oral tretinoin. Am J Hosp Pharm 1994 ; 51 : 2417-9.
56. Imcke E, Ruszczak Zb, Mayer-da-Silva A, Detmar M, Orfanos CE. Cultivation of human dermal microvascular endothelial cells in vitro: immunocytochemical and ultrastructural characterization and effect of treatment with three synthetic retinoids. Arch Dermatol Res 1991 ; 283 : 149-57.

23

Topical retinoids for the management of dysplastic epithelial lesions

Sylvie EUVRARD
Department of Dermatology, Hôpital Edouard-Herriot, Lyon, France.

Topical retinoids, mainly all-trans-retinoic acid (RA) and isotretinoin, have been largely used for many years in the treatment of acne and photoaging [1, 2]. The aim of this chapter is to present the main clinical data on their anticarcinogenic effect and their use for the treatment of dysplastic epithelial skin lesions in immunosuppressed and non-immunosuppressed patients, and to discuss the value of this treatment in organ transplant recipients.

Cutaneous dysplastic epithelial lesions in organ transplant recipients

Skin cancers, especially squamous cell carcinomas (SCC), represent the most frequent malignancy in organ transplant recipients involving half of these patients within 20 years following transplantation [3, 4]. The time lapse for the development of the lesions after transplantation is about 7 to 8 years after kidney transplantation and 3 years after heart transplantation [5]. This delay is shorter in older patients and in sunny countries. SCC are more aggressive than in non-immunosuppressed patients. They are complicated by local recurrences in 12% of cases and have a metastatic evolution in 8% of patients.

Carcinomas are usually preceded for some years by warts and various epithelial lesions such as premalignant keratoses, Bowen's disease and keratoacanthomas. All these lesions tend to be multiple, and after several years some patients may develop over 100 tumors. Multiplicity of SCC along with older age and cephalic location constitute clinical factors of unfavorable prognosis. An efficient treatment at the stage of warts and premalignant keratoses should decrease the incidence of SCC.

The most important factor for the development of skin carcinomas is sun exposure; indeed, warts and carcinomas appear preferentially on sun-exposed areas of light-skinned patients. UV light decreases the number of epidermal Langerhans cells (LC). This effect could be enhanced by the immunosuppressive treatment which also seems to alter LC [6, 7]; thus local cutaneous immunosuppression allows HPV proliferation and tumor promotion. HPV infections are associated with skin carcinomas as clinically suggested by the location of warts and cancers in the same areas and confirmed by the detection of HPV DNA in skin carcinomas [8]. A recent work concluded that the increased risk of skin cancer associated with immunosuppressive treatment is independent of the drugs used, being rather the result of the immunosuppression *per se* [4]. Surgical excision, which allows histological examination, represents the treatment of choice for both malignant and premalignant lesions. Cryotherapy can be applied to superficial basal cell carcinomas (BCC) and premalignant keratoses. However, when the lesions are multiple, repeated surgical excisions of neoplasms and sessions of cryotherapy are unsatisfactory since they induce numerous scars with an important esthetic damage, and therefore other therapeutic methods are required. Multiple lesions can be considered as a manifestation of overimmunosuppression, and a reduction of the immunosuppressive treatment should be considered; retinoids may also be useful [9].

Systemic retinoids and organ transplantation

The occurrence of multiple premalignant and malignant epithelial lesions in organ transplant recipients represents theoretically an ideal indication of systemic retinoids [10-12]. It has been shown that retinoic acid inhibits the growth of human papillomavirus-infected human keratinocytes more effectively as compared with normal keratinocytes, probably by suppressing the early transcription of HPV genes [13, 14]. These results provide a biochemical explanation for the role of retinoids in the chemoprevention of HPV-induced cancers. Several studies [15-25] have shown the benefit of systemic retinoids in organ transplant recipients with multiple skin dysplastic lesions. These agents generally induce a considerable reduction in the occurrence of dysplastic lesions and skin carcinomas and an improvement of solar keratoses. They do not interfere with cyclosporine nor do they induce graft rejection, any immunological changes that may occur being probably insignificant in patients who are already heavily immunosuppressed; however, retinoids invariably induce side effects, mainly mucocutaneous xerosis, hair loss, elevated serum lipids and arthralgias. Skeletal abnormalities, such as calcifications and hyperostotic axial skeletal lesions [26-29] have not been reported in transplant recipients since they occur after several years. Most of these side effects are dose-dependent. On the other hand, lower doses of systemic retinoids may not be effective. The usual relapse following discontinuation of retinoids raises the question of continuous treatments. Their long-term use may be limited by the side effects which cumulate with those of immunosuppressive treatment or the underlying pathology. Increase of serum lipids and osteoporosis are frequent in organ transplant patients, due to steroids. Hepatic dysfunction may be due to azathioprine or to chronic viral B or C hepatitis. Hence, systemic retinoids should be reserved to selected patients who develop a great number of lesions over short periods. Safer protocols have yet to be developed for the prevention of premalignant and malignant lesions in large groups of organ transplant recipients.

Topical all-trans-retinoic acid or tretinoin

Experimental studies

One of the effects of both ultraviolet (UV) light and immunosuppressive treatment is to deplete LC from the epidermis. Part of the anti-carcinogenic activity of retinoids may be due to their ability to protect LC during the early stages of carcinogenesis. Retinoic acid (RA) was shown to be effective on both chemical and UV-light-induced carcinogenesis [30, 31]. Topical application of RA prevents the tumor promoter 12-0-tetradecanoylphorbol-13-acetate (TPA) from depleting the density of LC in murine epidermis. Four weekly treatments with TPA reduced the LC density by 39%, and this effect was completely inhibited by RA. RA on its own does not influence LC density after one week treatment but increases LC density by 20% after 4 weeks treatment. Mice were irradiated with the minimal erythemal dose of UV light 5 days per week for 4 weeks. This UV procedure reduced the density of LC by about 62%. Topical application of RA 24 h prior to each UV irradiation completely prevented UV from depleting LC from murine epidermis. The mechanism by which retinoids inhibit TPA and UV-induced depletion of LC remains unclear.

Study of « normal » skin of kidney transplant recipients

The study of « normal » skin of kidney transplant recipients after application of topical tretinoin [32] during 6 months revealed upon histological and ultrastructural examination epidermal and dermal changes suggestive of an increased cellular metabolism in the treated sites.

Dysplastic lesions in non-immunosuppressed patients

After the initial report of Stüttgen in 1962 [33], several authors have experienced regression of BCC or actinic keratoses with topical tretinoin [34-38].

Basal cell carcinomas

In 1970, Bollag and Ott used 0.1% and 0.3% tretinoin ointments applied under occlusion once daily to treat 11 patients with 16 BCC on the face or the trunk for 3 to 5 weeks [34]. Complete responses were obtained in 3/6 tumors with 0.1% concentration and 2/10 tumors with 0.3% concentration. Two of them were followed by recurrences 8 and 10 months after treatment stopped. A three week-course with 1% tretinoin cream twice daily induced disappearance of a large recurrent BCC on the back without recurrence in a 2-year follow-up period [35]. Another patient with multiple arsenic-induced superficial BCC was treated with a concentration of 0.05% twice daily for 3 weeks followed by a 3-week interruption. After three cycles of treatment, histological examination of the lesional biopsies showed no evidence of tumor. However, 9 months later, all lesions relapsed [38].

Actinic keratoses

Sixty patients with multiple actinic keratoses were treated with 0.1% and 0.3% tretinoin ointment twice daily without dressing for 3 to 10 weeks [36]. Among 51 patients with facial keratoses, complete responses were obtained in 7/20 (35%) with the 0.1% and in 17/31 (55%) with the 0.3% concentration. In 20 of the remaining 27 patients a reduction greater than 50% was achieved. Complete responses were not obtained in actinic keratoses of the hands and forearms with any concentration, but 7/9 patients had a partial response.

Robinson and Kligman [39] evaluated 0.1% tretinoin cream applied once daily 8 to 14 days as adjunctive therapy to a 4-5 week topical 5-fluorouracil course. Combination therapy gave better results than each treatment alone: a complete response was obtained on the forearms for all 20 patients and on the hands in 18/20 patients, whereas 5-fluorouracil alone induced complete response in only 5/20 patients and no response on the hands. These results were confirmed subsequently by a three-month course of once daily application of 0.05% tretinoin cream [40].

The preventive effect on actinic keratoses was studied in a double-blind, bilateral paired comparison study [41]. Twenty-four patients with at least 5 and no more than 50 actinic keratoses on the face and arms were treated by 0.05% tretinoin cream or an emollient cream. The treatment was begun 2 weeks after cryotherapy of all keratoses and the patients were seen at 3-month intervals. Thirteen completed the one-year study. No difference in the development of actinic keratoses was noted between the two sides.

In all these studies, tretinoin treatment was accompanied by a more or less severe inflammatory reaction.

Dysplastic lesions in organ transplant recipients

Two studies have been performed in organ transplant patients. The first one [42] assessed the efficacy and safety of 0.05% tretinoin cream in the treatment of solar keratoses and warts on sun exposed areas in a controlled, double-blind randomized study with an intra-individual comparison. Twenty-five patients presenting with more than three lesions (warts or keratoses) on the forearms and/or hands on both sides were enrolled in the study. Patients applied once daily for three months the active cream on one side and the vehicle on the other side. A global count of all lesions (keratoses and warts) was performed. Twenty-two patients were evaluable at month 3 and 21 at month 6. The reduction of the number of lesions was higher with the tretinoin cream at months 3 (45% versus 23%) and 6 (29% versus 19%) (*Figure 39, page 223*). When the percent reduction of lesions from baseline was compared between treatments by a two-sided sign test (in intra-individual comparisons), a significant advantage was found for the active cream ($p < 0.05$). At month 6 this difference was maintained. Local tolerance was generally good. Furthermore, 17 patients with lesions on the face (median number: 10) applied only tretinoin cream. The median percentage of reduction when compared to baseline was significant ($p < 0.05$) at months 3 (55%) and 6 (51%) (*Figure 40, page 223*). There was no significant difference in the degree of evolution after treatment between months 3 and 6.

To avoid the toxicity of high-dose systemic retinoids, a second study combined topical tretinoin with low-dose etretinate (10 mg daily) for the treatment of multiple actinic keratoses, warts and squamous cell carcinomas in renal transplant recipients [21]. Eleven renal allograft recipients with multiple (more than 50) actinic keratoses, warts and squamous cell carcinomas were enrolled in a pilot study. Seven patients received combined tretinoin and etretinate therapy and 4 elected to use tretinoin alone. 0.025% tretinoin cream was applied to areas of actinically-damaged skin containing keratoses, warts and in some cases superficial SCC. After one month the concentration was increased to 0.05%. By 3 months of therapy, 9 of 11 patients (including 3 patients treated by tretinoin alone) exhibited at least a 25% decrease in the number of clinically apparent keratoses and a reduction of the size of warts. After 6 months, 6 of 8 evaluable patients (including 2 of 3 individuals receiving tretinoin alone) exhibited at least a 50% decrease in the number of the lesions. Three of 4 patients on the combined regimen and 2 of 3 receiving tretinoin alone for at least 9 months experienced a significant decrease in the rate of development of new SCC. At the onset of treatment, epidermal specimens were almost completely devoid of CD1+ LC, but their density increased greatly and in proportion to the duration of therapy. In one patient receiving tretinoin alone, epidermal LC showed more than a 7-fold increase after 6 months of treatment. None of the participants in this study experienced serious adverse effects of therapy.

Other topical retinoids

In non-immunosuppressed patients

Other topical retinoids have been used for the treatment of actinic keratoses in non-immunosuppressed patients.

The efficacy and tolerability of arotinoid methyl sulfone (Ro 14-9706) cream were compared with that of tretinoin in a study involving 25 patients with more than 3 lesions on each side of the face [43]. All patients applied each agent twice daily for 16 weeks as a 0.05% cream to opposite sides of the face. The mean percent decrease in the number of actinic keratoses was 37.8% for areas treated with Ro 14-9706 and 30.3% for areas treated with tretinoin. Each of these figures was significantly different from baseline but not from each other. Ro 14-9706 was better tolerated than tretinoin; local inflammation was slight or absent in most patients whereas tretinoin caused severe erythema and scaling in 50% and 23% of patients, respectively.

The efficacy and tolerability of isotretinoin 0.1% in the treatment of actinic keratoses were evaluated in a randomized, double-blind, placebo-controlled study [44]. One hundred patients were randomly assigned to treatment with 0.1% cream or vehicle twice daily for 6 months to the face, scalp and the upper extremities. On the face, the reduction in the number of lesions was significantly higher with isotretinoin. No effect was observed for lesions on the scalp or upper extremities. Mild to moderate local reaction occurred with isotretinoin.

Other topical retinoids such as retinaldehyde [45] could be useful but their action on actinic keratoses is not yet known.

In organ transplant recipients

Adapalene is a stable naphtoic acid derivative with potent retinoid pharmacology, controlling cell proliferation and differentiation [46]. We performed a randomized intra-individual study to assess the efficacy and safety of adapalene (0.1% and 0.3% gel, Galderma Research & Development) compared with adapalene gel vehicle in the treatment of actinic keratoses of organ transplant recipients (unpublished data). Forty patients with at least three actinic keratoses on each arm were randomized to apply either 0.1% or 0.3% gel on one side and the vehicle on the controlateral side once daily for 6 months. The face was also treated with the same concentration of adapalene as the treated arm. Eighteen patients were evaluable in the 0.1% group and 21 in the 0.3% group. The mean number of actinic keratoses located on the arms (11.5 in the 0.1% group and 10.5 in the 0.3% group) decreased significantly in the 0.3% adapalene group (32% *versus* 21 %, $p < 0.05$) but not in the 0.1% group. Only one case of (mild) skin irritation was observed in each group.

When to prescribe topical retinoids in organ transplant recipients

Topical retinoids represent probably the best way to control the proliferation of premalignant and malignant lesions. The majority of dysplastic epithelial lesions occur on sun-exposed areas but the location is different depending on the age at transplantation: before 40 years, 80% of the lesions are found on the dorsum of the hands, the forearms or the upper trunk, whereas after 40 years, 80% of the lesions develop on the head. It was shown in non-immunosuppressed patients that lesions of the face respond better than those of the forearms and the hands [36, 44]; we have no answer in organ transplant recipients, except from the fact that we obtained especially good results on lesions of the head (*Figure 39, page 223*).

All organ transplant recipients with multiple dysplastic epithelial lesions should be treated with topical retinoids. Until now, tretinoin proved to be the most efficient one. Local tolerance seems better than in non-immunosuppressed patients. The duration of the treatment has to be established depending on tolerance and efficacy. Relapses are observed after several months but it was shown that the benefit of a 3 month-course is maintained 3 months after treatment discontinuation. [42]. Three or 6 month-courses may be proposed and alternated with 3 or 6 month-discontinuation. Unfortunately, similarly with oral retinoids, some patients are « non-responders ». Each retinoid should be studied as an individual drug and the lack of response to one retinoid does not equate with unresponsiveness to other retinoids [10]. Etretinate was reported to be efficient in cases where acitretin had failed [47]. The efficacy may be related to the concentration of the retinoid in the cream, as we observed in the case of adapalene. In some cases, topical retinoids may be associated with low-dose systemic retinoids.

References

1. Kligman AM. The treatment of acne with topical retinoids: one man's opinions. *J Am Acad Dermatol* 1997 ; 36 : S92-5.

2. Kligman AM, Grove GL, Hirose R, Leyden JL. Topical tretinoin for photoaged skin. *J Am Acad Dermatol* 1986 ; 15 : 836-59.

3. Hartevelt MM, Bouwes Bavinck JN, Koote AMM, Vermeer BJ, Vandenbroucke JP. Incidence of skin cancer after renal transplantation in the Netherlands. *Transplantation* 1990 ; 49 : 506-9.

4. Bouwes-Bavinck JN, Hardie D, Green A, Cutmore S, MacNaught A, O'Sullivan B, Siskind V, Van der Voude FJ, Hardie IR. The risk of skin cancer in renal transplant recipients in Queensland, Australia. *Transplantation* 1996, 61 : 715-21.

5. Euvrard S, Kanitakis J, Pouteil-Noble C, Dureau G, Touraine JL, Faure M, Claudy A, Thivolet J. Comparative epidemiologic study of premalignant and malignant epithelial cutaneous lesions developing after kidney and heart transplantation. *J Am Acad Dermatol* 1995 ; 33 : 222-9.

6. Servitje O, Seron D, Ferrer I, Carrera M, Pagerols X, Peyri J. Quantitative and morphometric analysis of Langerhans cells in non-exposed skin in renal transplant patients. *J Cutan Pathol* 1991 ; 18 : 106-11.

7. Galvao MM, Sotto MN, Kihara SM, Rivitti EA, Sabbaga E. Lymphocyte subsets and Langerhans cells in sun-protected and sun-exposed skin of immunosuppressed renal allograft recipients. *J Am Acad Dermatol* 1998 ; 38 : 38-44.

8. Chardonnet Y, Viac J, Euvrard S. Warts and squamous cell carcinomas in organ transplant patients: is the human papillomavirus responsible for carcinogenesis? *Eur J Dermatol* 1997 ; 7 : 5-11.

9. Euvrard S, Kanitakis J, Thivolet J, Claudy A. Retinoids for the management of dermatological complications of organ transplantation. *Biodrugs* 1997 ; 3 : 176-84.

10. DiGiovanna JJ. Retinoids for the future: oncology. *J Am Acad Dermatol* 1992 ; 27 : S34-7.

11. Bollag W, Holdener E. Retinoids in cancer prevention and therapy. *Ann Oncol* 1992 ; 3 : 513-26.

12. Craven NM, Griffiths CEM. Retinoids in the management of non-melanoma skin cancer and melanoma. *Cancer Surv* 1996 ; 26 : 267-87.

13. Bartsch D, Boye B, Baust C, Zur Hausen H, Schwarz E. Retinoic acid mediated repression of human papillomavirus 18 transcription and different ligand regulation of the retinoic acid receptor beta gene in non-tumorigenic and tumorigenic Hela hybrid cells. *EMBO J* 1992 ; 11 : 2283-91.

14. Khan MA, Jenkins GR, Tolleson WH Creek KE, Pirisi L. Retinoic acid inhibition of human papillomavirus type 16-mediated transformation of human keratinocytes. *Cancer Res* 1993 ; 53 : 903-9.
15. Shuttleworth D, Marks R, Griffin PJA, Salaman J. Treatment of cutaneous neoplasia with Etretinate in renal transplant recipients. *Q J Med* 1988 ; 68 : 717-25.
16. McLelland J Chu AC. Skin tumours in renal allograft recipients. *J R Soc Med* 1988 ; 82 : 110-1.
17. Kelly JW, Sabto J, Gurr FW, Bruce F. Retinoids to prevent skin cancer in organ transplant recipients. *Lancet* 1991 ; 338 : 1407.
18. Vandeghinste N, de Bersaques J, Geerts ML Kint A. Acitretin as cancer chemoprophylaxis in a renal transplant recipient. *Dermatology* 1992 ; 185 : 307-8.
19. Euvrard S, Pouteil-Noble C, Kanitakis J, Ffrench M, Berger F, Delecluse HJ, D'Incan M, Thivolet J. Successive occurrence of T-cell and B-cell lymphomas after renal transplantation in a patient with multiple cutaneous squamous cell carcinomas. *N Engl J Med* 1992 ; 327 : 1924-7.
20. Glover MT, Niranjan N, Kwan JTC, Leigh I. Non-melanoma skin cancer in renal transplant recipients: the extent of the problem and a strategy for management. *Br J Plast Surg* 1994 ; 47 : 86-9.
21. Rook AH, Jaworsky C, Nguyen T, Grossman RA, Wolfe JT, Witmer WK, Kligman AM. Beneficial effect of low-dose systemic retinoid in combination with topical tretinoin for the treatment and prophylaxis of premalignant and malignant skin lesions in renal transplant recipients. *Transplantation* 1995 ; 59 : 714-9.
22. Bouwes Bavinck JN, Tieben LM, Van der Woude FJ, Tegzess AM, Hermans Jo, Ter Schegget J, Vermeer BJ. Prevention of skin cancer and reduction of keratotic skin lesions during acitretin therapy in renal transplant recipients, a double-blind, placebo-controlled study. *J Clin Oncol* 1995 ; 13 : 1933-8.
23. Yuan ZF, Davis A, MacDonald K Bailey RR. Use of acitretin for the skin complications in renal transplant recipients. *N Z Med J* 1995 ; 108 : 255-6.
24. Bellman BA, Eaglstein WH, Miller J. Low dose isotretinoin in the prophylaxis of skin cancer in renal transplant patients. *Transplantation* 1996 ; 61 : 173.
25. Gibson GE, O'Grady A, Kay EW, Murphy GM. Low-dose retinoid therapy for chemoprophylaxis of skin cancer in renal transplant recipients. *J Eur Acad Dermatol Venereol* 1998 ; 10 : 42-7.
26. McGuire J, Milstone L, Lawson J. Isotretinoin administration alters juvenile and adult bone. In : Saurat JH, ed. *Retinoids: new trends in research and therapy.* Basel : Krager, 1984 : 355-9.
27. DiGiovanna JJ, Helfgott RK, Gerber LH, Peck GL. Extraspinal tendon and ligament calcification associated with long-term therapy with Etretinate. *N Engl J Med* 1986 ; 315 : 1177-82.
28. Tangrea JA, Edwards BK, Taylor PR, Hartman AM, Peck GL, Salashe SJ, Menon PA, Benson PM, Mellette JR, Guill MA, Robinson JK, Guin JD, Stoll HL, Grabski WJ, Winton GB and other members of the Isotretinoin-basal cell carcinoma study group. Long-term therapy with low dose isotretinoin for prevention of basal cell carcinoma: a multicenter clinical trial. *J Natl Cancer Inst* 1992 ; 84 : 328-32.
29. Mork NJ, Kolbenstvedt A, Austad J. Efficacy and skeletal side effects of two years acitretin treatment. *Acta Derm Venereol* 1992 ; 72 : 445-8.
30. Halliday GM, Ho KKL, Barnetson RSC. Regulation of the skin immune system by retinoids during carcinogenesis. *J Invest Dermatol* 1992 ; 99 : 83-6.
31. Halliday GM, Dickinson JL, Muller HK. Retinoic acid protects Langerhans'cell from the effects of the tumour promotor 12-0-tetradecanoylphorbol 13-acetate. *Immunology* 1989 ; 67 : 298-302.
32. De Lacharrière O, Escoffier C, Gracia AM, Teillac D, Saint-Léger D, Berrebi C, Debure A, Levêque JL, Ducasse MF, Naret C, Kreis H, de Prost Y. Reversal effects of topical retinoic acid on the skin of kidney transplant recipients under systemic corticotherapy. *J Invest Dermatol* 1990, 95 ; 516-22.
33. Stüttgen G. Zur Lokalbehandlung von Keratosen mit Vitamin A-Säure. *Dermatologica* 1962 ; 124 : 65-80.
34. Bollag W, Ott F. Retinoic acid: topical treatment of senile or actinic keratoses and basal cell carcinomas. *Agents Actions* 1970 ; 1 : 172-5.
35. Peck GL. Hypertrophic scar after cryotherapy and topical tretinoin. *Arch Dermatol* 1973 ; 108 : 819-22.
36. Bollag W, Ott F. Vitamin A acid in benign and malignant epithelial tumours of the skin. *Acta Derm Venereol* 1975 ; 55 : S 74, 163-6.

37. Peck G. Topical tretinoin in actinic keratosis and basal cell carcinoma. *J Am Acad Dermatol* 1986 ; 15 : 829-35.

38. Brenner S, Wolf R, Dascalu DI. Topical tretinoin treatment in basal cell carcinoma. *J Dermatol Surg Oncol* 1993 ; 19 : 264-6.

39. Robinson TA, Kligman A. Treatment of solar keratoses of the extremities with retinoic acid and 5-fluorouracil. *Br J Dermatol* 1975 ; 92 : 703-6.

40. Bercovitch L. Topical chemotherapy of actinic keratoses of the upper extremity with tretinoin and 5-fluorouracil: a double-blind controlled study. *Br J Dermatol* 1987 ; 116 : 549-52.

41. Purcell SM, Pierre DK, Dixon SL, Spielvogel RL. Chemoprevention of actinic keratoses with topical all-trans-retinoic acid. *J Invest Dermatol* 1986 ; 86 : 501.

42. Euvrard S, Verschoore M, Touraine JL, Dureau G, Cochat P, Czernielewski J, Thivolet J. Topical retinoids for warts and keratoses in transplant recipients. *Lancet* 1992 ; 340 : 48-9.

43. Misiewicz J, Sendagorta E, Golebiowska A, Lorenc B, Czarnetzki BM, Jablonska S. Topical treatment of multiple actinic keratoses of the face with arotinoid methyl sulfone (Ro 14-9706) cream *versus* tretinoin cream: a double-blind, comparative study. *J Am Acad Dermatol* 1991 ; 24 : 448-51.

44. Alirezai M, Dupuy P, Amblard P, Kalis B, Souteyrand P, Frappaz A, Sendagorta E. Clinical evaluation of topical isotretinoin in the treatment of actinic keratoses. *J Am Acad Dermatol* 1994 ; 30 : 447-51.

45. Saurat JH, Didierjean L, Masgrau E, Piletta PA, Jaconi S, Chatellard-Gruaz D, Gumowski D, Masouyé I, Salomon D, Siegenthaler G. Topical retinaldehyde on human skin: biologic effects and tolerance. *J Invest Dermatol* 1994 ; 103 : 770-4.

46. Shroot B, Michel S. Pharmacology and chemistry of adapalene. *J Am Acad Dermatol* 1997 ; 36 : 96-103.

47. Bleiker TO, Bourke JF, Graham-Brown RAC, Hutchinson PE. Etretinate may work where acitretin fails. *Br J Dermatol* 1997 ; 136 : 368-70.

24

Porokeratosis

Jean KANITAKIS
Department of Dermatology, Edouard-Herriot Hospital, Lyon, France.

The term « porokeratosis » (PK) encompasses a group of uncommon hereditary or acquired diseases of keratinization of unknown aetiology, presenting with varying clinical aspects but sharing a common histopathological aspect, characterised by the presence of the « cornoid lamella ». PK was first described by Mibelli in 1893 [1]; several other clinical forms were subsequently identified. PK may appear in otherwise healthy persons but may also develop in the course of immunodeficiency states, among which organ transplantation seems to be the commonest. The general aspects of PK will first be dealt with, and the features that are particular to the forms appearing in the context of organ transplantation will then be discussed.

Porokeratosis: general features

Clinical manifestations

The primary lesion of PK is a dry brownish keratotic papule which spreads slowly in a centrifugal fashion. When the lesion is fully established, it presents as a well-demarcated irregular plaque with a slightly atrophic centre, bordered by a peripheral grooved keratotic ridge, from which a keratotic core projects at an obtuse angle. According to the number, size and distribution of the lesions the following clinical forms of PK have been described.

Classic (or Mibelli) porokeratosis

Classic (or Mibelli) porokeratosis (PKM) presents with one or a few annular plaques of large size (up to 20 cm). The lesions are usually unilateral but bilateral and symmetric lesions have been reported [2]. Giant lesions exist and comprise a highly raised peripheral border. In hereditary cases the lesions develop usually in childhood and enlarge slowly over the years, but in sporadic cases the lesions develop in adulthood. Men are more often afflicted than women (2.17:1). The lesions are usually asymptomatic and appear on the limbs but may be located on the face [3] (including the lips) [2], the palms and soles, and rarely the genitalia or the buccal mucosa [4].

Linear porokeratosis

Linear porokeratosis (LPK) consists of a unilateral, linear, systematized lesion extending over the limbs, reminiscent of an epidermal naevus, linear psoriasis or lichen striatus. The lesions may appear in the trunk with a zosteriform distribution. The disease becomes manifest in infancy or childhood but may exceptionally appear in the elderly [5]. There is a slight female preponderance (1.63:1).

Disseminated superficial actinic porokeratosis

Disseminated superficial actinic porokeratosis (DSAP) seems to be the commonest form of PK and would be more frequent in countries with high sun exposure. The lesions appear usually during the 3rd or 4th decade of life and are slowly progressive. A slight female preponderance has been noted (1.76:1), but is probably due to the fact that women are more likely to seek medical advice. DSAP manifests with several (up to hundreds of) small, dry, superficial annular lesions which characteristically appear in a bilateral and symmetric fashion on sun-exposed areas of the body, mainly the extensor surfaces of the limbs (Figures 41 and 42, page 224), shoulders and the back, more rarely the face. Individual lesions are less prominent than those of PKM and may thus be overlooked by the patients; they may be mistaken for actinic keratoses, flat seborrheic keratoses, stucco keratoses, annular lichen planus or granuloma annulare. At least half of the patients experience exacerbations during the summer months as a consequence of sun exposure [6] or after exposure to artifical light (UVA, UVB) [7-9], and one third of them experience pruritus or stinging sensations.

Disseminated superficial porokeratosis

Disseminated superficial porokeratosis (DSP) is clinically similar to DSAP, except that UV light does not act as an eliciting factor; the lesions are therefore located both in sun-exposed and sun-protected sites, and may be pruritic [10].

Porokeratosis palmaris, plantaris et disseminata

Porokeratosis palmaris, plantaris et disseminata (PPPD) is characterized by the development of symmetrical, bilateral red-brown keratotic papules resembling those of DSAP. It affects predominantly (2:1) males. The lesions appear in adolescence or early adulthood initially over the palms and soles but may later involve other body areas including sun-exposed and sun-protected sites (limbs and trunk) [11]. The buccal mucosa may be affected with small opalescent ring-like lesions [12].

Punctate porokeratosis

Punctate porokeratosis (PPK) is limited to the palms and soles and manifests with numerous punctate keratotic seed-like plugs that mimick « spines of an old-fashioned music box » [13]. This variant should be distinguished clinically from lesions of the naevoid basal-cell naevus syndrome, Darier's disease, palmoplantar lichen nitidus and hereditary punctate keratoderma. The lesions may be moderately tender to pressure. PPK may be associated with PKM or LPK.

Finally, some other varieties have been described, reflecting the clinical heterogeneity of PK, such as « reticulated » PK [14], and « eruptive pruritic » PK [15]. The relationship of PK with some other conditions, such as porokeratotic eccrine and ostial dermal duct naevus, porokeratosis punctata palmaris et plantaris, punctate porokeratotic keratoderma, is unclear.

Aetiology and pathogenesis

The aetiology and pathogenesis of PK are obscure but certainly complex and multifactorial. Many authors regard PK as a genodermatosis. It has been suggested that the lesions of PK result from the peripheral expansion of an abnormal, mutant clone of epidermal keratinocytes (that would be inherited) located at the base of the parakeratotic column [16]. This attractive hypothesis is supported by the cytological finding of abnormal DNA ploidy [17], the increased proportion of keratinocytes in the S and G2/M phases of the cell cycle [18], as well as by the overexpression of the p53 oncoprotein [19, 20] and of proliferation-associated antigens within keratinocytes in the vicinity of the cornoid lamella [20, 21]; it is in accordance with the results of experimental studies, showing that autotransplantation of normal skin into the border of a DSAP lesion results in the formation of a pathologic ridge within the graft, whereas this disappears from a lesion grafted onto normal-looking skin [6]. The following (eliciting or triggering) factors have been considered to play a role in the genesis of lesions.

Genetic factors

These are certainly important since several familial cases of PKM, DSAP, PPPD and PPK have been reported. The mode of inheritance is autosomal dominant with reduced penetrance [22]. The similarities in the clinical and histological appearance of all forms of PK and the possible coexistence of different forms within the same family [23] suggests that the various PK forms are different phenotypic expression of a common genetic defect. The sporadic cases reported could be due to somatic mutations. *In vitro* studies have shown chromosomal abnormalities in cultured fibroblasts and lymphocytes, concerning namely chromosome 3 (p12-14) [24].

Ultraviolet light

At least in the DSAP type, ultraviolet (UV) light plays a major role. This is suggested by clinico-epidemiological data (development of lesions on sun-exposed areas, exacerbation of the disease during the summer, PUVA-induced cases, predominance of DSAP in geographic areas with high sun exposure, appearance of the lesions in adulthood), and has been shown almost experimentally after UV exposure [7, 9]. However, *in vitro* studies have shown that cultured fibroblasts from PK patients are hypersensitive to X-ray but (curiously) not to UV irradiation [25], and one case of PK improved with PUVA treatment [26]; these facts, along with the scarcity of facial lesions in PK [27], cast some shadow on the predominant role of UV light in the genesis of lesions. On the other hand, electron-beam radiation also seems to act as a triggering factor [28].

Trauma

The development of PK in a burn scar [29] or the access region for haemodialysis [30] suggests that the isomorphic (Koebner) phenomenon could play a role in the development of lesions. However, attempts to deliberately induce lesions have failed [6].

Infectious agents

These were suspected because of the development of PK under immunosuppressive treatments, that could reactivate a putative virus [31]. However, attempts for animal inoculation have proven unsuccessful [6].

Immunosuppression

After the initial observation of PKM developing in a renal transplant recipient [31], several cases of PK have been reported in the course of immunodeficiency diseases (Table I). These include mainly organ transplantation [31-52] (see below), haemopoietic malignancies and lymphomas [28, 33, 49, 53-58], HIV infection [20, 59] and various inflammatory or autoimmune diseases usually treated with immunosuppressive drugs or chemotherapy [33, 60-71]. In several of these cases the course of PK paralleled the level of immunosuppression [31, 33, 34, 56, 59], and in two cases the disease regressed completely after discontinuation of immunosuppressive treatment [51, 65]. These observations clearly highlight the promoting role of immunosuppression, but its precise mode of action remains unknown. Immunosuppression could induce decreased immune surveillance, which would prevent pathologic keratinocyte clones from being recognised and immunologically rejected; alternatively, it could directly trigger the development and proliferation of a mutant clone of keratinocytes. On the other hand, (local) immunosuppression could probably also explain the promoting effect of UV light.

Table I. Immunodeficiency diseases (other than organ transplantation) associated with porokeratosis

Diseases	References	Diseases	References
Hodgkin's disease	[33, 53]	Ulcerative colitis	[33]
Leukaemia/Lymphoma	[33, 54-56]	Pemphigus vulgaris	[62]
Multiple myeloma	[33]	Pemphigus foliaceus	[63, 64]
Myelodysplastic syndrome	[57]	Dermatomyositis (paraneoplastic)	[65]
Mycosis fungoides	[27, 58]	Rheumatoid arthritis	[33]
Agammaglobulinaemia	[53]	Acute articular rheumatism	[33]
HIV infection	[20, 59]	Myasthenia gravis	[33]
Asthma	[33]	Liver cirrhosis	[66, 67]
Kala-azar	[60]	Chronic hepatitis	[32, 68, 69]
Hidradenitis suppurativa	[37]	Vitiligo	[69]
Multiple sclerosis	[33]	Cystic fibrosis	[70]
Crohn's disease	[61]	Lupus erythematosus	[71]

In summary, the most accepted theory explaining the development of PK is that the lesions are due to the expansion of a mutant clone of epidermal keratinocytes, that could be inherited. The abnormal clone could normally be controlled by immune mechanisms, and its expansion would be promoted by a number of triggering factors, such as UV light or immunosuppression (be it disease-related or iatrogenic). This hypothesis still needs unequivocal confirmation.

Histopathology

Histologically, the central part of PK lesions shows a hyperkeratotic, usually thin epidermis with flattened rete ridges. The epidermis may rarely be acanthotic. The underlying dermis usually harbours a mild perivascular mononuclear-cell infiltrate around dilated capillaries. The most characteristic changes are seen at the periphery of the lesion, at the level of the keratotic border: the horny layer is orthokeratotic and thickened, and contains a vertical stack of corneocytes containing pyknotic nuclei. This parakeratotic column (cornoid lamella) is seated on a dell of the underlying epidermis, extending downwards at an angle the apex of which points away from the centre of the lesion (*Figure 43, page 224*). At the level of the cornoid lamella the granular layer is usually interrupted; the malpighian layer contains cells with perinuclear oedema and cells with an eosinophilic cytoplasm (as a result of premature keratinization), *i.e.* dyskeratotic keratinocytes. The corresponding basal cell layer may show hydropic degeneration. The superficial dermis contains a mononuclear cell infiltrate of mild to moderate degree, that may come in contact with the basal cell layer of the epidermis, resulting in a lichenoid aspect; it consists predominantly of activated T-helper cells [72, 73]. Eosinophils [15], colloid bodies and amyloid deposits [10] may rarely be found in the papillary dermis, and rare cases showing eosinophilic spongiosis have been described [67]. The most pronounced changes are found in lesions of PKM; in the other forms (namely the DSAP) the cornoid lamella may be less prominent (the parakeratotic stack is usually smaller and the central invagination in which it is seated more shallow). Occasionally, the cornoid lamella corresponds to ostia of eccrine glands or hair-follicles, which led to the misnomer « porokeratosis »; however, this finding is fortuitous, since the peripheral border of PK lesions is moving centrifugally and therefore it cannot be permanently bound to epidermal adnexae (that are definite structures); moreover, the occurrence of lesions over mucous membranes further shows that PK lesions do not necessarily develop within epidermal adnexae.

The histologic aspect of PK is characteristic and allows confirmation of the diagnosis. It should be borne in mind, however, that the cornoid lamella is not absolutely specific of PK since it can be seen, although rarely, in premalignant keratoses, basal and squamous cell carcinoma, seborrheic keratosis and viral warts [74].

Electron microscopy reveals underneath the cornoid lamella a decrease of keratohyalin granules and lamellar bodies, a finding that could account for the defective desquamation of corneocytes. In the malpighian layer keratinocytes show signs of degeneration, such as cytoplasmic vacuoles and peripheral condensation of tonofilaments [20, 75]. Dyskeratotic cells contain aggregated tonofilaments [75]. The parakeratotic cells of the cornoid lamella contain pyknotic nuclei and an electron-dense cytoplasm due to the presence of degraded organelles and lipid droplets [20]. The expression of filaggrin is reduced, reflecting the decrease of the granular cell layer, but that of involucrin is increased [20, 21, 76]. Epidermal Langerhans cells may be present [72] but are usually diminished in number [20, 44].

Course

The lesions of PK progress slowly, increasing in size and number over the years; in rare occasions they may undergo inflammatory changes and regress spontaneously [15, 77]. As stated above, immunosuppression-asociated PK may fluctuate parallelly to the level of immunosuppression, and complete regressions have been reported after discontinuation of immunosuppressive treatment [51, 65]. In some cases, the lesions of PK may undergo malignant transformation to Bowen's disease, squamous cell and (more rarely) basal cell carcinoma [78-80]. A review of 281 cases of PK published in the English literature showed that malignant transformation occurs in 7.5% of patients [80]; remarkably, none of them occurred in immunosuppressed patients. Large lesions (namely of the extremities), those of long-standing duration and linear PK seem to be at greater risk, whereas DSAP has a much lower risk [27, 80]. Malignant lesions are usually single, but multiple tumours may develop in one third of cases. The duration of the disease is longer in patients presenting with malignancy (33.5 *versus* 13.7 years) [80]. Metastasis to lymph nodes and a fatal outcome have also been reported [81]. In Japanese patients the risk for malignant transformation would be even higher (11.6%) [79]. PK is therefore often considered as a premalignant condition. The finding that increased chromosomal instability is present not only in fibroblasts from non-affected skin but also in peripheral blood lymphocytes [24, 25] suggests the possibility of an increased susceptibility to malignancy in general.

Treatment

Several treatments have been proposed for PK but the response is variable and often disappointing; the treatment is therefore palliative rather than curative [82]. Locally, lubricating or keratolytic agents, 5-fluorouracil, tretinoin, and steroids can be tried. Recently, significant improvement was obtained in three patients with DSAP with topical calcipotriol [83]. Isolated lesions can be excised surgically or treated with cryotherapy, electrodessication, dermabrasion or CO_2 laser. Systemic retinoids can be tried in diffuse forms and may prove effective [84, 85]; however, relapses are common and exacerbations during this treatment have also been noted [86]. Photoprotection with sunscreens should be prescribed for patients with DSAP to prevent worsening of the lesions.

Porokeratosis after organ transplantation

Following the initial report of MacMillan and Roberts in 1974 [31], several cases of PK were reported after organ transplantation; our review of the literature revealed a total of 62 such cases, including kidney (n: 44), heart (n: 9), bone-marrow (n: 5), lung (n: 3) and liver (n: 1) transplantation (summarised in *Table II*). More than half of patients are men. PK associated with organ transplantation represents by far the commonest type of immunosuppression-associated PK, and could in the future outnumber cases of « idiopathic » PK.

The incidence of PK after organ transplantation varies considerably among the different series. In most retrospective studies it is usually low, having been estimated to 0.34% [86], 0.54% [36], 0.66% [40], 1.07% [33], 1.87% [48] or 3.4% [87]; however, a study performed prospectively in a series of renal-graft recipients [39] found a much higher incidence (10.68%). The difficulty in precisely estimating this incidence may be due to several reasons: firstly, the lesions may both be overlooked by patients (who seldom seek advice for them spontaneously) [39] and either pass unnoticed by physicians, or mistaken for solar keratoses [27]; secondly, as happens with other premalignant skin conditions, it can be speculated that the incidence of PK will increase with time after transplantation, so that the heterogeneity of the groups studied could account for the different results mentioned. Although the published series are small and do not allow definitive conclusions, it seems that patients having received organ transplants other than the kidney (lung or heart) develop PK relatively more often than kidney-transplant recipients [36, 37]; it can reasonably be speculated that this is because non-kidney transplant recipients receive more intensive immunosuppressive treatments.

The delay of appearance of PK following organ transplantation varies between 4 months and 14 years; in kidney-transplant recipients, who represent 72% of all reported organ-transplant recipients with PK, the average delay is around 4 years (one kidney-transplant recipient was reported to suffer from abrupt and extensive eruption of PK 2 weeks following transplantation,

Table II. Porokeratosis in organ-transplant recipients

Authors	Organ transplanted	Nb of patients/sex	Delay post graft	Clinical features	Associated skin lesions
Macmillan et al. [31]	K	1 W	2 weeks (exacerbation)	multiple lesions (legs)	herpes simplex, plane warts
Bouman et al. [34]	K	1 W	> 4 years	multiple lesions (arms, legs)	
Dodd et al. [35]	K	1 M	9 years	single lesion (leg)	warts, AK
Komorowski et al. [40]	K	1 M, 2 W	2-3 years	single lesion (leg)	
Manganoni et al. [44]	K	2 M, 2 W		DSAP	
Wilkinson et al. [42]	K	1 M	6-7 years	single lesion (leg)	warts, AK, SCC
Raychaudhuri et al. [37]	K	2 M	?	single lesion (arm, leg)	
Sudoh et al. [43]	K	1 M	5 years	Mibelli	
Chun et al. [38]	K	1 M	11 years	DSP	warts, DEA
Bencini et al. [33]	K	8 M, 5 W	mean: 2.5 years	mainly legs	warts, condylomas, AK, SCC
Euvrard et al. [36]	K	2 W, 1 M	mean: 10 years	2 single, 1 multiple (legs)	warts, AK, SCC
Matsushita et al. [41]	K	1 M	3 years	DSAP	
Herranz et al. [39]	K	5 M, 6 W	mean: 3.5 years	Mibelli or DSP	
Legoux et al. [45]	K	1 W	> 3 months	DSAP	warts
Auslaender et al. [46]	H	1 M	1 year	?	?
Raychaudhuri et al. [37]	H	5 M	0.5-3 years	3 single lesions 2 multiple	
Rothman et al. [47]	H	1 M	2 years	single (thigh)	
O'Connell et al. [48]	H	2	?	?	
Euvrard et al. [36]	L	2 W, 1 M	mean: 22 months	1 single, 2 multiple (legs ± arms)	warts, AK, BD, BCC
Komorowski et al. [40]	Li	1 M	2 years	multiple lesions (legs)	
Lederman et al. [50]	BM	1 M	some months	multipe lesions (legs/buttocks)	
Ghigliotti et al. [49]	BM	1 M	18 months	multiple lesions (legs)	
Raychaudhuri et al. [37]	BM	1 M	?	single (arm)	
Gilead et al. [51]	BM	1 M	some months	multiple lesions (legs, buttock, flank)	moll. contagiosum, penile condyloma
Rio et al. [52]	BM (autologous)	1 M	5 years	DSP	intraepithelial carcinoma

AK: actinic keratosis; BD: Bowen's disease; BCC: basal cell carcinoma; BM: bone marrow; DEA: disseminated epidermolytic acanthoma; DSP: disseminated superficial porokeratosis; H: heart; L: lung; Li: liver; M: man; SCC: squamous-cell carcinoma; W: woman; ?: not precisely known.

but this patient had probably preexisting PK so that this case most likely represents exacerbation of preexisting disease rather than *de novo* development) [31]. The delay of appearance is shorter (usually less than 3 years) after transplantation of other organs (liver, lung, heart and bone-marrow), a finding that would further highlight the promoting role of immunosuppression.

Clinically, PK in organ-transplant recipients manifests with multiple and more rarely single lesions, located on the legs in the majority of cases. The prevalent clinical forms therefore correspond either to DSP or to PKM. Histologically, immunosuppression-associated PK shows no significant differences from cases appearing in immunocompetent individuals [37].

From a pathogenetic point of view, genetic factors do not seem to be of major importance in immunosuppression-associated PK, since none of the reported transplant recipients with PK had family history of the disease. A decreased expression of HLA-DR antigens by epidermal Langerhans cells has been observed within PK lesions of renal-transplant recipients, and it has been speculated that this defective expression could account for failure of local immunosurveillance, contributing to the development of abnormal keratinocyte clones [44]. In one study it was suggested that exposure to sunlight was not a major factor for the development of PK, contrasting with PK developing in non-immunosuppressed patients [33]; however cases of renal-transplant recipients developing lesions under the influence of sun-exposure have also been reported [39, 41].

As in « idiopathic » cases, the course of PK in the setting of immunosuppression is slowly progressive. Usually more lesions continue to appear in affected areas but lesions do not develop in previously unaffected areas [33]. Substitution of cyclosporine A by azathioprine and steroids has resulted in one case in partial regression of the lesions [34], but there is no firm evidence to suggest that any of the commonly used immunosuppressive drugs is more likely to induce the development of PK than another. In one bone-marrow graft recipient the disease regressed completely after discontinuation of the immunosuppressive treatment [51], highlighting the important role of immunosuppression. Curiously, another patient who received a liver transplant (performed for end-stage liver disease) experienced regression of PK [68]; however it seems likely that in this case PK had been induced by liver dysfunction that was restored after transplantation. No long-term follow-up of this particular patient has been reported, but it can be anticipated that PK would recur under long-term immunosuppressive treatment.

The fact that so far no malignant degeneration in immunosuppression-associated PK has been observed is puzzling, all the more so that transplant recipients are at highly increased risk for developing cutaneous malignancies as compared with the general population. A possible explanation could be the relatively short follow-up time, since malignant transformation occurs in classical PK after an average of 33.5 years [80]; furthermore, DSAP, representing one of the most frequent forms of PK in organ-transplant recipients, has a low-risk for malignant transformation. Therefore, and despite the fact that lesions may be resistant to treatment, we recommend that lesions of PK in organ-transplant recipients should be removed surgically or destroyed (*e.g.* by cryotherapy). The development of PK in an organ-transplant recipient should prompt a close dermatologic surveillance [88] since these patients develop (more or less concomitantly) other cutaneous premalignant (actinic keratoses, Bowen's disease) and malignant lesions (basal and squamous cell carcinomas).

References

1. Mibelli V. Contributo allo studio della ipercheratosi dei canali sudoriferi. *Gior Ital Mal Ven* 1893 ; 28 : 313-55.

2. Kanitakis C, Ktenides M, Tsoitis G. Porokératose de Mibelli des lèvres bilatérale et symétrique. *Dermatologica* 1981 ; 163 : 1-4.

3. Mehregan A, Khalili H, Fazel Z. Mibelli's porokeratosis of the face. A report of seven cases. *J Am Acad Dermatol* 1980 ; 3 : 394-6.

4. Mikhail G, Wertheimer F. Clinical variants of porokeratosis (Mibelli). *Arch Dermatol* 1968 ; 98 : 124-31.

5. Bogaert M, Hogan D. Linear porokeratosis in a 74-year-old woman. *J Am Acad Dermatol* 1991 ; 25 : 338.

6. Chernosky M, Freeman R. Disseminated superficial actinic porokeratosis (DSAP): clinical studies and experimental production of lesions. *Arch Dermatol* 1967 ; 96 : 611-24.

7. Chernosky M, Anderson D. Disseminated superficial actinic porokeratosis. Clinical studies and experimental production of lesions. *Arch Dermatol* 1969 ; 99 : 401-7.

8. Cockerell C. Induction of disseminated superficial actinic porokeratosis by phototherapy for psoriasis. *J Am Acad Dermatol* 1991 ; 24 : 301-2.

9. Neumann R, Knobler R, Metze D, Jurecka W, Gebhart W. Disseminated superficial actinic porokeratosis: experimental induction and exacerbation of skin lesions. *J Am Acad Dermatol* 1989 ; 21 : 1182-8.

10. Hill MP, Balme B, Gho A, Perrot H. Porokératose disséminée superficielle avec amylose dermique. *Ann Dermatol Venereol* 1992 ; 119 : 651-4.

11. Guss S, Osbourn R, Lutzner M. Porokeratosis palmaris, plantaris et disseminata: a third type of porokeratosis. *Arch Dermatol* 1971 ; 104 : 366-73.

12. Patrizi A, Passarini B, Minghetti G, Massina M. Porokeratosis palmaris, plantaris et disseminata: an unusual clinical presentation. *J Am Acad Dermatol* 1989 ; 21 : 415-8.

13. Lestringant G, Berge T. Porokeratosis punctata palmaris et plantaris. A new entity? *Arch Dermatol* 1989 ; 125 : 816-9.

14. Helfman R, Poulos E. Reticulated porokeratosis: a unique variant of porokeratosis. *Arch Dermatol* 1985 ; 121 : 1542-3.

15. Kanzaki T, Miwa N, Kobayashi T, Ogawa S. Eruptive pruritic papular porokeratosis. *J Dermatol* 1992 ; 19 : 109-12.

16. Reed R, Leone P. Porokeratosis: a mutant clonal keratosis of the epidermis. *Arch Dermatol* 1970 ; 101 : 340-7.

17. Otsuka F, Shima A, Ishibashi Y. Porokeratosis as a premalignant condition of the skin. Cytologic demonstration of abnormal DNA ploidy in cells of the epidermis. *Cancer* 1989 ; 63 : 891-6.

18. Otsuka F, Iwata M, Watanabe R, Chi H, Ishibashi Y. Porokeratosis: clinical and cellular characterization of its cancer-prone nature. *J Dermatol* 1992 ; 19 : 702-6.

19. Magee J, McCalmont T, LeBoit P. Overexpression of p53 tumor suppressor protein in porokeratosis. *Arch Dermatol* 1994 ; 130 : 187-90.

20. Kanitakis J, Misery L, Nicolas JF, Lyonnet S, Chouvet B, Haftek M, Faure M, Claudy A, Thivolet J. Disseminated superficial porokeratosis in a patient with AIDS. *Br J Dermatol* 1994 ; 131 : 284-9.

21. Gray M, Smoller B, McNutt N. Carcinogenesis in porokeratosis: evidence for a role relating to chronic growth activation of keratinocytes. *Am J Dermatopathol* 1991 ; 13 : 438-44.

22. Anderson D, Chernosky M. Disseminated superficial actinic porokeratosis. Genetic aspects. *Arch Dermatol* 1969 ; 99 : 408-12.

23. Commens C, Schumack S. Linear porokeratosis in two families with disseminated superficial actinic porokeratosis. *Pediatr Dermatol* 1987 ; 4 : 209-14.

24. Sacppaticci S, Limbiase S, Orecchia G, Fraccaro M. Clonal chromosome abnormalities with preferential involvement of chromosome 3 in patients with porokeratosis of Mibelli. *Cancer Genet Cytogenet* 1989 ; 43 : 89-94.

25. Watanabe R, Ishibashi Y, Otsuka F. Chromosomal instability and cellular hypersensitivity to X-ray irradiation of cultured fibroblasts derived from patients with porokeratotic patients' skin. *Mutat Res* 1990 ; 230 : 273-8.

26. Schwartz T, Seiser A, Gschnait F. Disseminated superficial 'actinic' porokeratosis. *J Am Acad Dermatol* 1984 ; 11 : 724-30.

27. Shumack S, Commens C. Disseminated superficial actinic porokeratosis: a clinical study. *J Am Acad Dermatol* 1989 ; 20 : 1015-22.

28. Halper S, Medinica M. Porokeratosis in a patient treated with total electron beam radiation. *J Am Acad Dermatol* 1990 ; 23 : 754-5.

29. Nova M, Goldberg L, Mattison T, Halperin A. Porokeratosis arising in a burn scar. *J Am Acad Dermatol* 1991 ; 25 : 354-6.

30. Nakazawa A, Matsuo I, Ohkido M. Porokeratosis localized to the access region for hemodialysis. *J Am Acad Dermatol* 1991 ; 21 : 338-40.

31. Macmillan A, Roberts S. Porokeratosis of Mibelli after renal transplantation. *Br J Dermatol* 1974 ; 90 : 45-51.

32. Bencini PL, Crosti C, Sala F. Porokeratosis: immunosuppression and exposure to sunlight. *Br J Dermatol* 1987 ; 116 : 113-6.

33. Bencini PL, Tarantino A, Grimalt R, Ponticelli C, Caputo R. Porokeratosis and immunosuppression. *Br J Dermatol* 1995 ; 132 : 74-8.

34. Bouman T, van de Kerkhof P, Happle R. Disseminierte Porokeratosis nach Nierentransplantation. In : Gollnick H, Stadler R, eds. *Dia-Klinik Fallvorstellungen anlässlich des 17. Weltkongresses für Dermatologie*. Stuttgart : Schattauer, 1987 : 49-50.

35. Dodd H, Sarkany I. Porokeratosis of Mibelli following renal transplantation. *Br J Dermatol* 1988 ; 119 : 101-2.

36. Euvrard S, Kanitakis J, D'Incan M, Lefrançois N, Mornex JF, Pouteil-Noble C, Faure M, Claudy A. Porokératoses et greffe d'organe. *Nouv Dermatol* 1996 ; 15 : 208.

37. Raychaudhuri S, Smoller B. Porokeratosis in immunosuppressed and non-immunosuppressed patients. *Int J Dermatol* 1992 ; 31 : 781-2.

38. Chun SI, Lee JS, Kim NS, Park KD. Disseminated epidermolytic acanthoma with disseminated superficial porokeratosis and verruca vulgaris in an immunosuppressed patient. *J Dermatol* 1995 ; 22 : 690-2.

39. Herranz P, Pizarro A, De Lucas R, Robayana M, Rubio F, Sanz A, Contreras F, Casado M. High incidence of porokeratosis in renal transplant patients. *Br J Dermatol* 1997 ; 136 : 176-9.

40. Komorowski RA, Clowry L. Porokeratosis of Mibelli in transplant recipients. *Am J Clin Pathol* 1989 ; 91 : 71-4.

41. Matsushita S, Kanekura T, Kanzaki T. A case of disseminated superficial actinic porokeratosis subsequent to renal transplantation. *J Dermatol* 1997 ; 24 : 110-2.

42. Wilkinson S, Cartwright P, English J. Porokeratosis of Mibelli and immunosuppression. *Clin Exp Dermatol* 1991 ; 16 : 61-2.

43. Sudoh H, Yokote R, Takigawa M, Iwatsuki K. A case of porokeratosis of Mibelli after renal transplantation. *Hifu Rinsyou* 1993 ; 35 : 50-1.

44. Manganoni A, Facchetti F, Gavazzoni R. Involvement of epidermal Langerhans cells in porokeratosis of immunosuppressed renal transplant patients. *J Am Acad Dermatol* 1989 ; 21 : 799-801.

45. Legoux A, Maître F, Estève E. Porokératose actinique superficielle disséminée inflammatoire chez une greffée rénale. 2e Symposium *Peau et greffes d'organe*, Lyon, 23/10/98.

46. Auslaender S, Barzilay A, Trau H. Porokeratosis of the skin in an immunosuppressed patient. *Harefuah* 1994 ; 127 : 303-5.

47. Rothman I, Wirth P, Klaus M. Porokeratosis of Mibelli following heart transplant. *Int J Dermatol* 1992 ; 31 : 52-4.
48. O'Connell B, Abel E, Nickoloff B, Bell B, Hunt S, Theodore J. Dermatologic complications following heart transplantation. *J Heart Transplant* 1986 ; 5 : 430-6.
49. Ghigliotti G, Nigro A, Gambini C, Farris A, Burroni A, De Marchi R. Porokératose de Mibelli après une greffe de moelle. *Ann Dermatol Venereol* 1992 ; 119 : 968-70.
50. Lederman J, Sober A, Lederman G. Immunosuppression: a cause of porokeratosis? *J Am Acad Dermatol* 1985 ; 13 : 75-9.
51. Gilead L, Guberman D, Zlotogorski A, Vardy D, Klaus S. Immunosuppression-induced porokeratosis of Mibelli : complete regression of lesions upon cessation of immunosuppressive therapy. *J Eur Acad Dermatol Venereol* 1995 ; 5 : 170-2.
52. Rio B, Magana C, Le Tourneau A, Bachmeyer C, Levy V, Hamont N, Diebold J, Zittoun R. Disseminated superficial porokeratosis after autologous bone marrow transplantation. *Bone Marow Transplant* 1997 ; 19 : 77-9.
53. Nicolas JF, Fauvet N, Kanitakis J, Hermier C, Thivolet J. Porokératose «actinique» superficielle disséminée et immunosuppression : à propos de deux cas. *Nouv Dermatol* 1990 ; 9 : 187-8.
54. Fields L, White C, Maziarz R. Rapid development of disseminated superficial porokeratosis after transplant induction therapy. *Bone Marrow Transplant* 1995 ; 15 : 993-5.
55. Vire G, Latour D, King L. Porokeratosis and immunosuppression. *J Am Acad Dermatol* 1986 ; 14 : 683.
56. Zenarola P, Melillo L, Lomuto M, Carotenuto M, Enzo Gomes V, Marzocchi W. Exacerbation of porokeratosis: a sign of immunodepression. *J Am Acad Dermatol* 1993 ; 29 : 1035-6.
57. Luelmo-Aguilar J, Gonzalez-Castro U, Mieras-Barcelo C, Castells-Rodellas A. Disseminated porokeratosis and myelodysplastic syndrome. *Dermatology* 1992 ; 184 : 289.
58. Puissant A, Venencie JY. In : Lederman J, Sober A, Lederman G. Porokeratosis and immunosuppression. *J Am Acad Dermatol* 1986 ; 14 : 683-4.
59. Rodriguez E, Jakubowicz S, Chinchilla D, Carril A, Viglioglia P. Porokeratosis of Mibelli and HIV infection. *Int J Dermatol* 1996 ; 35 : 402-4.
60. Velez A, Del Rio A, Fuente C, Belinchon I, Martin N, Sanchez Yus E. Disseminated superficial actinic porokeratosis and immunosuppression. *Eur J Dermatol* 1992 ; 2 : 336-8.
61. Morton C, Shuttleworth D, Douglas WS. Porokeratosis and Crohn's disease. *J Am Acad Dermatol* 1995 ; 32 : 894-7.
62. Feverman E, Sandbank M. Disseminated superficial porokeratosis in a patient with pemphigus vulgaris treated with steroids. *Acta Derm Venereol (Stockh)* 1974 ; 48 : 59-61.
63. Neumann R, Knobler R, Metze D, Jurecka W. Disseminated superficial porokeratosis and immunosuppression. *Br J Dermatol* 1988 ; 119 : 375-80.
64. Leibovici V, Zeidenbaum M, Goldenhersch M. Porokeratosis and immunosuppressive treatment for pemphigus foliaceus. *J Am Acad Dermatol* 1988 ; 19 : 910-1.
65. Tsambaos D, Spiliopoulos T. Disseminated superficial porokeratosis: complete remission subsequent to discontinuation of immunosuppression. *J Am Acad Dermatol* 1993 ; 28 : 651-2.
66. Tatnall F, Sarkany I. Porokeratosis of Mibelli in an immunosuppressed patient. *Br J Dermatol* 1988 ; 119 : 100-1.
67. Park BS, Moon SE, Kim JA. Disseminated superficial porokeratosis in a patient with chronic liver disease. *J Dermatol* 1997 ; 24 : 485-7.
68. Hunt S, Sharra W, Abell E. Linear and punctate porokeratosis associated with end-stage liver disease. *J Am Acad Dermatol* 1991 ; 25 : 937-9.
69. Dippel E, Haas N, Czarnetzki B. Porokeratosis of Mibelli associated with active chronic hepatitis and vitiligo. *Acta Derm Venereol (Stockh)* 1994 ; 74 : 463-4.
70. Klapholtz L, Goldenhersh M, Sherman Y, Leibivici V. Superficial actinic porokeratosis and cystic fibrosis. *Acta Derm Venereol (Stockh)* 1991 ; 71 : 440-1.
71. Grattan C, Christopher A. Porokeratosis and immunosuppression. *J R Soc Med* 1987 ; 80 : 597-8.

72. Jurecka W, Neumann R, Knobler R. Porokeratoses: immunohistochemical, light and electron microscopic evaluation. *J Am Acad Dermatol* 1991 ; 24 : 96-101.

73. Shumack S, Commens C, Kossard S. Disseminated superficial actinic porokeratosis. A histological review of 61 cases with particular reference to lymphocytic infiltration. *Am J Dermatopathol* 1991 ; 23 : 26-31.

74. Wade T, Ackerman B. Cornoid lamellation: a histologic reaction pattern. *Am J Dermatopathol* 1980 ; 2 : 5-15.

75. Sato A, Anton-Lamprecht I, Schnyder U. Ultrastructure of inborn errors of keratinization: porokeratosis Mibelli and disseminated superficial actinic porokeratosis. *Arch Dermatol Res* 1976 ; 255 : 271-84.

76. Ito M, Fujiwara H, Maruyama T, Oguro K, Ishihara O, Sato Y. Morphogenesis of the cornoid lamella: histochemical, immunohistochemical and ultrastructural study of porokeratosis. *J Cutan Pathol* 1991 ; 18 : 247-56.

77. Tanaka M, Terui T, Kudo K, Tagami H. Inflammatory disseminated superficial porokeratosis followed by regression. *Br J Dermatol* 1995 ; 132 : 153-5.

78. Otsuka F, Huang J, Sawara K, Asahina A, Ishibashi Y. Disseminated porokeratosis accompanying multicentric Bowen's disease. Characterization of porokeratotic lesions progressing to Bowen's disease. *J Am Acad Dermatol* 1990 ; 23 : 355-9.

79. Otsuka F, Someya T, Ishibashi Y. Porokeratosis and malignant skin tumors. *J Cancer Res Clin Oncol* 1991 ; 117 : 55-60.

80. Sasson M, Krain A. Porokeratosis and cutaneous malignancy. A review. *Dermatol Surg* 1996 ; 22 : 339-42.

81. Brodkin R, Rickert R, Fuller W, Saporito C. Malignant disseminated porokeratosis. *Arch Dermatol* 1987 ; 123 : 1521-6.

82. Schamroth JM, Zlotogorski A, Gilead L. Porokeratosis of Mibelli. Overview and review of the literature. *Acta Derm Venereol (Stockh)* 1997 ; 77 : 207-13.

83. Harrison P, Stollery N. Disseminated superficial actinic porokeratosis responding to calcipotriol. *Clin Exp Dermatol* 1994 ; 19 : 95.

84. Hacham-Zadeh S, Holubar K. Etretinate in the treatment of disseminated porokeratosis of Mibelli. *Int J Dermatol* 1985 ; 24 : 258-60.

85. Danno K, Yamamoto M, Yokoo T. Etretinate treatment in disseminated porokeratosis. *J Dermatol* 1988 ; 15 : 440-4.

86. Knobler R, Neumann R. Exacerbation of porokeratosis during etretinate therapy. *Acta Derm Venereol (Stockh)* 1990 ; 70 : 319-22.

87. Cohen E, Komorowski R, Clowry L. Cutaneous complications in renal transplant recipients. *Am J Clin Pathol* 1987 ; 88 : 32-7.

88. Ponticelli C, Bencini P. Disseminated porokeratosis in immunosuppressed patients. *Nephrol Dial Transplant* 1996 ; 11 : 2353-4.

25

Cutaneous complications in bone marrow transplant recipients

Sélim ARACTINGI
Department of Dermatology, Tenon Hospital, Paris, France.

Bone marrow transplantation (BMT) is no more restricted to a few highly specialized centres, and since the mortality of patients treated with this therapeutic modality has been largely reduced, one may speculate that dermatologists will increasingly observe in their private or hospital practice BMT recipients seeking advice for cutaneous lesions. The present review will highlight the most frequent cutaneous disorders occurring in this patient population, including mainly graft-*versus*-host disease (GVHD), skin tumours and skin infections.

Cutaneous graft-*versus*-host disease

The definition of GVHD given in 1966 by Billingham [1] is still accurate. GVHD encompasses a group of manifestations occurring when the following three conditions are met: 1) an organ containing immunologically-competent cells has been transplanted to 2) a recipient whose tissue antigens are different from those of the donor, and 3) this recipient is unable to clear the cells of the donor. Since BMT is preceded by an intensive myeloablative regimen, leading to a deep immunodeficiency of the recipient, and since the marrow contains many mature lymphocytes, BMT is the selective circumstance giving rise to GVHD. GVHD is classified into an acute and a chronic form, according to whether the manifestations occur respectively before or after day 100 following BMT.

Acute GVHD

Pathogenesis

Acute GVHD has generated during the past 20 years a huge amount of literature directed toward a better understanding of this disorder. Human tissues were studied, but a large number of animal models were carried out especially in mice and less frequently in dogs. It is beyond the scope of this review to provide the state of the art concerning GVHD pathogenesis, however some relevant data in this domain will be summarised here. Marrow depletion experiments have demonstrated in humans as well as in animals that acute GVHD is a disease induced by mature T cells [2, 3]. CD4 as well as CD8 cells may induce GVHD [2] and the severity of the disease parallels the amount of T cells transplanted to the recipient. The disease is due to the recognition of host-specific antigens by mature donor T cells. Several experiments have indeed shown the presence of host-specific helper and cytotoxic T cells in the blood as well as in the skin of these patients [4, 5]. These host T cells are specific for an HLA antigen, in the case of an HLA mismatch between the donor and the host. Most BMT are now performed with an HLA geno-identical donor, but GVHD still occurs in 35% of these patients. This situation led to the discovery of tissue antigens different from those of the HLA system, which may also behave as targets of T cell allorecognition [6, 7]. These peptides, called « minor antigens » (MiAg) [8], had been known in mice since the mid-seventies, but it was only in 1996 that the sequence of the first human MiAg was unravelled [6, 7]. MiAg do not generate B cell responses, and when GVHD develops in a recipient HLA geno-identical to his donor, the T cells are specific for one or more MiAg. Acute GVHD is therefore a reaction induced by donor T cells recognizing host cells. This reaction is amplified by other pathways, especially IL1α and TNFα produced by macrophages, T cells or epithelial cells but also by the expression of CD54 (ICAM1) which allows epithelial cells to « retain » lymphocytes in the involved tissue [9, 10].

Risk factors

As previously mentioned, the mean frequency of GVHD in adults receiving an HLA-identical graft is 35%; however the frequency varies greatly between 6% and 90% depending on age, HLA type and the prevention protocols applied. Multivariate analysis of cohorts of BMT recipients has demonstrated that the main risk factors for developing this disease are the older recipients' ages, a sex mismatch with the donor being female (especially transfused or multigravida women) and the recipient male, a mismatch in HLA antigens, the use of irradiation in the conditioning regimen and a suboptimal dose of immunosuppressive drugs.

Acute GVHD presents as a disseminated maculo-papular eruption

The disease usually begins after day 7, and is sometimes preceded by a feeling of pain or itch in the skin. The lesions present as a disseminated maculopapular eruption of sudden onset and variable extent (*Figure 44, page 225*). Some authors consider the presence of perifollicular lesions as very useful for establishing the diagnosis. Other useful signs are the presence of palmo-plantar erythema, a violaceous colour of the ears and initial involvement of the cheeks or the sides of the neck. Oral lesions (erythema and erosions) are frequent. However, it is usually impossible to distinguish oral acute GVHD from chemotherapy-induced mucositis. In 6% of cases, epidermal necrosis occurs. In these cases, Nikolsky's sign is positive and epidermal detachment is noted [11]. Depending on the extent of involvement, cutaneous GVHD is classified into four grades that are correlated to prognosis (*Table 1*). Extracutaneous manifestations of acute GVHD concern the gut and the liver; these usually occur in association with cutaneous signs, but may occasionally be isolated.

Table I. Clinical grading of acute GVHD

Stage	Skin	Liver	Gut
+	Maculopapular rash involving < 25% of the body surface	Bilirubin 2-3 mg/dl	Diarrhea 500-1000 ml/day
++	Maculopapular rash involving > 25% of the body surface	Bilirubin 3-6 mg/dl	Diarrhea 1000-1500 ml/day
+++	Generalized erythroderma	Bilirubin 6-15 mg/dl	Diarrhea > 1500 ml/day
++++	Toxic epidermal necrolysis (TEN)-like appearance	Bilirubin > 15 mg/dl	Pain or ileus

Histopathology of cutaneous acute GVHD lacks specificity

Histological examination of a skin biopsy shows a lymphocytic infiltrate in the superficial dermis, with moderate epidermal exocytosis. Focal or diffuse vacuolisation of basal cells of the epidermis and of hair follicles is present. Characteristically, clustered lymphocytes around dyskeratotic/necrotic keratinocytes are observed, a phenomenon referred to as « satellite cell necrosis ». In grade IV GVHD necrosis of the basal cell layer results in dermal-epidermal separation. Recent studies in murine as well as human acute GVHD have focused on hair-follicle involvement; they showed that the infiltrate selectively affects the bulge region of anagen hair follicles [12, 13], before invasion of the neighbouring interfollicular dermis. Because stem-cell density is higher in these sites, it had been suggested that epidermal stem cells could represent selective cytotoxicity targets in acute GVHD. After having reviewed retrospectively a series of acute GVHD in humans, Sale and Beauchamp [14] reported similar findings with involvement of the follicular bulge in all 38 patients who could be evaluated.

In situ studies confirmed that necrosis of keratinocytes in mice [15] and man [16] occurs *via* apoptosis. Finally, as for clinical manifestations, histological signs are classified into four grades, ranging from simple vacuolisation of basal layer keratinocytes (grade I) to epidermal necrosis and sloughing (grade IV). Direct immunofluorescence has shown granular deposits of IgM and/or C3 at the dermal-epidermal junction in 39% of biopsies from patients with acute GVHD, *versus* only 11% in recipients without GVHD [17].

The phenotype of infiltrating cells is controversial

Many studies have been conducted to determine which lymphocyte subpopulations are found in the acute GVHD skin, but their results are controversial. Briefly, the infiltrate is composed of T lymphocytes, with either both CD4+ and CD8+ cells, or with one of these subsets predominating. Two investigations claimed that NK lymphocytes were present in acute GVHD skin lesions [18, 19]. B cells were not found, while cells expressing the TCRγδ receptor represented a small minority.

The differential diagnosis is a difficult problem

Chemotherapy or radiation therapy, adverse drug reaction and even some viral infections can produce eruptions similar to acute GVHD. Using 13 criteria, three pathologists blindly evaluated tissue sections from patients considered as having GVHD, eruptions attributed to the conditioning regimen, and eruptions from patients that could not possibly have GVHD (autografts or allografts from a monozygotic twin) [20]. Keratinocyte vacuolisation, pyknosis, eosinophilic bodies and satellite-cell necrosis were similarly found in all groups, and a consensus among the three pathologists was reached in only 31% of the cases. A french group analysed nine cases of grade IV acute GVHD; four of them had no extracutaneous involvement and therefore could correspond to a drug reaction [11]. Finally, Yoshikawa et al. [21] showed that, after BMT, up to 48% of patients had evidence of infection with Human herpesvirus type 6 (HHV6), with one third of these patients presenting disseminated eruptions; this finding suggests that at least some cutaneous eruptions developing after BMT could in fact represent HHV6 infections and not acute GVHD. Therefore, no absolute diagnostic criteria of acute GVHD exist so far. The presence of extracutaneous involvement may help in supporting the diagnosis. In the absence of such symptoms, the attitude adopted varies among the different BMT units, and takes into account the benefit/risk ratio of introducing immunosuppressive treatment. All too often, chronologically and symptomatologically compatible eruptions are considered as GVHD. This pragmatic approach, when applied, probably leads to an overestimation of the frequency of acute GVHD.

Chronic GVHD

Pathogenesis

The pathogenesis of chronic GVHD in humans is less clearly understood than that of acute GVHD. This may be explained by the fact that animal models do not reproduce well the human disease and also by the difficulties in obtaining large series of chronic GVHD specimens; indeed, this disease occurs at various delays after BMT, at times when patients are likely to be followed by different practitioners. As for the acute form, chronic GVHD is characterised by the presence of T cells specific for host antigens. This was shown long ago by several groups [22, 23] and has recently been confirmed by the analysis of the frequency of host-specific T helper-cell precursors (Thp) [24]; however, autoimmune phenomena may also be involved. Indeed, antibodies targeting donor cell lines (such as lymphocytes and platelets) have been found in chronic GVHD [25, 26]. Antibodies targeting ubiquitous antigens, common to the donor and host (such as antinuclear, antinucleolar and antithyroid antibodies) have been also shown in the same setting. Finally, CD4 autoreactive clones have been demonstrated in mice with « chronic » GVHD [27]. All these data, as well as the close resemblance between chronic GVHD and some autoimmune diseases (scleroderma, lichen planus, Sjögren's syndrome) led several authors to suggest that chronic GVHD could be due not only to alloimmune but also to autoimmune mechanisms.

Risk factors

The incidence of chronic GVHD is significantly higher in patients who had prior moderate or severe acute GVHD [28]. Besides the main role of prior acute GVHD, multivariate analysis has identified recipient's age (> 20 years), a female donor (having received transfusions or been pregnant) for a male recipient and non-T cell-depleted BM as other risks for chronic GVHD.

Cutaneous manifestations

Chronic GVHD occurs in 25-50% of patients surviving more than 6 months after BMT [29]. The skin is the main target organ of chronic GVHD, since it is involved in almost all patients presenting this complication, whereas the mouth is involved in 90% of them [29]. Chronic GVHD appears either in continuity with acute GVHD, after a variable period in patients with a (resolved) acute GVHD, or more rarely *de novo*. Chronic cutaneous GVHD can develop spontaneously or be « induced » (isomorphic phenomenon) by several agents, namely ultraviolet irradiation, physical trauma or herpes zoster [30].

The two main types of cutaneous manifestations are lichen planus-like and sclerodermoid lesions. Lichenoid lesions consist in erythematous papules or plaques (*Figure 45, page 225*) [31, 32]. The most frequently affected sites include the periorbital region, the ears and the palms and soles. Lichen planus-like GVHD can also occur selectively around hair follicles [33]. Rarely, the lesions become generalized resulting in erythroderma. Less typical forms exist, including red papules with central vesicles resembling dysidrosis on palms or soles. Lichenoid GVHD can also affect the nails, with atrophy and pterygion. Recently, cases of lichenoid GVHD restricted to one or several dermatomes have been reported [34]. The authors postulated that these individuals presented epidermal mosaicism with different expressions of some histocompatibility antigens in a dermatome, leading to GVHD restricted to this site.

Chronic GVHD can also present with sclerodermoid lesions [35]. These are indurated, sclerotic, shiny, white-yellow plaques with poorly-defined contours, usually with an early patchy hyperpigmentation or a poikiloderma-like aspect. As with the lichen planus-like form, the lesions can be localized or generalized (*Figure 46, page 225*). On the legs, the skin can become so tightly adherent to deeper layers that mechanical ulcers may develop. Peripheral axonal neuropathy, linked to fibrotic trapping of nerve endings has been reported in the same region as the sclerosis [36]. When the plaques are located over the joints, tendon retraction may occur.

Diffuse hyperpigmentation and fasciitis constitute rare but well-established manifestations of chronic GVHD [37, 38]. As in Shulman's syndrome (eosinophilic fasciitis), the presentation of fasciitis in chronic GVHD is characterized by initial cellulitis followed by hardening and retraction of the involved area. The flanks and the proximal part of the limbs are preferentially involved. Fasciitis is remarkably resistant to treatment.

Oral involvement is very frequent

Any site of the oral mucosa may be affected; the lesions are characterized by redness, usually with atrophy [39]. Lichenoid reticular or hyperkeratotic lesions may develop anywhere in the mouth. These lesions are usually interspersed within the atrophic erythematous areas. In severe forms ulcerative lesions may develop. The severity of these abnormalities usually parallels that of the systemic chronic GVHD. Xerophtalmia and xerostomia are almost invariably present.

Extracutaneous involvement should always be sought

Chronic GVHD may involve many other organs in addition to the skin, although more rarely [29]. It is therefore important to search for the presence of ocular lesions (conjunctivitis or keratitis secondary to the sicca syndrome), respiratory troubles (dyspnea linked to bronchiolitis obliterans), jaundice due to liver and biliary GVHD and gastrointestinal disease manifesting with diarrhoea.

Histological examination is not mandatory

GVHD is classified in two phases. The « early » phase is seen in biopsies of lichen-planus like lesions and the histological aspect resembles that of acute GVHD. The epidermis is thickened with acanthosis, parakeratotic hyperkeratosis and hypergranulosis; it includes variable degree of keratinocyte necrosis, sometimes with satellite-cell necrosis. A lymphoid infiltrate of the superficial dermis with moderate exocytosis is present. The « late » phase specimens show marked epidermal atrophy and superficial collagen fibrosis. A few basal keratinocytes are vacuolated or apoptotic. Pericapillary sclerosis is absent [40]. Importantly, histological and ultrastructural examination show that there are several differences between sclerotic GVHD and scleroderma. A lupus band test is found in 86% of the biopsies of chronic GVHD [17].

Treatment of GVHD

Prevention of acute GVHD is mandatory and relies on the systematic association of methotrexate (given 3 or 4 times starting on the day of BMT) and cyclosporine (administered for 6 months) [41]. The use of such regimens decreases the incidence of acute GVHD by 15% to 40%, but not that of chronic GVHD. Curative therapy of acute GVHD includes mainly high-dose steroids (1-3 mg/kg/d), usually given intravenously. Cyclosporine, cyclophosphamide, antithymocyte globulins, antibodies to IL2R or TNFα may be proposed in steroid-resistant cases [42]. If skin detachment is present, hydration, cutaneous antisepsis and balanced diet are needed.

The treatment of chronic GVHD relies on the association of steroids and cyclosporine. Addition of azathioprine does not seem useful. In isolated cutaneous chronic GVHD, PUVA therapy has shown efficacy in more than 50% of patients with lichen-planus like lesions [43]. PUVA has also occasionally been used successfully in steroid-resistant GVHD; by contrast, extracutaneous chronic GVHD (especially hepatic) showed no benefit. The efficacy of PUVA therapy for sclerodermoid chronic GVHD is much more controversial. The beneficial effect of high-dose thalidomide (200-800 mg/d) on chronic GVHD has been reported in small series [44], but remains difficult to assess. Recently, extracorporeal photopheresis has also shown efficacy in steroid-resistant and even in sclerodermoid GVHD. Finally, topical steroids are frequently needed.

Skin and mucous membrane malignant tumours

Several recent studies have now demonstrated an increased risk of squamous cell carcinoma, connective tissue tumours and of melanoma in BMT recipients. In a European study of 748 severe aplastic anaemia patients who had received BMT, there was an increased risk of secondary solid tumours with a ratio of observed to expected cancers of 5.74 [45]. The main observed malignancies concerned head and neck tumours. Three factors were associated with this increased risk: male sex, age at diagnosis (with risk increasing with age) and use of a radiation-based conditioning regimen. By contrast, in a control cohort of patients with the same disease treated only with immunosuppressive regimens, no significant increase in solid tumours was noted. These results were confirmed and expanded by more recent studies, particularly by a large series including almost 20,000 recipients of allogeneic BMT [46]. The results of this study demonstrated a ratio of observed to expected cases of 11.1 for cancers of the oral cavity, 8 for sarcomas (fibrosarcomas, rhabdomyosarcomas...), and 5 for melanoma. Increased ratios for brain and thyroid tumours were also found. Of note, the risk for cancers of the oral cavity tended to be higher five or more years after BMT whereas the risk for melanomas and sarcomas was increased throughout the follow-up period. Multivariate analysis for patients who survived at least one year after BMT demonstrated a striking role of limited-field irradiation as part of the conditioning regimen; however, analysis for individual sites of cancers showed that high total body irradiation doses induced a significant increase in the risk for melanoma, and that limited-field irradiation and chronic GVHD were associated with elevated risks of oral cancers. Finally, in another study, cutaneous squamous cell carcinomas were observed, and chronic GVHD appeared as a risk factor for these [47]. All these results are consistent with what has been learned from renal allograft recipients. Therefore, BMT recipients should be subjected to regular dermatological examination so that these tumours can be detected early. In addition, one should be aware of these risks when using PUVA for the treatment of diseases such as chronic GVHD.

Cutaneous infections

There is an increased risk of skin infections in BMT recipients [48, 49]. The major factor associated with the occurrence of infections developing 6 months after transplantation is the presence of chronic GVHD [48, 49]. The immunodeficiency state induced by chronic GVHD, with CD4+ lymphocytopenia and hypogammaglobulinaemia, as well as the immunosuppressive regimens given for the treatment of GVHD are responsible for this increased risk. In addition, other factors associated with chronic GVHD could promote infections. These include:
– the presence of mucosal atrophy and xerostomia which decrease mouth lubrication and therefore also the clearance of local pathogens,
– the presence of skin or mucous membranes hard-to-heal erosions,
– IgA decrease.

Micro-organism identification in a series of 114 infected patients showed the presence of a virus – mainly varicella-zoster – in 42% of cases, of bacteria (*S. pneumoniae* and *S. aureus*) in 33% and *Candida* in 23% [48]. Other target organs for infections in BMT recipients are the ear, eye-nose and throat (34% of the cases) and lungs (25%) followed by the skin (20%) [49].

References

1. Billingham R. The biology of graft-*versus*-host reactions. *Harvey Lect* 1966 ; 62 : 21-73.
2. Korngold R, Sprent J. T cell subsets in graft-*versus*-host disease. In : Ferrara J, Deeg J, Burakoff S, eds. *Graft-versus-host disease*. New York : Marcel Dekker, 1991 : 31-49.
3. Champlin R, Jansen J, Ho W. Retention of graft-*versus*-leukemia using selective depletion of CD8-positive T lymphocytes for prevention of graft-*versus*-host disease following bone marrow transplantation for chronic myelogenous leukemia. *Transplant Proc* 1991 ; 23 : 1695-6.
4. Kasten-Sportes C, Masset M, Varrin F, Devergie A, Gluckman E. Phenotype and function of T lymphocytes infiltrating the skin during graft-*versus*-host disease following allogeneic bone marrow transplantation. *Transplantation* 1989 ; 47 : 621-4.
5. Gaschet J, Mahé B, Milpied N, Devilder MC, Dréno B, Bignon JD, Davodeau JP, Bonnet MM, Bonneville M, Vié H. Specifity of T cells invading the skin during acute graft-*versus*-host disease after semiallogeneic bone marrow transplantation. *J Clin Invest* 1993 ; 91 : 12-20.
6. Goulmy E, Schipper R, Pool J, Blokland L, Frederik Falkenburg JH, Vossen, J, Gratwohl, A, Vogelsang GB, van Houwelingen HC, van Rood JJ. Mismatches of minor histocompatibility antigens between HLA identical donors and recipients and the development of graft-*versus*-host disesase after bone marrow transplantation. *N Engl J Med* 1996 ; 334 : 281-5.
7. den Haan J, Sherman N, Blokland E, Huczko E, Koning F, Wooter Drijfoot JW, Skipper J, Shabanowitz J, Hunt DF, Engelhard VH, Goulmy E. Identification of a graft-*versus*-host disease-associated human minor histocompatibility antigen. *Science* 1995 ; 268 : 1476-80.
8. Perreault C, Décary F, Brochu S, Gyger M, Bélanger R, Roy D. Minor histocompatibility antigens. *Blood* 1990 ; 76 : 1269-80.
9. Ferrara J. Cytokines other than growth factors in bone marrow transplantation. *Curr Opin Oncol* 1994 ; 6 : 127-34.
10. Ferrara J. Cytokine dysregulation as a mechanism of graft-*versus*-host disease. *Curr Opin Immunol* 1993 ; 5 : 794-9.
11. Villada G, Roujeau J, Cordonnier C, Bagot M, Kuentz M, Wechsler J, Vernant JP. Toxic epidermal necrolysis after bone marrow transplantation: study of nine cases. *J Am Acad Dermatol* 1990 ; 23 : 870-5.
12. Murphy G, Whitaker D, Sprent J, Korngold R. Characterization of target injury of murine acute graft-*versus*-host disease directed to multiple minor histocompatibility antigens elicited by either CD4+ or CD8+ effector cells. *Am J Pathol* 1991 ; 138 : 983-90.

13. Murphy G, Lavker R, Whitaker D, Korngold R. Cytotoxic folliculitis in acute graft-*versus*-host disease: evidence of follicular stem cell injury and recovery. *J Cutan Pathol* 1990 ; 18 : 309-14.
14. Sale G, Beauchamp M. The parafollicular hair bulge in human GVHD: a stem cell rich primary target. *Bone Marrow Transplant* 1993 ; 11 : 223-5.
15. Gilliam A, Whitaker-Menezes D, Korngold R, Murphy G. Apoptosis is the predominant form of epithelial target cell injury in acute experimental graft-*versus*-host disease. *J Invest Dermatol* 1996 ; 107 : 377-83.
16. Langley R, Walsch N, Nevill T, Thomas L, Rowden G. Apoptosis is the mode of keratinocyte death in cutaneous graft-*versus*-host disease. *J Am Acad Dermatol* 1996 ; 35 : 187-90.
17. Tsoi M, Storb R, Jones E, Weiden PF, Shulman H, Witherspoon R, Atkinson R, Thomas ED. Deposition of IgM and complement at the dermoepidermal junction in acute and chronic cutaneous graft-*versus*-host disease in man. *J Immunol* 1978 ; 120 : 1485-92.
18. Elliott C, Sloane J, Pallett C, Sanderson K. Cutaneous leucocyte composition after human allogeneic bone marrow transplantation: relationship to marrow purging, histology and clinical rash. *Histopathology* 1988 ; 12 : 1-16.
19. Acevedo A, Aramburu J, Lopez J, Fernandez-Herrera J, Fernandez-Ranada J, Lopez-Botet M. Identification of natural killer (NK) cells in lesions of human cutaneous graft-*versus*-host disease: expression of a novel NK-associated surface antigen (Kp43) in mononuclear infiltrates. *J Invest Dermatol* 1991 ; 97 : 659-66.
20. Sale G, Lerner K, Barker E, Shulman H, Thomas E. The skin biopsy in the diagnosis of acute graft-*versus*-host disease in man. *Am J Pathol* 1977 ; 89 : 621-36.
21. Yoshikawa T, Suga S, Asano Y, Nakashima T, Yasaki T, Sobue R, Hirano M, Kojima S, Matsuyama T. Human herpes virus 6 infection in bone marrow transplantation. *Blood* 1991 ; 78 : 1381-4.
22. Tsoi M, Storb R, Dobbs S, Medill L, Thomas D. Cell-mediated immunity to non-HLA antigens of the host by donor lymphocytes in patients with chronic graft-*versus*-host disease. *J Immunol* 1980 ; 125 : 2258-62.
23. Van Els C, Bakker A, Zwinderman A, Zwaan F, Van Rood JJ, Goulmy E. Effector mechanisms in graft-*versus*-host disease in response to minor histocompatibility antigens. Absence of correlation with cytotoxic effector cells. *Transplantation* 1990 ; 50 : 62-6.
24. Bunjes D, Theobald M, Nierle T, Arnold R, Heimpel H. Presence of host-specific interleukin 2-secreting T helper cell precursors correlates closely with active primary and secondary chronic graft-*versus*-host disease. *Bone Marrow Transplant* 1995 ; 15 : 727-32.
25. Anasetti C, Rybka W, Sullivan K, Banaji M, Slichter S. Graft-*versus*-host disease is associated with autoimmune-like thrombocytopenia. *Blood* 1989 ; 73 : 1054-8.
26. Graze P, Gale R. Chronic graft-*versus*-host disease: a syndrome of disordered immunity. *Am J Med* 1979 ; 66 : 611-20.
27. Parkman R. Clonal analysis of murine graft-*versus*-host disease. I Phenotypic and functional analysis of T lymphocyte clones. *J Immunol* 1986 ; 136 : 3543-8.
28. Storb R, Prentice R, Buckner C, Clift LA, Appelbaum F, Deeg HJ, Doney K, Mason M, Sanders E, Singer J, Sullivan J, Witherspoon R, Thomas ED. Graft-*versus*-host disease and survival in patients with aplastic anemia treated by marrow grafts from HLA identical siblings. *N Engl J Med* 1983 ; 98 : 461-6.
29. Atkinson K. Chronic graft-*versus*-host disease. *Bone Marrow Transplant* 1990 ; 5 : 69-82.
30. Shulman H, Sale G, Lerner K, *et al*. Chronic cutaneous graft-*versus*-host disease in man. *Am J Pathol* 1978 ; 92 : 545-70.
31. Saurat J, Gluckman E, Bussel A, Didierjean L, Puissant A. The lichen planus-like eruption after bone marrow transplantation. *Br J Dermatol* 1975 ; 92 : 675-81.
32. Touraine R, Revuz J, Dreyfus B, Rochant H, Mannoni P. graft-*versus*-host reaction and lichen planus. *Br J Dermatol* 1975 ; 92 : 589.
33. Saurat J. Cutaneous manifestations of graft-*versus*-host disease. *Int J Dermatol* 1981 ; 20 : 249-56.
34. Beers B, Kalish R, Kaye V, Dahl M. Unilateral linear lichenoid eruption after bone marrow transplantation: an unmasking of tolerance to an abnormal keratinocyte clone? *J Am Acad Dermatol* 1993 ; 28 : 888-92.

35. Chosidow O, Bagot M, Vernant J, Touraine R, Cordonnier C, Revuz J. Sclerodermatous chronic graft-*versus*-host disease. *J Am Acad Dermatol* 1992 ; 26 : 49-55.

36. Aractingi S, Socié G, Devergie A, Dubertret, Gluckman E. Localized scleroderma-like lesions on the legs in bone marrow transplant recipents: association with polyneuropathy in the same distribution. *Br J Dermatol* 1993 ; 129 : 201-3.

37. Aractingi S, Janin A, Devergie A, Bourges M, Socié G, Gluckman E. Histochemical and ultrastructural study of diffuse melanoderma after bone marrow transplantation. *Br J Dermatol* 1996 ; 134 : 325-31.

38. Janin-Mercier A, Socié G, Devergie A, Aractingi S, Esperou H, Verola O, Gluckman E. Fasciitis in chronic graft-*versus*-host disease. *Ann Intern Med* 1994 ; 120 : 993-8.

39. Schubert M, Sullivan K, Morton T, Izutsu KT, Peterson DE, Flournoy L, Truelove El, Sale GE, Buckner D, Storb R, Thomas ED. Oral manifestations of chronic graft-*versus*-host disease. *Arch Intern Med* 1984 ; 144 : 1591-5.

40. Janin-Mercier A, Saurat J, Bourges J, Sohier J, Jean L, Gluckman E. The lichen planus like and sclerotic phases of the graft-*versus*-host disease in man: an ultrastructural study of six cases. *Acta Derm Venereol (Stockh)* 1981 ; 61 : 187-93.

41. Storb R, Prentice R, Buckner CD, Clift, LA, Appelbaum, F, Deeg, HJ, Doney, K, Mason, M, Sanders, E, Singer, J, Sullivan, K, Witherspoon, R, Thomas, ED. Graft-*versus*-host disease and survival in patients with aplastic anemia treated by marrow grafts from HLA identical siblings. *N Engl J Med* 1983 ; 98 : 431-66.

42. Anasetti C, Martin PM, Hansen JA. Treatment of acute graft-*versus*-host disease with humanized anti Tac: an antibody that binds to IL2 receptor. *Blood* 1994 ; 84 : 1320-7.

43. Vogelsang G, Farmer E, Hess A, Altamonte, V, Beschorner, WE, Jabs, DA, Corio, RL, Levin, LS, Colvin, OM, Wingard, JM. Thalidomide for the treatment of chronic graft-*versus*-host disease. *N Engl J Med* 1992 ; 326 : 1055-8.

44. Volc-Platzer B, Hönigsmann H, Hinterberger W, Wolff K. Photochemotherapy improves chronic cutaneous graft-*versus*-host disease. *J Am Acad Dermatol* 1990 ; 23 : 220-8.

45. Socié G, Henry-Amar M, Bacigalupo A, Hous J, Tichelli A, Ljungran P, McCann SR, Frickoffen R, Van'tveer-Korhoff E, Gluckman E. Malignant tumors occurring after treatment of aplastic anemia. European bone marrow transplantation severe aplastic anemia working party. *N Engl J Med* 1993 ; 329 : 1152-7.

46. Curtis R, Rowlings P, Deeg H, Shriner DA, Socié G, Travis LB, Horowitz MM, Witherspoon R, Hoover RN, Sobincki KA, Fraumeni JF, Boice D. Solid cancers after bone marrow transplantation. *N Engl J Med* 1997 ; 336 : 897-904.

47. Lowsky R, Lipton J, Fyles G, Minden M, Meharchand J, Tepkar I, Atkins H, Sutcliffe S, Messner H. Secondary malignancies after bone marrow transplantation in adults. *J Clin Oncol* 1994 ; 12 : 2187-92.

48. Atkinson K, Farewell V, Tsoi M, Sullivan KR, Witherspoon R, Thomas ED, Storb R. Analysis of late infections after human bone marrow transplantation. Role of non-specific suppressor cells in patients with chronic graft-*versus*-host disease and genotypic non identity between marrow donor and recipient. *Blood* 1982 ; 60 : 714-20.

49. Atkinson R, Storb R, Prentice R, Weiden PL, Witherspoon R, Sullivan K, Noel D, Thomas ED. Analysis of late infections in 89 long-term survivors of bone marrow transplantation. *Blood* 1979 ; 53 : 720-31.

26

Graft-*versus*-host disease after solid organ transplantation

Beth A. DROLET, Jennifer S. PETERSON, Nancy B. ESTERLY
Department of Dermatology, Medical College of Wisconsin, Milwaukee WI, USA.

Although graft-*versus*-host disease (GVHD) is a frequent complication after allogenic bone marrow transplantation (BMT), it can also, less commonly, manifest after transfusion of non-irradiated blood products to immunocompromised patients, and after solid organ transplantation. In 1986, Deierhoi *et al.* [1] reported the first case of GVHD after solid organ transfer, occurring after a pancreas-spleen transplantation. GVHD has since been described after liver, kidney-pancreas, heart-lung, and small bowel transplantation [2-6].

Pathogenesis

GVHD following solid organ transplantation is presumed to be mediated by immunocompetent T-lymphocytes harbored within the donor graft. Lymphatics and lymph node tissue are retained within solid organ grafts, and the majority of the reactive donor lymphocytes are thought to be derived from these tissues. The donor lymph tissue and the graft itself have been shown to hypertrophy after transplant into the recipient, analogous to proliferation in a two-way culture of mixed lymphocytes [7, 8]. Even after cold perfusion of donor livers at the time of procurement, a substantial number of lymphocytes (25-40%) may still reside within the parenchyma of the liver graft [9]. After engrafting into the host, these lymphocytes recognize and attack the recipient's epithelial tissues. This attack is usually directed against minor antigens that differ between recipient and donor cells. The recipient is unable to mount an adequate immune response against these attacking donor cells, resulting in destruction of host tissues. The attacking donor cells have been identified as immunocompetent cytotoxic T-lymphocytes (CD8+) and lymphokine-secreting T-helper lymphocytes (CD4+) [10].

If immunocompetent allogenic cells are transfused into a healthy recipient, these cells are normally removed quickly by the recipient's circulating lymphocytes. The donor lymphocytes spread by vascular routes to the recipient's lymphoid tissue. This process leads to a mixture of donor and recipient cells throughout the patients body, which is termed chimerism [7]. Thus, those allografts with large numbers of migratory lymphocytes such as bone marrow, spleen, and small bowel would produce significant chimerism in the patient's tissue and peripheral blood samples. These allografts with a large lymphocyte load have also shown the highest incidence of GVHD [11, 12]. The postulated order for risk of GVHD following solid organ transplantation is: spleen > small bowel > heart-lung > liver > kidney > heart [11]. Due to the large lymphoid load involved in splenic transplantation, pre-operative irradiation of the spleen and post-transplantation immunosuppression of the recipient have been successfully used to prevent GVHD [13]. Irradiation is not an option before small bowel transplantation due to the vulnerable nature of intestinal tissue.

Chimerism is seen following all types of allogenic organ transplantation [7, 14]. Chimerism can be viewed as a balancing act between donor and recipient cells. The two cell populations oppose each other, and ideally should cancel each other out immunologically. If an equilibrium between the two cell populations is not achieved, this results in a state of unstable chimerism. Unstable chimerism leads most frequently to graft rejection, but can also induce GVHD [14]. A number of factors are important in determining the final outcome. Although chimerism occurs to some extent after all solid organ transplantation, not all transplant recipients experience the signs and symptoms of GVHD.

GVHD following solid organ transplantation is rare and is most likely the result of a compilation of extraordinary circumstances. The donor lymphocytes may be unusually numerous or extremely sensitized. The recipient's HLA phenotype may be highly immunogenic to the donors immune cells. Ironically, if the HLA match is too similar (*i.e.* related donors), the recipient may be unable to detect donor lymphocytes as foreign, and thus be unable to destroy them. The recipient may be immunosuppressed, leaving the donor immune cells at an advantage [15]. Pre-operative immunosuppression is fairly common in patients undergoing solid organ transplantation. The nature of most illnesses that require a solid organ transplant are such that the recipients are chronically ill, and thus immunosuppressed prior to the surgery. Pre-transplant immunosuppression may also be the result of medications required to control the underlying medical condition, particularly autoimmune diseases. It should also be noted from BMT experience that the presence of active cytomegalovirus (CMV) infection may play a role in the induction of GVHD [16].

Clinical features

GVHD after solid organ transplantation occurs one to six weeks post-transplant, and is manifest by a characteristic set of signs and symptoms. Fever, diarrhea, pancytopenia, and a cutaneous eruption occur during the course of the disease. In all reported cases, fever was noted as the initial sign. Pancytopenia is the sole finding that differentiates GVHD after solid organ transplantation from GVHD after BMT. Extensive pancytopenia evidenced in GVHD after solid organ transplantation results from the destruction of the recipient's bone marrow by the immunogenic donor cells attacking the host cells. This differs from BMT, in which there is only one cell population inhabiting the bone marrow, as the recipient's own cells have been eradicated prior to the transfusion. Liver abnormalities, similar to those seen after BMT may be present in patients who have received solid organ transplantation, however, they are notably absent after allograft liver transplantation. The liver is not affected due to the fact that the liver is not sensed as foreign tissue. The reactive lymphocytes are derived from the liver, and thus recognize the donor liver as self [15].

The non-specific nature of these early presenting characteristics makes the diagnosis of GVHD a difficult one. Post-transplant fever can be attributed to numerous causes, including infection or acute graft rejection. Diarrhea can be secondary to infection, altered bile metabolism, food intolerance, drugs, or fluid and electrolyte imbalances. Pancytopenia can occur as the result of hypersplenism, myelodepression from drug toxicity (usually azathioprine), viral infections (usually CMV) or sepsis [17]. Thus, the cutaneous manifestations of GVHD may play an important role in the early diagnosis and treatment of this disorder. The presence of these clinical findings is associated with a very high mortality rate. Of the 19 reported cases of GVHD after liver transplantation, 15 were fatal, a mortality rate of 78% [2, 8, 9, 15-25]. Early, severe involvement of the recipient bone marrow resulting in pancytopenia is a set up for infections, and results in the major cause of mortality from GVHD.

The cutaneous eruption of GVHD after solid organ transplantation is similar to cutaneous GVHD seen after BMT. It usually presents as an asymptomatic to mildly pruritic erythematous, edematous maculopapular rash involving the face, ears, back, chest, palms, and soles (*Figure 47, page 225*). In many cases the eruption becomes confluent, resulting in diffuse erythroderma. GVHD after solid organ transplantation can also manifest with mucositis, conjunctivitis, and vesiculobullous lesions that progress to extensive denudation of the skin with full thickness epidermal necrosis. In one reported case after liver allograft transplant, a maculopapular eruption on the trunk and limbs progressed to lichenoid papules involving the palms and hard palate [22].

The differential diagnosis of the cutaneous eruption of solid organ GVHD involves the same spectrum of diagnoses seen after BMT, and must include toxic drug eruption, viral exanthem, erythema multiforme and toxic epidermal necrolysis. A skin biopsy obtained from the involved area may aid in the diagnosis of GVHD. The usual histologic features of GVHD after solid organ transplantation include dyskeratosis of epidermal cells, basal cell layer vacuolization with necrotic keratinocytes, and a limited mononuclear and lymphocytic infiltrate (*Figure 48, page 225*). These histologic findings are identical to those seen in GVHD after BMT. Toxic drug eruptions demonstrate a similar histologic picture, however, definitive diagnosis of GVHD can be achieved by the demonstration of pronounced chimerism in peripheral lymphocytes or bone marrow aspirate.

Treatment

The current treatment for GVHD following solid organ transplant is enhanced immunosuppression in the recipient in an attempt to halt donor cells from attacking recipient tissues. This can be done with high-dose steroids, cyclosporine, antithymocyte globulin (ATG), antilymphoblast globulin (ALG), or OKT3. These drugs are often used in combination to achieve the desired effect of immunosuppression. Granulocyte-macrophage colony stimulating factor (GM-CSF) may shorten the duration of the neutropenic period and provide some antimicrobial activity [21]. The high mortality rates associated with GVHD after solid organ transplant can be attributed to infection as the result of severe pancytopenia and immunosuppression of the recipient. It is for this reason that once the diagnosis of GVHD is made, it has been recommended that the patient immediately be started on broad spectrum antibiotic, antifungal, and antiviral coverage in an attempt to evade infection [22, 23]. As the response to therapy for GVHD is unpredictable, it is important to focus on preventative measures. Prophylaxis for GVHD could involve: immunosuppression of the donor, pretransplant perfusion of the organ graft with ALG, irradiation of the organ prior to transplantation, or surgical removal of excess lymphatic tissue prior to transplantation. The efficacy and plausibility of these measures is as yet unknown. For successful treatment of GVHD, the importance of early diagnosis must be stressed.

References

1. Deierhoi MH, Sollinger HW, Bozdech MJ, Belzer FO. Lethal graft-*versus*-host disease in a recipient of a pancreas-spleen transplant. *Transplantation* 1986 ; 41 : 544-5.
2. Burdick JF, Vogelsang GB, Smith WJ, Farmer ER, Bias WB, Kaufmann SH. Horn TJ, Colombani PM, Pitt HA, Perler BA, Merritt WT, Williams GM, Boitnott JK, Herlong HF. Severe graft-*versus*-host disease in a liver-transplant recipient. *N Engl J Med* 1988 ; 318 : 689-91.
3. Wood H, Higenbottam T, Joysey J, Wallwork J. Graft-*versus*-host disease after human heart-lung transplantation. International Congress of the Transplantation Society 1990 ; 364.
4. McAlister V, Wall W, Ghent C, Zhong GR, Duff J, Grant D. Successful small intestine transplantation. *Transplant Proc* 1992 ; 24 : 1236-7.
5. Ingham Clark CL. The immune response in small bowel transplantation. *Ann R Coll Surg Engl* 1996 ; 78 : 97-102.
6. Kimball P, Ham J, Eisenberg M, King A, Fisher R, Rhodes C, Posner M. Lethal graft-*versus*-host disease after simultaneous kidney-pancreas transplantation. *Transplantation* 1997 ; 63 : 1685-8.
7. Starzl TE, Demetris AJ, Murase N, Ildstad S, Ricordi C, Trucco M. Cell migration, chimerism, and graft acceptance. *Lancet* 1992 ; 339 : 1579-82.
8. Marubayashi S, Matsuzaka C. Fatal generalized acute graft-*versus*-host disease in a liver transplant recipient. *Transplantation* 1990 ; 50 : 709.
9. Mazzaferro V, Andreola S, Regalia E, Poli F, Doci R, Bozzetti F, Gennari L. Confirmation of graft-*versus*-host disease after liver transplantation by PCR HLA-typing. *Transplantation* 1993 ; 552 : 423-5.
10. Lazarus HM, Vogelsang GB, Rowe JM. Prevention and treatment of acute graft-*versus*-host disease: the old and the new. *Bone Marrow Transplant* 1997 ; 19 : 577-600.
11. Jamieson NV, Joysey V, Friend PJ, Markus R, Ramcbottom S, Baglin T, Johnston PS, Williams R, Calne RY. Graft-*versus*-host disease in solid organ transplantation. *Transplant Int* 1991 ; 4 : 67-71.
12. Llull R, Murase N, Demetris AJ, Starzl TE. Chimerism, graft-*versus*-host disease, rejection, and their association with reciprocal donor-host immune reactions after cell, organ, and composite tissue transplantation. *Transplant Proc* 1997 ; 29 : 1203-4.
13. Booster MH, Wijnen RMH, VanHooff JP, Tiebosch ATMG, Peltenburg HG, Van Pen Berg-Loonen PM, Van Kroonenburgh MJPG, Verschuren T, Hofstra L, Kootstra G. The role of the spleen in pancreas transplantation. *Transplantation* 1993 ; 56 : 1098-102.
14. Starzl TE, Demetris AJ, Rao AS, Thomson AW, Trucco M, Murase N, Zeevi A, Fontes P. Spontaneous and iatrogenically augmented leukocyte chimerism in organ transplant recipients. *Transplant Proc* 1994 ; 26 : 3071-6.
15. Collins RH, Cooper B, Nikaein A, Klintmalm G, Fay JW. Graft-*versus*-host disease in a liver transplant patient. *Ann Intern Med* 1992 ; 116 : 391-2.
16. Cattral MS, Langnas AN, Wisecarver JL, Harper JC, Rubocki RJ, Stevenson Bynon J, Fox IJ, Heffron TG, Shaw BW. Survival of graft-*versus*-host disease in a liver transplant recipient. *Transplantation* 1994 ; 57 : 1271-4.
17. Redondo P, Espana A, Herrero JI, Quiroga J, Cienfuegos JA, Azanza JR, Prieto J. Graft-*versus*-host disease after liver transplantation. *J Am Acad Dermatol* 1993 ; 29 : 314-7.
18. Roberts JP, Ascher NL, Lake J, Capper J, Purohit S, Garoroy M, Lynch R, Ferrell L, Wright T. Graft-*versus*-host disease after liver transplantation in humans: a report of four cases. *Hepatology* 1991 ; 14 : 274-81.
19. Connors J, Drolet BA, Walsh J, Crosby DL, Esterly NB. Morbilliform eruption in a liver transplantation patient. *Arch Dermatol* 1996 ; 132 : 1161-3.

20. Pageaux GP, Perigault PF, Fabre JM, Portales P, Souche B, Dereure O, Eliaou JF, Larrey D, Domergues J, Michel H. Lethal acute graft-*versus*-host disease in a liver tansplant recipient: relations with cell migration and chimerism. *Clin Transplant* 1995 ; 9 : 65-9.

21. Sanchez-Izquierdo JA, Lumbreras C, Colina F, Martinez-Laso J, Jimenez C, Gomez R, Garcia I, Alvarez M, Arnaiz-Villena A, Moreno E. Severe graft-*versus*-host disease following liver transplantation confirmed by PCR-HLA-B sequencing: report of a case and literature review. *Hepatogastroenterology* 1996 ; 43 : 1057-61.

22. Bhaduri BR, Tan KC, Humphreys S, Williams R, Donaldson P, Vergani D, Mowat AP, Mieli-Vergani G. Graft-*versus*-host disease after orthotopic liver transplantation in a child. *Transplant Proc* 1990 ; 22 : 2378-80.

23. Joysey VC, Wood H, Ramsbottom S, Morgan H, Ford C, Horsford J, Jamieson N, Friend P, Alexander G, Caine RY. Lymphocyte chimaerism after organ transplantation. *Transplant Proc* 1992 ; 24 : 2519-22.

24. Neumann UP, Kaisers U, Langreh JM, Muller AR, Blimhardt G, Bechstein WO, Lobeck H, Riess H, Zimmermann, Neuhaus P. Fatal graft-*versus*-host disease : a grave complication after orthotopic liver transplantation. *Transplant Proc* 1994 : 26 ; 3616-7.

25. Rosen CB, Moore SB, Batts KP, Santrach PJ, Noel P, Wiesner RH, Krom RAF. Clinical and pathologic features of graft-*versus*-host disease after liver transplantation. *Clin Transplant* 1993 ; 7 : 52-8.

General guidelines

Sylvie EUVRARD
Department of Dermatology, Hôpital Edouard-Herriot, Lyon, France.

Most of the dermatological complications developing in organ transplant recipients have been dealt with in the various chapters of this book. The aim of this chapter is to assist the physician to manage with practical aspects of dermatological care and to provide some important guidelines to treat these patients. For most cutaneous disorders, the deeper the level of immunosuppression, the more widespread are the lesions and the more difficult is the treatment especially for human papillomavirus (HPV) infections. Some long-term immunosuppressed patients may present with common dermatological disorders which do not need to be cared for differently as compared with nonimmunosuppressed patients. The most important point is to know when to treat in a different manner.

The assessment of the level of immunosuppression

The management of organ transplant recipients must take into consideration features of immunosuppression such as the level of immunosuppressive treatment, its duration and the function of the graft. The various immunosuppressive treatments are regulated according to standard criteria such as blood levels and tolerance. Despite the advances of immunology, there are still no satisfactory methods to accurately assess the correct dosage of the immunosuppressive drugs. The ideal level of immunosuppression corresponds to the minimal dosage of immunosuppressive drugs allowing good graft tolerance without inducing adverse effects. A disease is regarded to be linked to overimmunosuppression if it improves after decrease of the treatment. Physicians treating graft recipients give priority to the good function of the graft and rather tend to prescribe higher doses of immunosuppressive treatments than required. Skin disorders may be the occasion to initiate a decrease of the immunosuppressive treatment.

In practice, the first step in the dermatological management of organ transplant recipients is to consider the dosages of the immunosuppressive treatment. Patients could be classified in three groups according to the level of the immunosuppressive treatments: low, medium and strong. The low level corresponds to the association of two drugs including steroids ≤ 10 mg + azathioprine ≤ 100mg or cyclosporine ≤ 4 mg/kg. The medium level corresponds to these three drugs at similar dosages. The strong level comprises the three drugs at higher dosages or new potent drugs such as mycophenolate mofetil or FK 506. This classification should be merely regarded as a practical help since some patients with a medium level treatment may be deeply immunosuppressed. There are differences in individual susceptibility for the various drugs and especially recent studies have shown that the metabolism of azathioprine depends on a genetic factor [1].

Generally, the dosages of the immunosuppressive treatments are higher for heart, lung and multiorgan as compared to kidney transplant recipients. In long-term liver transplant recipients very low dose treatments may be sufficient and after five years a complete weaning of immunosuppression may be achieved in 27% of them [2].

The past history of acute rejections or the existence of chronic rejection should be also registered since in these patients tapering of the immunosuppressive treatment is hazardous.

How to manage skin disorders reflecting deep immunosuppression? When to treat in a special way?

Infections

Cytomegalovirus (CMV) infection is one of the main complications of severe immunosuppression [3]. If CMV skin lesions are very rare, CMV infection is often associated with *Herpes simplex* infections [4] and the occurence of *Herpes simplex* in the first weeks following transplantation or after the treatment of acute rejection should invariably prompt work-up for an underlying CMV co-infection.

Herpes simplex and *herpes zoster* can be treated with oral acyclovir or valacyclovir at the usual dosages if the treatment is started early. However, the duration and the mode of treatment can be modified according to the course. If lesions become especially extensive and painful, intravenous acyclovir is required to prevent systemic complications.

Multiple *molluscum contagiosum* lesions can be observed especially in the pubis, beard or other areas where shaving may favour their spreading (*Figure 49, page 226*). They occur more frequently in heart or lung transplant recipients. They should be removed as soon as they occur to prevent uncontrollable extension. In our experience, topical retinoids can be useful.

Human papillomavirus infections
When a cutaneous wart presents with an inflammatory aspect, it should be removed and examined histologically because of the high frequency of pre-epitheliomatous keratoses or keratoacanthomas or squamous cell carcinomas which may mimick them clinically (*Figure 50, page 226*).

Systemic retinoids can be useful when warts are numerous [5] even though their effect is only temporary (*Figure 51, page 227*).

Histological examination of lesions presenting as condylomata acuminata is also strongly recommended since bowenoid papulosis or *in situ* carcinoma may clinically simulate these lesions.

Fungal infections
Tinea versicolor develops in about 20% of patients; repeated topical treatments are useful to prevent frequent recurrences. Extensive dermatophytosis often requires systemic antifungal treatment.

Tumours: the tricks

The excision of any tumoral lesion in a transplant recipient should be followed by an histological examination due to the increased frequency of malignant and rare tumours (*Figure 52, page 227*) or opportunistic infections (*Figure 53, page 228*). Cultures of all suppurative lesions should be performed to isolate the causative agent [6].

Which therapeutic precautions to respect?

Drug interactions and graft survival

Many drugs may interfere with the metabolism of cyclosporine or FK 506 (Tacrolimus). Those prescribed by dermatologists which may increase the risk of toxicity include mainly macrolids (*e.g.* erythromycin) and antifungal agents (fluconazole, ketoconazole, itraconazole). Some other drugs increase their catabolism and reduce their immunosuppressive effect (rifampicin, phenobarbital, phenytoin). When one of these drugs must be introduced for a long period (for exemple to treat an opportunistic infection), the dosages of cyclosporine or FK 506 should be regularly adjusted according to the blood levels. The use of interferon α should be limited in transplant recipients due to the risk of acute rejection [7].

Surgical treatments

Physicians who perform surgery in transplant recipients should be careful since the rate of hepatitis B or C is still high especially among kidney transplant recipients. Wound healing occurs normally in organ transplant recipients when the immunosuppressive treatment is stable. However, surgical excision or electrocautery of warts in the weeks following a steroid pulse should better be avoided. Firstly, healing may be complicated by superinfection and secondly the risk of recurrence of warts is very high. Many transplant patients take anticoagulation therapy. If surgery is required, an adaptation of the anticoagulation treatment should be performed according to each case (short discontinuation some days before the surgery or replacement by heparin treatment).

Chemotherapy

Chemotherapy can be helpful in the treatment of metastatic squamous cell carcinomas [8] or Kaposi's sarcoma [9] but the immunosuppressive effect of chemotherapy should be balanced.

Radiotherapy

Radiotherapy for the treatment of skin malignancies should be generally avoided because of its carcinogenic effect. We have observed in several patients recurrences of squamous cell carcinoma after surgery during complementary radiotherapy, and sarcomas have been reported after this treatment [10]. Exceptionally, radiotherapy could be performed after surgery for metastases to the parotid gland [11].

When a decrease or a change of the immunosuppressive treatment should be recommended?

Decrease of the doses

The reduction of the immunosuppressive treatment is an important measure which may be responsible for graft rejection. It should be suggested and discussed only under strict circumstances. Each patient behaves differently. Whatever the reason of the decrease, the best candidate is a long-term transplant patient who has never experienced graft rejection and whose treatment was not changed for several years.

It has been shown that the increased risk of skin cancer associated with immunosuppression is independent of the agent used but is rather the result of the immunosuppression *per se* [12]. The new agents such as FK 506 are also associated with the risk of cancer [13, 14].

Infectious disorders

Infectious disorders may justify a reduction of the immunosuppressive treatment if they are extensive and resistant to the usual treatments; this is especially true for HPV infections because of the possible progression towards malignancy. Patients with extensive and chronic long-standing anogenital condylomas were cured after the immunosuppressive treatment was tapered or discontinued [15].

Opportunistic infections may also justify this measure, especially those due to atypical mycobacteria [16].

Malignancy

Kaposi's sarcoma

The reduction of the immunosuppressive treatment is admitted widely as the first treatment step. This results in partial or complete regression of the lesions which can occur within some weeks.

Squamous cell carcinomas

Squamous cell carcinomas when they become multiple or if they develop local recurrences or metastases can benefit of the reduction of the immunosuppressive treatment. Because of the relatively slow appearance several years after transplantation and since UV light shares with the immunosuppressive treatment the responsability in carcinogenesis, this measure is more controversial. It is now largely admitted in France and proposed also abroad [17, 18]. We have seen many patients developing aggressive squamous cell carcinomas that did not recur after reduction of the immunosuppressive treatment without rejection even after several years [19, 20]; however, patients with multiple squamous cell carcinomas with a previous heavy sun exposure exist who continue to develop new lesions even after returning to dialysis.

Melanoma

The prognosis of *de novo* melanoma is poor since at least 30% of patients die of their tumour [21]. As in immunocompetent hosts, the prognosis depends on tumor thickness (Breslow index). Although no precise data are currently available, we feel that, along with wide surgical excision, the immunosuppressive treatment should be reduced.

Patients with melanoma transmitted from donors having cerebral metastases of melanoma (when the cause of death had been misdiagnosed as primary brain tumour or cerebral hemorrhage) may experience complete remission of their tumour following transplant nephrectomy and discontinuation of immunosuppressive treatment.

Other rare malignant tumours
Although the experience is limited, we also think that the reduction of the immunosuppressive is advisable. One of our patients with atypical fibroxanthoma developed several recurrences until his immunosuppressive treatment was tappered [22].

Multiple types of malignancies
Patients with skin carcinomas seem to have also an increased risk for other types of malignancies such as melanoma [21], non-Hodgkin's lymphoma [19, 23], malignant fibrous histiocytoma [23], atypical fibroxanthoma [22] and anogenital cancers [24]. In these cases, the reduction of the treatment is especially recommanded.

Changes of the drugs

The usual immunosuppressive drugs may be responsible for undesirable effects: steroids (even at low doses) induce sometimes a major cushingoid aspect and cyclosporine frequently induces hypertrichosis and gingival hyperplasia. When these side-effects become severe and/or cosmetically inacceptable, conversion to FK 506 may prove beneficial [25].

Which dermatological conditions may contraindicate transplantation?

The following conditions are relative contraindications for transplantation:
– Kaposi's sarcoma: despite limited data, it seems that patients with previous posttransplantation Kaposi's sarcoma are at a high risk of recurrence [26, 27];
– melanoma: posttransplant recurrences occur in 20% of cases even when the primary lesion had appeared 10 years before transplantation; therefore, except from *in situ* or very thin melanomas, a waiting period of five years before undertaking transplantation is advised [21];
– multiple cutaneous *squamous cell carcinomas* may also represent a contraindication to a second transplantation.

Prevention of malignancies in the future

A better prevention could be done to avoid the development of the two main skin malignancies in organ transplant recipients, *i.e.* squamous cell carcinomas and Kaposi's sarcoma. The compliance of these patients concerning sun protection is still insufficient [28] and efforts should be made towards a more efficient information. Along with investigation of donors for other viral infections (HIV, EBV, CMV, HBV, HCV, HTLV...), serologic screening for Kaposi's sarcoma-associated herpesvirus may be necessary to avoid the transmission of the virus to negative recipients [29, 30]. All organ transplant recipients should have a dermatological examination at least once a year.

References

1. Chocair PR, Duley JA, Simmonds HA, Cameron JS. The importance of thiopurine methyltransferase activity for the use os azathioprine in transplant recipients. *Transplantation* 1992 ; 53 : 1051-6.
2. Ramos HC, Reyes J, Abu-Elmagd K, Zeevi A, Reinsmoen N, Tzakis A, Demetris A, Fung JJ, Flynn B, McMichael J, Ebert F, Starzl TE. Weaning of immunosuppression in long-term liver transplant recipients. *Transplantation* 1995 ; 59 : 212-7.

3. Pouteil-Noble C, Megas F, Chapuis F. Cytomegalovirus prophylaxis by ganciclovir followed by high-dose acyclovir in renal transplantation: a randomized controlled trial. *Transplant Proc* 1996 ; 28 : 2811.

4. Mora-Fernandez C, Navarro JF, Garcia-Perez J. *Herpes simplex* virus as a sentinel lesion for cytomegalovirus. *Nephrol Dial Transplant* 1997 ; 12 : 853.

5. Euvrard S, Kanitakis J, Thivolet J, Claudy A. Retinoids for the management of dermatological complications of organ transplantation. *Biodrugs* 1997 ; 3 : 176-84.

6. Abel E. Cutaneous manifestations of immunosuppression in organ transplant recipients. *J Am Acad Dermatol* 1989 ; 21 : 167-79.

7. Magnone M, Holley J, Shapiro R, Scantlebury V, McCauley J, Jordan M, Vivas C, Starzl T, Johnson J. Interferon-α induced acute renal allograft rejection. *Transplantation* 1994 ; 59 : 1068-70.

8. Benisovich VI, Silverman L, Slifkin R, Stone N, Cohen E. Cisplatin-based chemotherapy in renal transplant recipients. *Cancer* 1996 ; 77 : 160-3.

9. Shepherd FA, Maher E, Cardella C, Cole E, Greig P, Wade JA, Levy G. Treatment of Kaposi's sarcoma after solid organ transplantation. *J Clin Oncol* 1997 ; 15 : 2371-7.

10. Penn I. Sarcomas in organ allograft recipients. *Transplantation* 1995 ; 60 : 1485-90.

11. Christiansen TN, Freije JE, Neuburg M, Roza A. Cutaneous squamous cell carcinoma metastatic to the parotid gland in a transplant patient. *Clin Transplant* 1996 ; 10 : 561-3.

12. Bouwes-Bavinck JN, Hardie D, Green A, Cutmore S, MacNaught A, O'Sullivan B, Siskind V, Van der Voude FJ, Hardie IR. The risk of skin cancer in renal transplant recipients in Queensland, Australia. *Transplantation* 1996 ; 61 : 715-21.

13. Kadry Z, Bronsther O, Van Thiel DH, Randhawa P, Fung JJ, Starzl TE. Kaposi's sarcoma in two primary liver allograft recipients occurring under FK 506 immunosuppression. *Clin Transplant* 1993 ; 7 : 188-94.

14. Jonas S, Rayes N, Neumann U, Neuhaus R, Bechstein WO, Guckelberger O, Tullius SG, Serke S, Neuhaus P. De novo malignancies after liver transplantation using tacrolimus-based protocols or cyclosporine-based quadruple immunosuppression with an interleukin 2 receptor antibody or antithymocyte globulin. *Cancer* 1997 ; 80 : 1141-50.

15. Euvrard S, Kanitakis J, Chardonnet Y, Pouteil-Noble C, Touraine JL, Faure M, Thivolet J, Claudy A. External anogenital lesions in organ transplant recipients. *Arch Dermatol* 1997 ; 133 : 175-8.

16. Patel R, Roberts GD, Keating M, Paya CV. Infections due to nontuberculous mycobacteria in kidney, heart and liver transplant recipients. *Clin Infect Dis* 1994 ; 19 : 263-73.

17. Blohmé I, Larkö O. Premalignant and malignant skin lesions in renal transplant patients. *Transplantation* 1984 ; 37 : 165-7.

18. Fernandez-Gonzalez A, Espana A, Redondo P. Solid tumors after heart transplantation. *Ann Thorac Surg* 1996 ; 62 : 943-4.

19. Euvrard S, Pouteil-Noble C, Kanitakis J, French M, Berger F, Delecluse HJ, D'Incan M, Thivolet J, Touraine JL. Successive occurrence of T-cell and B-cell lymphomas after renal transplantation in a patient with multiple cutaneous squamous cell carcinomas. *N Engl J Med* 1992 ; 327 : 1924-7.

20. Euvrard S, Kanitakis J, Pouteil-Noble C, Disant F, Dureau G, Finaz de Villaine, Claudy A, Thivolet J. Aggressive squamous cell carcinomas in organ transplant recipients. *Transplant Proc* 1995 ; 27 : 1767-8.

21. Penn I. Malignant melanoma in organ allograft recipients. *Transplantation* 1996 ; 61 : 274-8.

22. Kanitakis J, Euvrard S, Montazeri A, Garnier JL, Faure M, Claudy A. Atypical fibroxanthoma in a renal graft recipient. *J Am Acad Dermatol* 1996 ; 35 : 262-4.

23. Barroso-Vicens E, Ramirez G, Rabb H. Multiple primary malignancies in a renal transplant patient. *Transplantation* 1996 ; 61 : 1655-6.

24. Arends MJ, Benton EC, McLaren KM, Stark LA, Hunter JAA Bird CC. Renal allograft recipients with high susceptibility to cutaneous malignancy have an increased prevalence of human papillomavirus DNA in skin tumours and a greater risk of anogenital malignancy. *Br J Cancer* 1997 ; 75 : 722-8.

25. Distant D, Navarro J, Akoad M, Singh A, Baqi N, Sumrani N, Hong J, Sommer B. Successful Tacrolimus rescue in cyclosporine treated pediatric renal transplant recipients. *Pediatr Transplant* 1998 ; 2 S1 62.

26. Doutrelepont JM, De Pauw L, Gruber SA, Dunn DL, Qunibi W, Kinnaert P. Renal transplantation exposes patients with previous Kaposi's sarcoma to a high risk of recurrence. *Transplantation* 1996 ; 62 : 463-6.

27. Al-Sulaiman MH, Mousa DH, Dhar JM, Al-Khader AA. Does regressed posttransplantation Kaposi's sarcoma recur following reintroduction of immunosuppression? *Am J Nephrol* 1992 ; 12 : 384-6.

28. Seukeran DC, Newstead CG, Cunliffe WJ. The compliance of renal transplant recipients with advice about sun protection measures. *Br J Dermatol* 1998 ; 138 : 301-3.

29. Parravicini C, Olsen SJ, Capra M, Poli F, Sirchia G, Gao SJ, Berti E, Nocera A, Rossi E, Bestetti G, Pizzuto M, Galli M, Moroni M, Moore PS, Corbellino M. Risk of Kaposi's sarcoma-associated herpes virus transmission from donor allografts among Italian posttransplant Kaposi's sarcoma patients. *Blood* 1997 ; 90 : 2826-9.

30. Bottalico D, Santabosti Barbone G, Giancaspro V, Bignardi L, Arisi L, Cambi V. Post-transplantation Kaposi's sarcoma appearing simultaneously in same cadaver donor renal transplant recipients. *Nephrol Dial Transplant* 1997 ; 12 : 1055-7.

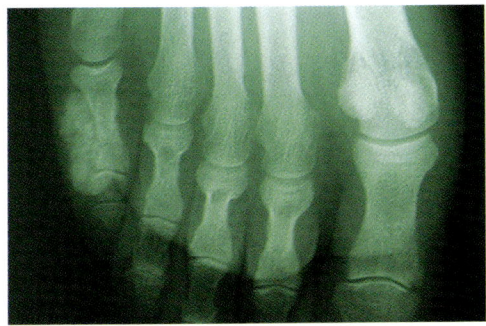

Figure 1. Cutaneous calcifications in chronic renal failure.

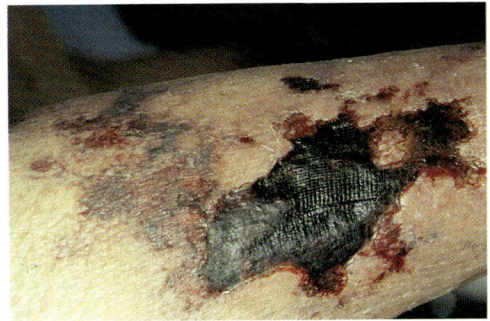

Figure 2. Calciphylaxis: cutaneous necrosis in a patient on hemodialysis.

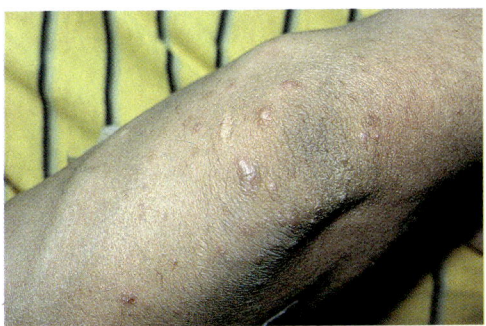

Figure 3. Acquired perforating disease of chronic renal failure: hyperkeratotic papules.

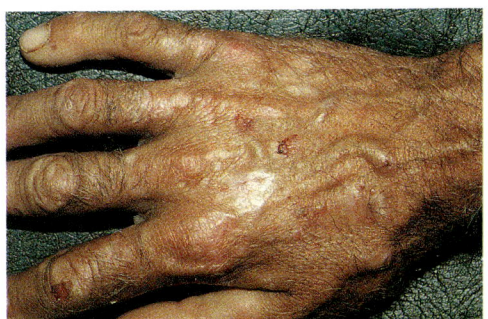

Figure 4. Pseudo-porphyria cutanea tarda of hemodialysis.

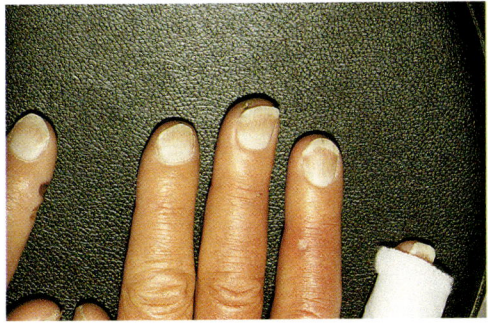

Figure 5. Half-and-half nail syndrome in chronic renal failure.

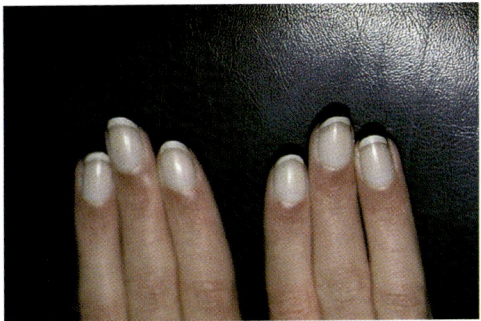

Figure 6. Leuconychia in chronic renal failure.

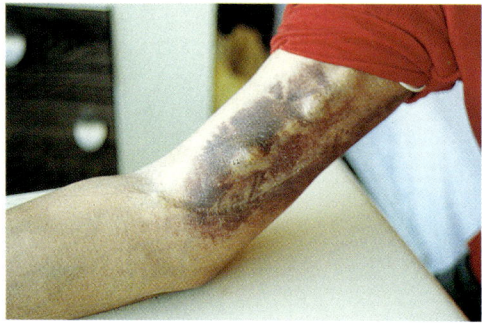

Figure 7. Arterio-venous shunt: blood extravasation.

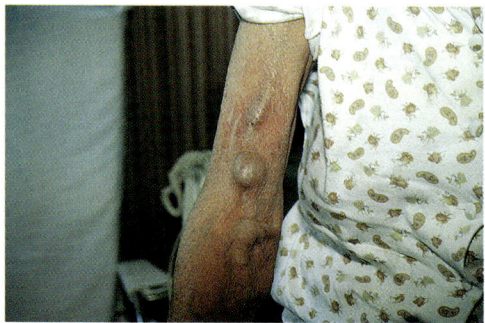

Figure 8. Arterio-venous shunt: aneurysm.

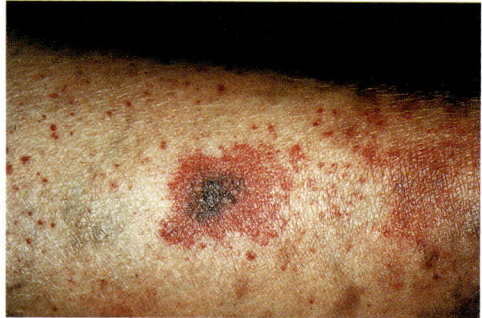

Figure 9. Mixed cryoglobulinemia associated with HCV infection: purpuric lesions of lower limbs.

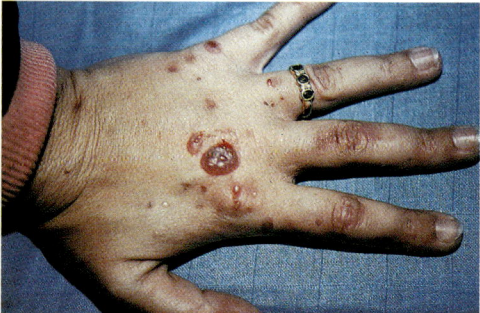

Figure 10. Porphyria cutanea tarda associated with HCV infection: bullous lesions on the dorsa of the hands.

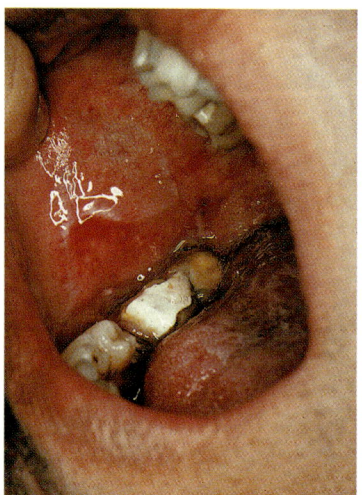

Figure 11. Oral lichen planus associated with HCV infection: reticular and erosive lesions.

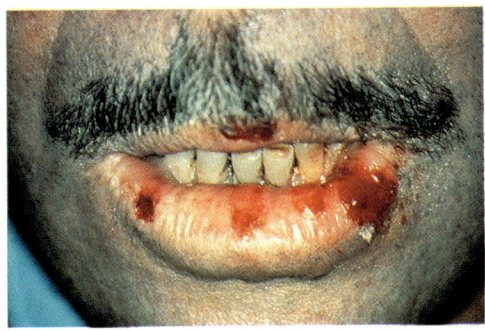

Figure 12. Extensive herpetic labial erosions developing some days after kidney transplantation.

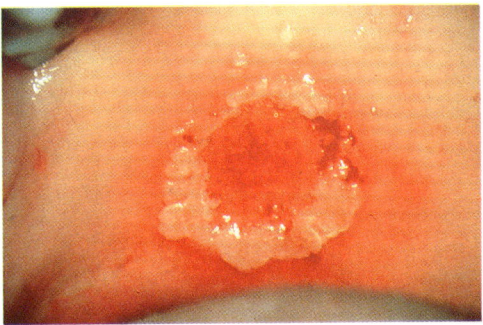

Figure 13. Typical lesions of *Herpes simplex* on the hard palate (same patient as in figure 12).

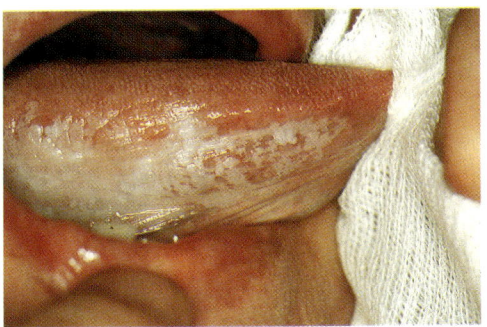

Figure 14. Clinical aspect of OHL.

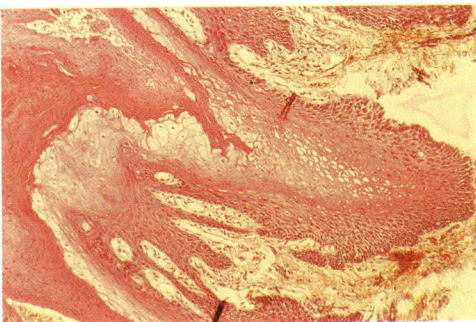

Figure 15. Histologic aspect of lesional tissue in OHL: parakeratotic hyperkeratosis and acanthosis.

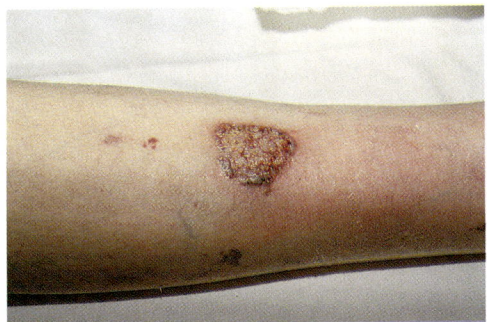

Figure 17. Cutaneous alternariosis in a kidney transplant recipient.

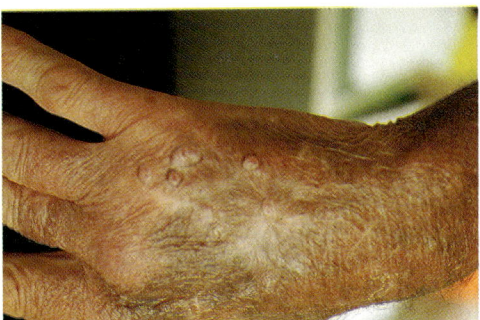

Figure 18. Cutaneous alternariosis in a kidney transplant recipient.

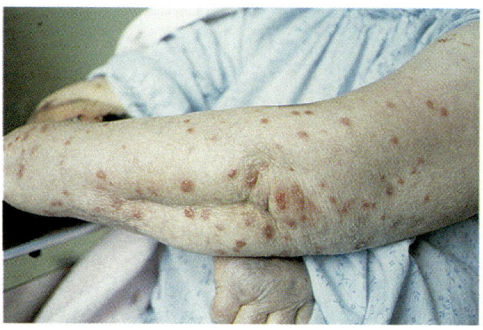

Figure 19. Cutaneous alternariosis in a kidney transplant recipient.

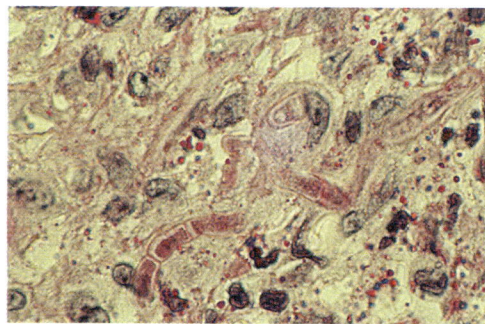

Figure 20. Histological aspect of alternariosis.

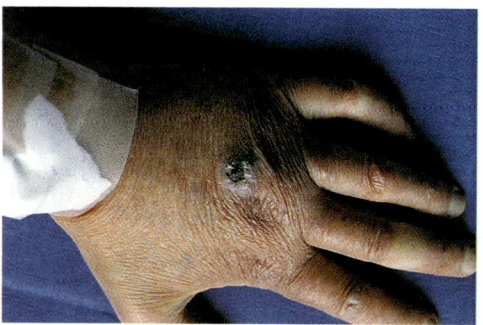

Figure 21. Chronic verrucous lesion due to *Exophiala janselmei* in a kidney transplant recipient.

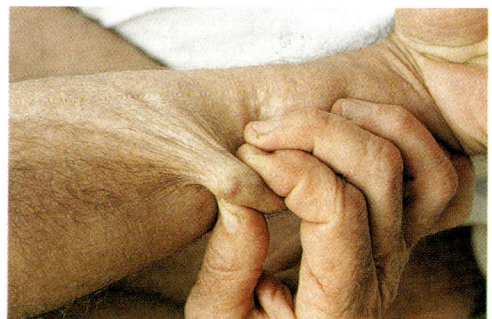

Figure 22. Numerous subcutaneous cysts due to *Exophiala janselmei* in a liver and kidney transplant recipient.

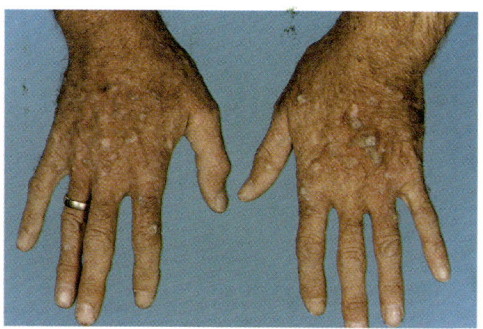

Figure 23. Extensive keratotic skin lesions on the hands of a kidney transplant recipient.

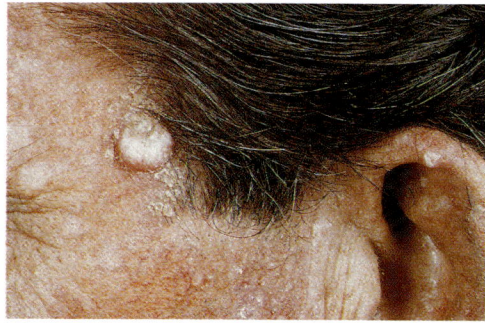

Figure 24. Squamous cell carcinoma on the temple of a kidney transplant recipient.

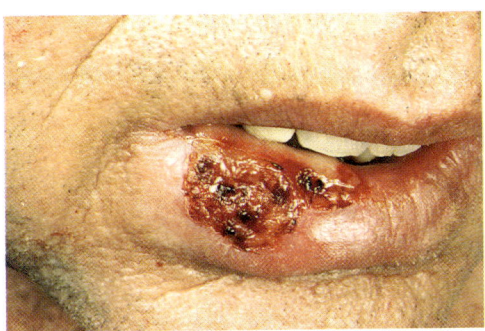

Figure 26. Squamous cell carcinoma of the lip in a kidney transplant recipient.

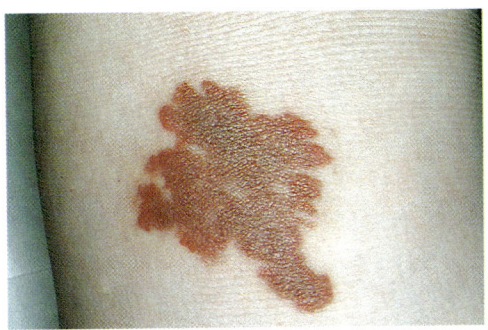

Figure 27. Large plaque of Kaposi's sarcoma on the leg of a kidney transplant recipient.

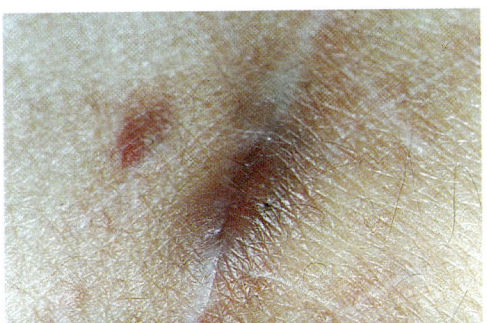

Figure 28. Nodular lesions of Kaposi's sarcoma on the transplantation's scar (liver).

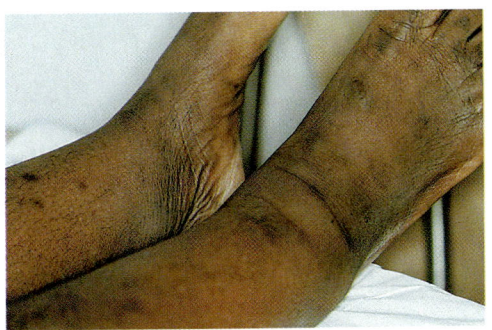

Figure 29. Edema of the right leg with bilateral pigmented papules of Kaposi's sarcoma on the legs of a kidney transplant recipient.

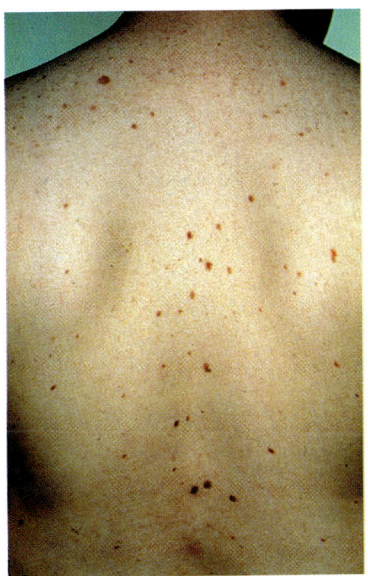

Figure 30. Kidney transplant recipient aged 16 years who developed large numbers of benign and dysplastic-looking melanocytic nevi within two years of immunosuppressive therapy.

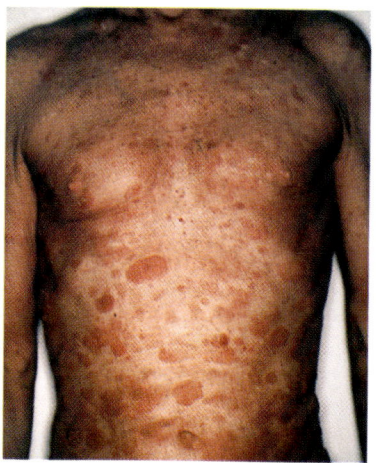

Figure 31. Sézary syndrome in a kidney transplant recipient presenting with multiple infiltrated plaques.

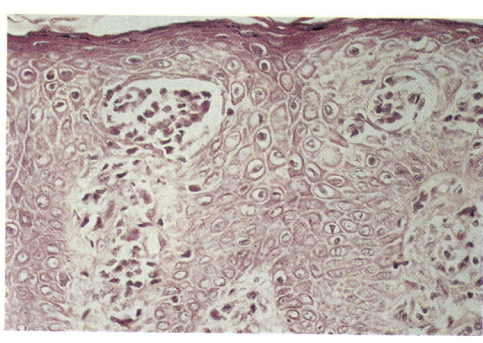

Figure 32. Histologic aspect of the lesions of patient shown in figure 31: an epidermotropic infiltrate of lymphocytes with convoluted nuclei is seen.

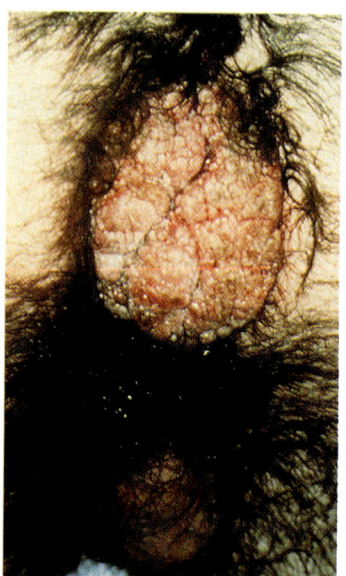

Figure 33. Giant cauliflower-like tumour (condyloma) of the anus in a liver transplant recipient.

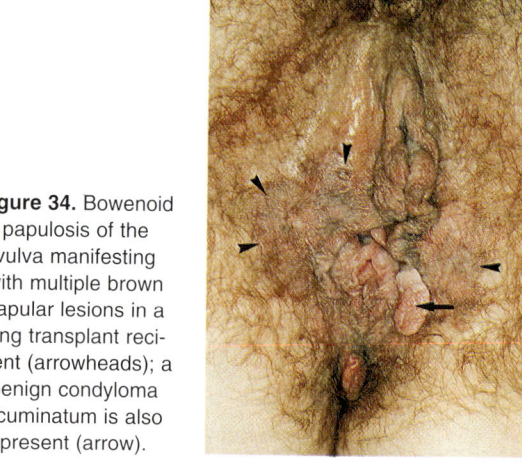

Figure 34. Bowenoid papulosis of the vulva manifesting with multiple brown papular lesions in a lung transplant recipient (arrowheads); a benign condyloma acuminatum is also present (arrow).

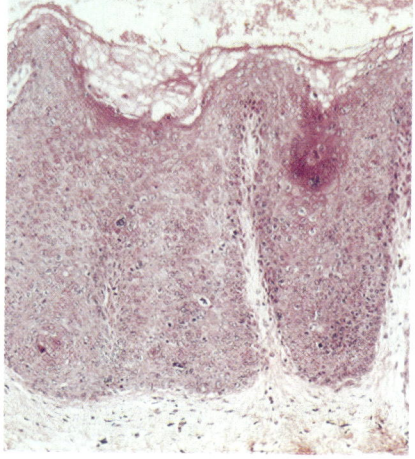

Figure 35. Histological aspect of bowenoid papulosis: disorderly arrangement of keratinocytes within the epidermis, atypical, mitotic, multinucleated and dyskeratotic keratinocytes are seen.

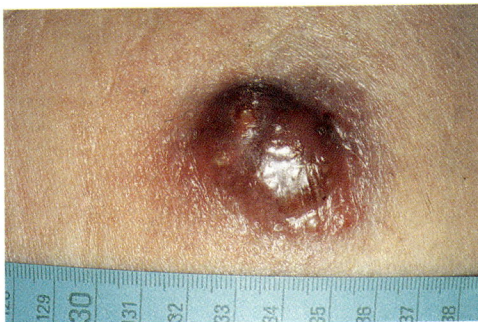

Figure 36. Merkel cell carcinoma in a kidney transplant recipient.

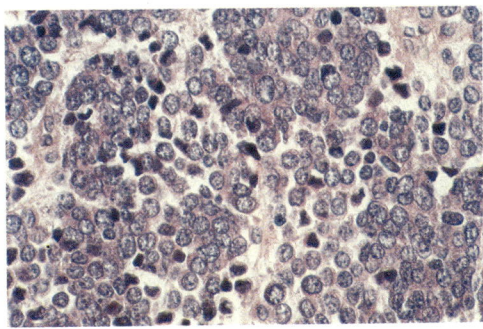

Figure 37. Histological aspect of Merkel cell carcinoma.

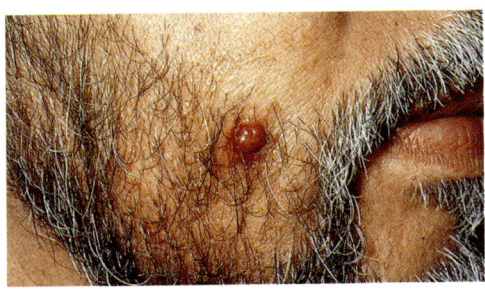

Figure 38. Pyogenic granuloma in a kidney transplant recipient.

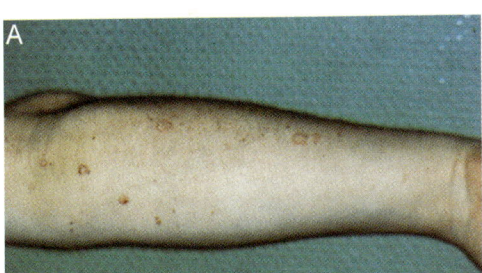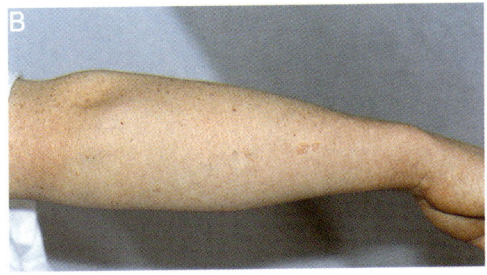

Figure 39. A. Multiple warts and keratoses on the forearm in a twenty-year old kidney transplant recipient. B. Considerable reduction of the number of the lesions after a three-month course of topical tretinoin.

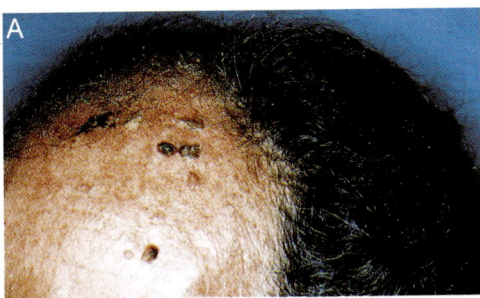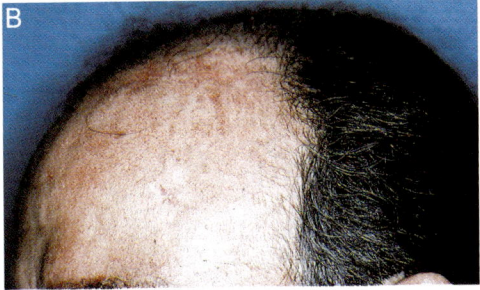

Figure 40. A. Multiple keratoses on the face and the scalp in a 61-year old kidney transplant recipient. B. Obvious improvement after a three-month course of topical tretinoin.

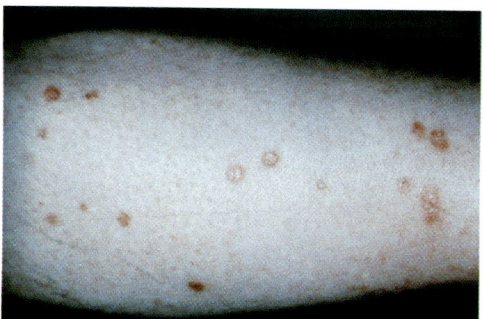

Figure 41. Disseminated superficial porokeratosis in a lung-transplant recipient: typical annular, hyperkeratotic lesions on the leg.

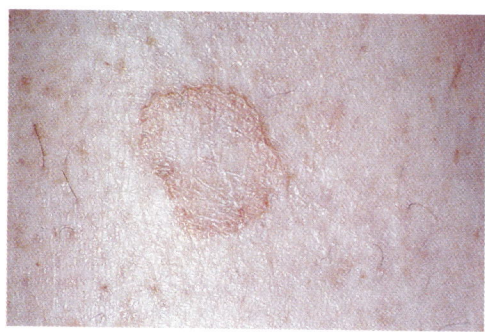

Figure 42. Close-up view of the lesions of the same patient: the peripheral keratotic border is visible.

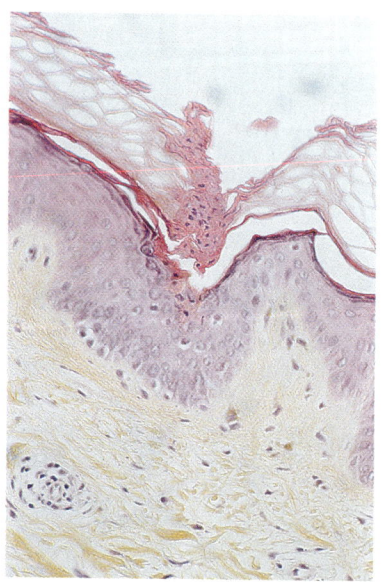

Figure 43. Histopathology of porokeratosis: the cornoid lamella, a vertical stack of parakeratotic corneocytes, is seen invaginating within the epidermis.

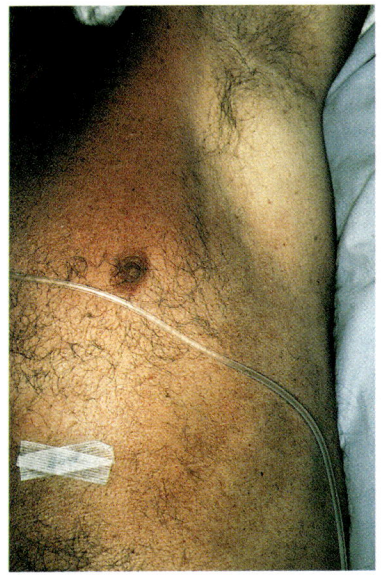

Figure 44. Maculo-papular eruption in acute GVHD.

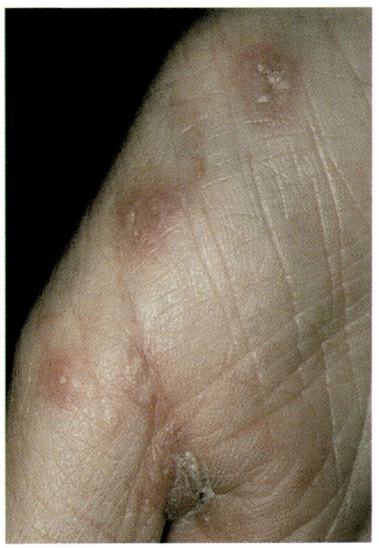

Figure 45. Lichen planus-like lesions in chronic GVHD.

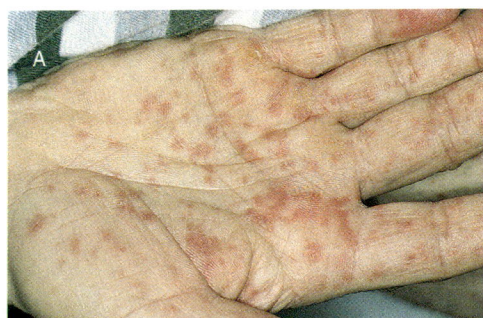

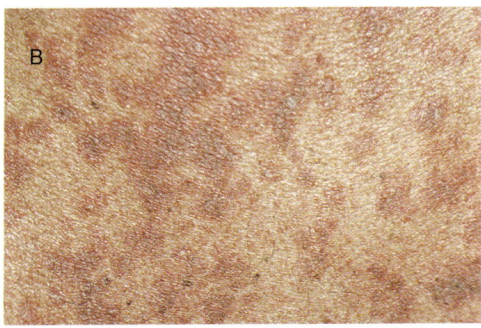

Figure 47. GVHD after liver transplantation: maculopapular rash on the palm (A) and the back (B).

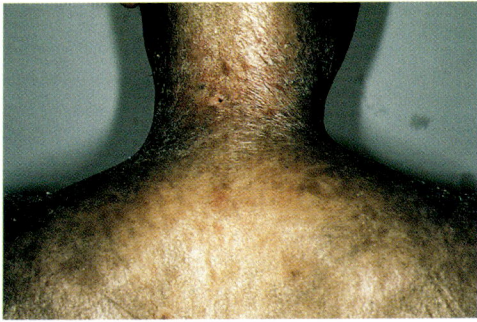

Figure 46. Disseminated sclerotic GVHD.

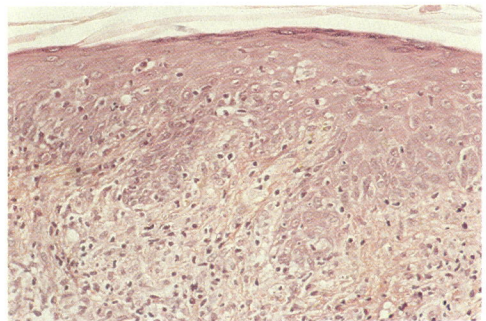

Figure 48. Histological aspect of GVHD after liver transplantation: hydropic degeneration of basal cells, necrotic epidermal keratinocytes and exocytosis of lymphocytes in the epidermis.

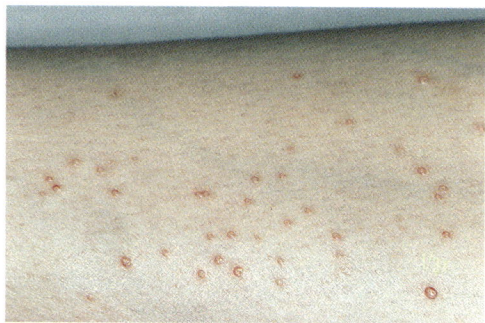

Figure 49. Multiple molluscum contagiosum lesions on the legs (spreading favoured by shaving) in a female lung transplant recipient.

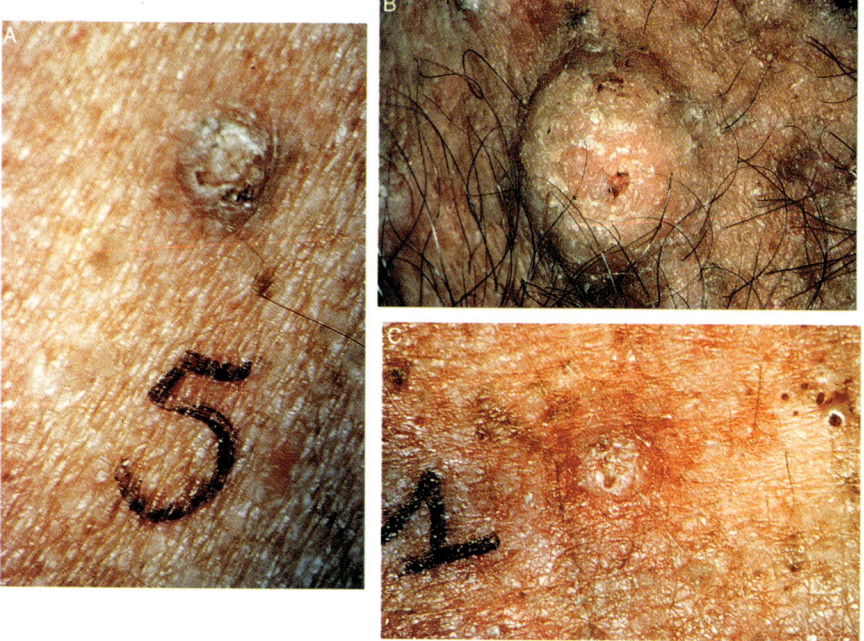

Figure 50. Similar warty aspects of A) common wart, B) keratoacanthoma, C) squamous cell carcinoma in a kidney transplant recipient.

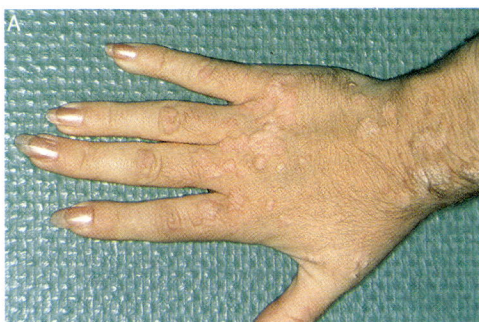
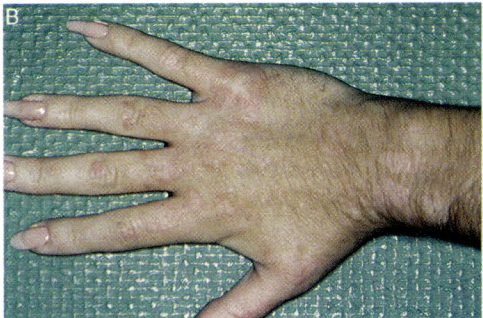

Figure 51. A. Extensive warts in a kidney transplant recipient. B. Considerable improvement after a one-month course of acitretin.

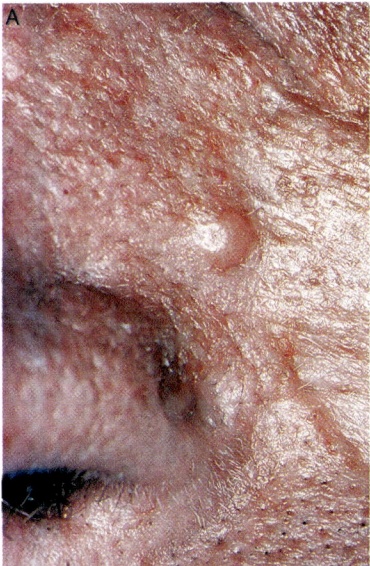
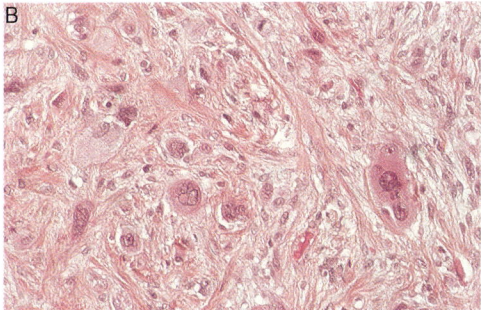

Figure 52. A. Recurrent atypical fibroxanthoma which had been initially removed without histological examination in a kidney transplant recipient. B. Histology shows a dermal infiltration of atypical mesenchymal cells.

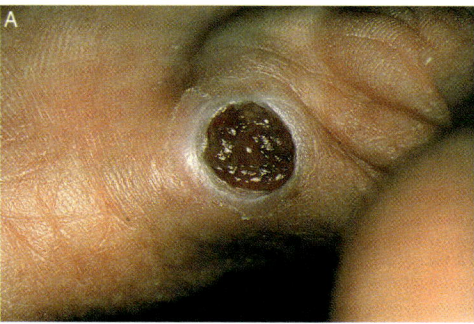
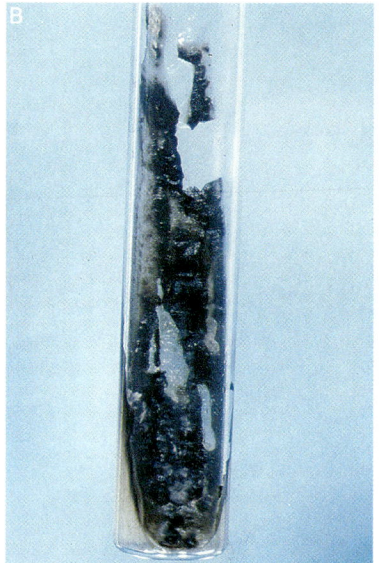

Figure 53. A. Opportunistic infection due to *Exophiala janselmei* mimicking pyogenic granuloma in a heart transplant recipient. B. Growth of the black fungi on Sabouraud's dextrose agar.

Index

13-*cis*-retinoic acid, 37, 169, 171

Acyclovir, 25, 82, 89-93, 97, 119, 146, 147, 210
Acitretin, 41, 171, 180
Acne, 19, 21, 41, 82, 83, 175
Actinic keratoses, 54, 75, 124, 127, 156, 159, 163, 164, 171, 177-179, 184, 189, 190
Actinomycosis, 106
Adapalene, 41, 168, 169, 179, 180
All-*trans* retinoic acid, 38
Allergic cutaneous manifestations, 46
Alopecia areata, 84
Alternariosis, 109
Amyloidosis, 45, 80
Angiosarcoma, 75, 118, 156
Anogenital lesions, 150-152
Antigen-presenting cells, 9, 18, 26
Antioxidants, 163
Arotinoid-methyl-sulfone, 179
Arterio-venous shunt dermatitis, 47
Aspergillosis, 103, 108
Atopic dermatitis, 11, 12, 40, 86
Atypical fibroxanthoma, 156, 213
Atypical mycobacterial infections, 104
Autoimmune diseases, 30, 84, 186, 198, 205
Azathioprine, 2, 8, 9, 11, 13, 17, 18, 20, 22, 26, 83, 86, 119, 124, 126, 145, 147, 156, 176, 190, 200, 206, 210

B cell lymphoma (*see also* Lymphoma), 74, 147
Bacillary angiomatosis, 106, 155
Bacterial infections, 3, 12, 25, 103, 106
Bartonellosis, 106
Basal cell carcinoma, 11, 29, 54, 75, 122, 123, 125, 157, 159, 161, 169, 170, 172, 176, 177, 187, 189
Bone marrow transplant, 5, 89, 90, 91, 142
Bone marrow tranplantation, 66, 89, 99, 107, 195, 204
Botryomycosis, 106
Bowenoid papulosis, 151, 210
Brequinar sodium, 2, 17, 23
Bullous dermatosis, 45, 81

Calcification, 44, 170, 176

Calciphylaxis, 44, 80
Cancer, 29, 30, 33, 51-57, 83, 113-120, 122, 125, 140, 145, 150, 161, 176, 200, 212, 213
Cancer prevention, 167
Candidiasis, 81, 97, 107
Carcinogenesis, 51-53, 55-57, 124, 177, 212
Carcinoma, 9, 12, 13, 44, 52, 54-56, 62, 65, 82, 113-119, 122, 125, 135, 145, 150-152, 154-156, 159-161, 163, 175, 176, 189, 210, 213
Chemotherapy, 92, 120, 135, 140, 148, 155, 157, 186, 196, 197, 211
Chromoblastomycosis, 109
Chronic renal failure, 3, 20, 43-47, 80
Coccidioidomycosis, 104, 109
Condyloma, 82, 118, 151, 189, 212
Contact hypersensitivity, 30
Cornoid lamella, 183, 185, 187
Cryoglobulin, 63, 64
Cryptococcus, 104, 107
Cutaneous infections, 81, 105, 108, 201
Cutaneous lymphomas, 76, 145-148
Cutaneous tumor, 29, 52, 54, 119, 170
Cyclosporin (or cyclosporine, or CSA), 2, 8, 9, 11, 13, 17-21, 38, 40, 83, 89, 92, 95, 105, 124, 126, 133, 145, 147, 155, 157, 176, 190, 200, 206, 210, 211, 213
Cytokines, 12, 13, 18, 19, 21-23, 25, 31, 32, 38, 39, 55-57, 72
Cytomegalovirus, 71, 90, 102, 104, 205, 210
Cytotoxic lymphocytes, 55

Dematiaceous fungi, 107, 109
Deoxyspergualin, 2, 17, 23
Dermatofibrosarcoma protuberans, 156
Dermatomyositis, 67, 186
Dermatophytosis, 81, 108, 211
Dialysis, 3, 20, 45-47, 81, 83, 85, 119, 136, 141, 212
Dimorphic fungi, 107, 109
Dysplastic epithelial lesions, 175, 180

E6 oncoprotein, 55, 160
E7 oncoprotein, 52, 55, 160
Ecthyma gangrenosum, 103, 104, 110
Epidermodysplasia verruciformis, 52, 124
Epstein-Barr virus, 72, 91, 95, 115, 146
Erythema multiforme, 67, 206
Erythema nodosum, 67, 109
Etretinate, 40, 86, 148, 169-172, 178, 180

Extracutaneous tumors, 113-120

FK506, *see* Tacrolimus
Fungal infections, 103, 106, 211

Genital warts, 118, 151
Giant condyloma, 151
Graft *versus* host disease (GVHD), 66, 195-201, 204-207

Half-and-half nail, 46, 80
Heart transplant, 82, 97, 98, 106, 110, 122, 145
Heart transplantation, 84, 85, 131, 133, 134, 146, 150, 155, 156, 175
Hemodialysis, 43-47, 81, 117
Hepatitis C virus, 45, 62-67, 85, 86
Hepatoma, 118
Herpes simplex virus, 31, 81, 82, 89, 210
Herpes zoster, 92, 104, 198, 210
Histoplasmosis, 104, 109
Human herpes virus 8 (HHV8), 71-76, 91, 132-136
Human papillomavirus (HPV), 51-57, 71, 81, 82, 122, 124-126, 150-152, 159, 160, 176, 209, 210, 212

Immune response, 8, 17, 29, 30, 37-41, 84, 86, 87, 125, 126, 142, 146, 160, 205
Immunogenetics, 55, 125
Immunosuppression, 5, 6, 17, 29, 31-33, 40, 54, 55, 57, 62, 74, 75, 80-84, 89-92, 95, 99, 102, 119, 124, 134, 135, 139-143, 151, 152, 155, 156, 160, 163, 176, 186-188, 190, 205-207, 209, 210, 212
Immunosuppressive therapy, 2, 4, 5, 17-26, 29, 54, 63, 83, 84, 87, 105, 116, 117, 119, 126, 131, 146, 148, 157, 159, 160, 170
Infections, 8, 9, 13, 18, 19, 21, 25, 39, 44, 45, 52, 54-57, 62-67, 73-75, 80-82, 86, 89-93, 95-97, 99, 102-110, 113, 115, 118-120, 122, 124, 125, 133, 134, 140, 151, 159, 160, 176, 186, 195, 197, 198, 201, 205-207, 209, 210, 212, 213
Interferon, 39, 55, 72, 85, 119, 170-172, 211
Isotretinoin, 83, 168, 169-172, 175, 179

Kaposi's sarcoma, 38, 47, 71, 74-76, 83, 91, 113, 114, 116, 131-136, 132, 155, 156, 172, 211-213

KSHV, 71, 91, 132
Kidney transplant, 2, 9, 11, 85, 102, 109, 110, 115, 155, 169, 177, 188, 210, 211
Kidney transplantation, 4, 44, 45, 80, 81, 90, 103, 145, 157, 175
Kyrle's disease, 45

Langerhans cells, 8, 9, 30, 32, 33, 40, 57, 96, 99, 176, 187, 190
Leflunomide, 17, 23
Lichen planus, 11, 62, 65, 66, 86, 97, 184, 198, 199
Lichen planus - like GVHD, 199
Linear IgA bullous dermatosis, 84
Liver transplant, 9, 62, 90, 92, 98, 106, 133, 155, 190, 210
Liver transplantation, 62, 64, 81, 87, 92, 131, 133, 155, 206
Lung transplant, 92, 210
Lung transplantation, 145
Lymphocyte, 8-11, 17, 18-20, 22-24, 38-40, 55, 66, 85, 89, 97, 116, 125, 145, 147, 185, 188, 195-198, 204-206
Lymphoma, 12, 71, 74-76, 91, 113-117, 119, 133, 134, 145-149, 156, 172, 186, 213
Lymphoproliferative disorders, 21, 24, 63, 74, 84, 95, 115, 146, 147

Malakoplakia, 67, 106
Malignancy, 30, 51, 52, 54, 56, 82, 83, 99, 113-116, 118, 119, 142, 155, 157, 163, 167, 170, 171, 175, 186, 188, 190, 200, 211-213
Malignant fibrous histiocytoma, 156, 213
Melanoderma of Bright, 46
Melanoma, 33, 54, 56, 76, 83, 84, 115, 125, 126, 139, 141-143, 154, 159-161, 163, 171, 200, 212, 213
Merkel cell carcinoma, 115, 154, 155
Mibelli, 183, 189
Molluscum contagiosum, 107, 109, 210
Monoclonal antibodies, 3, 17, 24-26, 31
Mucormycosis, 107, 110
Mycetoma, 105, 108, 109
Mycophenolate mofetil (MMF), 2, 8, 17, 22, 26, 119, 210
Mycosis fungoides, 76, 116, 148, 186

Naevus, 83, 139, 140, 142, 143, 184, 185
Necrolytic acral erythema, 67
Nested PCR, 54, 57, 75

Neuroendocrine carcinoma, 155
NK cells, 13, 55
Nocardiosis, 105

OKT3, 17, 24, 25, 89, 91, 92, 145, 155, 206
Onychomycosis, 81
Opportunistic fungi, 106, 107
Opportunistic infections, 102-105, 133, 135, 211, 212
Oral hairy leukoplakia, 91, 95-99
Organ shortage, 3-6
Organ transplantation, 1-6, 10, 13, 19, 23, 75, 80, 82, 83, 85, 86, 102, 106, 131-133, 135, 139-141, 143, 145, 146, 148, 152, 159, 164, 176, 183, 186, 188, 205
Overimmunosuppression, 24, 176, 209

p53, 51-53, 55-57, 72, 73, 156, 160, 169, 185
Pancytopenia, 205, 206
Perforating disorders, 45
Peritoneal dialysis, 43, 45, 46
Phaeohyphomycosis, 109
Pharmacokinetics, 20, 21, 23
Photoprotection, 159-164, 188
Phototypes, 160
Polyarteritis nodosa, 64
Polyclonal antibodies, 17, 23
Porokeratosis, 154, 183-194
Porphyria, 87
Porphyria cutanea tarda, 62, 64, 65, 81
pRb, 51-53
Premalignant keratoses, see also Actinic keratoses, 175
Prophylaxis, 17, 23, 25, 89-93, 145, 207
Prototheca, 104, 110
Pruritus, 43-47, 67, 80, 170, 184
Pseudomonas aeruginosa, 103, 104
Pseudoporphyria cutanea tarda, 45
Psoriasis, 11, 12, 38, 40, 41, 85, 86, 184
PUVA, 55, 57, 185, 200
Pyogenic granuloma, 75, 155

Radiotherapy, 135, 147, 148, 155-157, 211
Rapamycin/e (RPM), see Sirolimus
Rejection, 8, 17, 18, 20-26, 82-86, 89, 91, 92, 102, 103, 105, 113, 116, 117, 119, 126, 135, 145, 147, 155, 156, 176, 205, 206, 210-212
Renal carcinomas, 113, 117
Retinaldehyde, 179
Retinoic acid, 37-41, 44, 168, 176, 177

Retinoids, 10, 37-41, 45, 97, 127, 167-172, 175-177, 179, 180, 210
Retinoid receptors, 38, 40, 168, 169
Sarcoma, 113-115, 117, 118, 156, 157, 200, 211
Sézary syndrome, 76, 148
Sirolimus, 2, 17, 22, 26
Skin cancer, 5, 9, 21, 29, 30, 33, 52-54, 56, 57, 83, 84, 113-115, 119, 122-127, 139, 142, 159-161, 163, 164, 167-170, 172, 175, 176, 212
Skin immune system, 8-13
Solid organ transplant, 30, 142, 205, 206
Solid organ transplantation, 106, 204-206
Squamous cell carcinoma, 12, 53, 75, 115, 122-125, 154, 159, 167, 169-172, 175, 178, 187, 190, 200, 210-213
Steroids, 9, 13, 17-20, 23-26, 37, 45, 56, 82-86, 89, 92, 147, 148, 168, 176, 188, 190, 200, 206, 210, 211, 213
Sun protective factor, 161
Sunscreen, 126, 160-164, 188
Sweat gland carcinoma, 157
Syringomatous carcinoma, 157
Systemic retinoids, 167, 170-172, 176, 178, 180, 188, 210

Tacrolimus, 17, 21, 22, 210, 211
T cell lymphoma (see also Lymphoma), 76, 148, 172
Tinea versicolor, 81, 211
Tolerance, 5, 6, 25, 26, 30, 32, 33, 178, 180, 209
Tretinoin, 171, 172, 177-180, 188
Trichosporonosis, 108
Tumor necrosis factor alpha, 30, 39, 73, 200

Ultraviolet B light, 29-33
Ultraviolet radiation, 57, 139, 160, 185
Urticaria, 46, 63, 67

Valaciclovir, 93, 210
Varicella-zoster virus, 90
Vasculitis, 63, 64, 91, 108
Viral warts, 122, 169, 187, 210
Vitamin A, 37-40, 44, 167, 169

Xenotransplantation, 23
Xerosis, 43, 44, 80, 176

Zygomycetes, 110

Achevé d'imprimer par Corlet, Imprimeur, S.A.
14110 Condé-sur-Noireau (France)
N° d'Imprimeur : 34427 - Dépôt légal : octobre 1998

Imprimé en U.E.